MEDICAL PROCEDURES, TESTING AND TECHNOLOGY

# TRADITIONAL MEDICINE

## NEW RESEARCH

## MEDICAL PROCEDURES, TESTING AND TECHNOLOGY

Additional books in this series can be found on Nova's website under the Series tab.

Additional e-books in this series can be found on Nova's website under the e-books tab.

## PUBLIC HEALTH IN THE 21ST CENTURY

Additional books in this series can be found on Nova's website under the Series tab.

Additional e-books in this series can be found on Nova's website under the e-books tab.

MEDICAL PROCEDURES, TESTING AND TECHNOLOGY

# TRADITIONAL MEDICINE

## NEW RESEARCH

YOSHIHARU MOTOO
EDITOR

NOVA BIOMEDICAL

*New York*

**Library of Congress Cataloging-in-Publication Data**

ISBN: 978-1-62257-448-3

Library of Congress Control Number: 2012941952

*Published by Nova Science Publishers, Inc. † New York*

# Contents

# Preface

Traditional Medicine (TM) is currently used widely in the world. However, TM is not as universal and standard as Western Medicine (WM). Each TM has its unique characters, and such diversity reflects its history of utilization in each country or region. Traditional East Asian Medicine (TEAM) is the TM, which originated from ancient Chinese Medicine and later developed to Kampo Medicine (Traditional Japanese Medicine), Traditional Korean Medicine (Korean Oriental Medicine), Traditional Vietnamese Medicine, etc. Kampo, with its high-quality finished products and the health insurance coverage, is well incorporated into a modern Westernized medical system in Japan. In China and Korea, TM is basically independent of WM, but recently combination of both TM and WM has been examined.

In this book, there are various unique chapters from molecular, pharmacognostic, pharmacoeconomic, and clinical viewpoints. Especially, several chapters focused on cancer patient care, regarding TM as an important supportive measure. We have other interesting issues such as ethics for East Asian Medicine and perspectives for TM systems. These new researches will surely stimulate future studies on TM.

I wish to thank all the authors and the Nova Science Publishers, Inc.

March, 2012

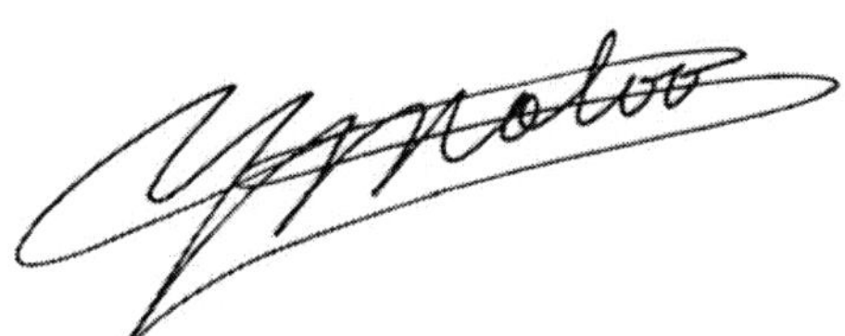

Yoshiharu Motoo, MD, PhD, FACP
Department of Medical Oncology
Kanazawa Medical University
Uchinada, Ishikawa 920-0293
Japan

In: Traditional Medicine: New Research
Editor: Yoshiharu Motoo

ISBN: 978-1-62257-448-3


*Chapter 1*

# Kampo for Cancer Care: Significance as Supportive Measures

***Keiko Ogawa-Ochiai[1,*], Masao Ogawa[2] and Yoshiharu Motoo[3]***

[1]Department of Oto-rhino-laryngology and Clinic of Japanese Oriental (Kampo) Medicine, Kanazawa University Hospital, Kanazawa, Japan

[2]Department of Anesthesiology

[3]Department of Medical Oncology, Kanazawa Medical University, Ishikawa, Japan

## Abstract

Kampo is the Japanese traditional herbal medicine. The aim of Kampo therapy is to improve patients' condition whatever their diseases are. Kampo Medicine plays more and more important roles in closing the gap between modern Western Medicine and demand of patients, especially for the cancer patient. It is also expected to solve the problems such as the side effects of chemotherapy or radiotherapy, appetite loss, and various types of general fatigue or malaise. For instance, rikkunshito (RKT) is the most frequently used and has been proved to be effective for CINV and anorexia. Hangeshashinto (HST) effectively prevents CPT-11-induced delayed diarrhea in animal experiments and in humans. Although Kampo methodology for diagnosis and treatment is referred to as "formulation corresponding to [sho]", some routine treatments as above have produced fruitful results, which were better than expected. In this chapter, we introduce some formulas and recent clinical research on Kampo supportive therapy for the following symptoms of cancer patients. However, it is important to understand that the concept of Kampo medicine is to improve the general condition of patients. The integration of western medicine and Kampo medicine would make new progress in cancer supportive therapy.

* E-mail: ikkandoo@gmail.com.

## Abbreviation of Kampo Formulas

| | |
|---|---|
| Rikkunshito | RKT |
| Hangekobokuto | HKT |
| Goreisan | GRS |
| Hangeshashinto | HST |
| Orengedokuto | OGT |
| Daikenchuto | DKT |
| Shokenchuto | SHKT |
| Mashiningan | MNG |
| Goshajinkigan | GJG |
| Hochuekkito | HET |
| Ninjinyoeito | NYT |
| Juzentaihoto | JTT |

## Introduction

Kampo — Japanese traditional herbal medicine — is the most frequently used alternative and complementary medicine in Japan. The aim of Kampo therapy is to improve patients' condition whatever their diseases are. In this concept, Kampo medicine plays a more and more important role in closing the gap between Western Modern Medicine and demands of patients. In Japan, Kampo can be used easily for cancer patient because it is covered by the national health insurance system. It is also expected to relieve the symptoms such as the side effects of chemotherapy and radiotherapy, and various types of general fatigue or malaise. However, Kampo might have an adverse effect against the cytotoxic effects of chemotherapy. It must be continually examined by laboratory data, physical examination, and history of patients.

Although Kampo methodology for diagnosis and treatment is referred to as "formulation corresponding to sho", some routine treatments have been producing better results than expected. This leads to rising expectations for Kampo medicine. An increasing number of reports or studies have been made on Kampo medicine in cancer supportive therapy, from basic research to clinical studies. In this chapter, we introduce some formulas and recent clinical researches on Kampo supportive therapy for cancer patients and the concept of Kampo Medicine in supportive therapy.

## 1. Chemotherapy-induced Nausea, Vomiting, and Anorexia

Chemotherapy-induced nausea and vomiting (CINV) is potentially the most severe and the most distressing, which sometimes makes completion of chemotherapy impossible. Quite a few Kampo formulas are used to improve CINV and anorexia, for example, rikkunshito (RKT), hangekobokuto (HKT), or goreisan (GRS). Among these Kampo formulas, RKT is the most frequently used and has been proved to be effective for CINV and anorexia. In this section, we introduce recent clinical and basic research on RKT.

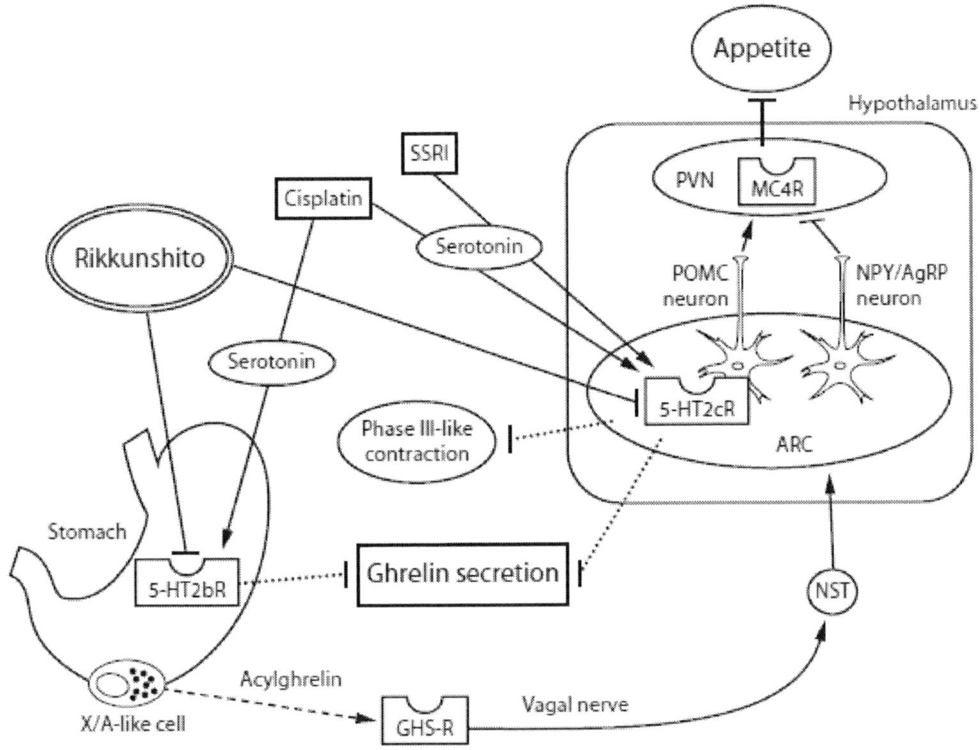


Figure1. Schematic diagram of action mechanisms of rikkunshito on appetite. (revised from [7]).

RKT is composed of eight crude drugs: Atractylodis Lanceae Rhizoma, Ginseng Radix, Pinelliae Tuber, Hoelen, Zizyphi Fructus, Aurantii Nobilis Pericarpium, Glycyrrhizae Radix and Zingiberis Rhizoma. RKT is the most popular Japanese traditional medicine for various gastrointestinal tract disorders, and has been used for patients with hypofunctional constitution and anorexia, heaviness of stomach, and stomach discomfort. In a double-blind controlled study, RKT significantly ameliorated dysmotility-like dyspepsia and upper gastric symptoms such as nausea and anorexia [1] [2]. Several studies in rats have proved the enhanced gastric emptying and a protective effect on gastric mucosa injury with RKT administration. These findings show that RKT might be useful for treatment of anorexia and may provide a new strategy for improvement of upper gastrointestinal dysfunction in cancer patients.

Ghrelin is the key factor of the mechanism of RKT. Ghrelin is a 28-amino-acid orexigenic hormone that stimulates growth hormone release and enhances feeding and weight gain to regulate energy homeostasis [3]. It has recently been shown that RKT ameliorates cisplatin-induced anorexia by an increase of the circulating ghrelin concentration. Cisplatin causes a significant decrease in plasma ghrelin and appetite loss in rodents, and intravenous injection of exogenous acylated ghrelin inhibits the appetite loss after cisplatin administration. It is also reported that RKT suppresses cisplatin-induced anorexia in rat via 5-HT2 receptor antagonism [4]. Moreover, rat models with decreased contractions of the antrum and duodenum induced with a selective serotonin reuptake inhibitor were reversed by RKT via enhancement of the circulating ghrelin concentration [5]. It is also demonstrated that RKT improves anorexia of aging via inhibiting reduced hypothalamic ghrelin receptor reactivity [6]. RKT inhibits peripheral 5-HT2B and central 5-HT2C receptor and stimulates secretion of ghrelin from the stomach (Figure 1) [7]. Moreover, RKT also enhances ghrelin receptor reactivity via PDE3 inhibition. These studies show RKT is effective in treating anorexia in cancer patients.

In Kampo medicine, formulas that expel dampness are often used for patients with CINV. GRS is one of the most major formulas that expel dampness. GRS includes five crude drugs: Alismatis Rhizoma, Poria, Polyporus, Atractylodis macrocephalae Rhizoma, and Cinamomoni Cortex. GRS promotes urination, which is the principal way to expel dampness from the body. It is especially effective for severe vomiting immediately after drinking water, which is called "water rebellion disorder".

HKT is an important formula that can be used for many disorders with somatic and psychoemotional symptoms. It is also used to treat functional dyspepsia [8]. Since most of cancer patients feel anxiety, fear, or discomfort for their disease, their symptoms are often influenced by their emotion. Moreover, it is classically considered one of the representative formulations to improve abdominal bloating, which includes an excess of abdominal gas in its pathophysiology. Therefore, HKT seems to be very effective for CINV of patients with an excess of abdominal gas and anxiety.

## 2. Chemotherapy-induced Diarrhea

Irinotecan hydrochloride (CPT-11) possesses a wide antitumor spectrum against lung cancer, colon cancer, malignant lymphoma, and so on. It is a semisynthetic derivative of camptothecin and an anticancer drug which inhibits nucleic acid synthesis by topoisomerase I inhibition [9]. The leading side effects of CPT-11 include diarrhea, which occurs in 63–79% of the patients. This side effect is the main reason for discontinuing administration. There are two types of CPT-11-induced diarrhea: acute diarrhea that occurs during the early stages of drug administration, and delayed diarrhea that occurs during later stages. The former is thought to be caused by the anticholinesterase actions of CPT-11. It is mostly transient in nature, and can be treated effectively with anticholine drugs [10]. The latter sometimes develops into severe diarrhea, which is difficult to control. For this reason, other patients drop out from taking CPT-11 [10]. The mechanism of CPT-11-induced delayed diarrhea is as follows. CPT-11 is metabolized to 7-ethyl-10-hydroxycamptothecin (SN-38) in the liver, and inactivated by glucuronate conjugation as SN-38 glucuronide. It is deconjugated by β-glucuronidase of intestinal bacteria, and returns as SN-38 in the bile [11]. Activated SN-38 directly damages the intestinal mucous membrane and induces delayed diarrhea.

HST, containing baicalin, serves as a β-glucuronidase inhibitor, which prevents the deconjugation of inactive SN-38. Experiments with rats have shown that it effectively prevents CPT-11-induced delayed diarrhea [12], and HST can effectively prevent diarrhea caused by CPT-11 [13]. Moreover, a randomized comparative trial in combination therapy with cisplatin and CPT-11 in advanced non-small-cell lung carcinoma (NSCLC) showed that HST reduces the rate of CPT-11-induced severe diarrhea (grade3 and 4) [14].

HST contains seven crude drugs: Pinellaiae Tuber, Scutellariae Radix, Glycyrrhizae Radix, Zizyphi Fructus, Ginseng Radix, Coptitis Rhizoma, and Zingiberis Siccatum Rhizoma. In Kampo medicine, HST is indicated for focal distention caused by clumping of constrained heat and fluids in the epigastrium. In this concept, it is used for nausea, emesis, diarrhea, acute and chronic gastroenteritis, or dysfunction of all digestive systems.

In a colitis animal model, HST down-regulates the pro-inflammatory prostaglandins. HST effectively prevents CPT-11-induced delayed diarrhea in animal experiments [12, 15]. Moreover, one of the main ingredients of HST, Coptis Rhizome, contains berberin. Berberine inhibits butyrate-induced colonic epithelial cell death. The other important ingredient, Scutellariae Radix, contains baicalin, which is an inhibitor of β-glucuronidase.

# 3. Chemotherapy-induced Oral Mucositis

Chemotherapy induced oral mucositis (COM) is a common adverse effect associated with cytotoxic cancer chemotherapy. COM results in severe discomfort and impairment of patients' ability to eat, swallow, or speak. COM sometimes demands an unfavorable modification or reduction of chemotherapy, which may affect the survival rate. Chemotherapy-induced myelosuppression places patients at significant risk of bacteremia and sepsis from oral microorganisms resulting in increased COM[16]. Factors that exacerbate COM also activate the cyclooxygenase pathway that mediates ulcer and pain through the upregulation of pro-inflammatory prostaglandins [17].

It is shown that hangeshashinto (HST) downregulates the pro-inflammatory prostaglandins, such as prostaglandin E2 in colitis animal models [18, 19]. As mentioned in diarrhea section, berberine in HST has broad-spectrum antibacterial activity and inhibits butyrate-induced colonic epithelial cell death [20, 21]. Repeated topical application of HST improved the COM symptoms in the majority of patients [22]. It is also noted that two-thirds of patients on FOLFIRI (leucovorin, 5FU, and irinotecan) treatment developed COM. Mucosal lesions typically appear between 7 and 14 days after the initiation of chemotherapy, mainly on the movable mucosa and rarely affecting the dorsum of the tongue, the hard palate, or the gingiva [22]. Compounds like berberine might be responsible for the antimicrobial and anti-inflammatory effects, suppression of prostaglandins, and alleviation of COM symptoms by HST. In Kampo medicine, oral mucositis is caused by excess heat in the chest and diaphragm. Those that clear heat in the chest and diaphragm are called "shashinto" group, which means "Drain the Heart". HST is the representative formula in this group. The other important formula in this group is orengedokuto (OGT). "Shashinto"s resolves anxiety, malaise, or pain. HST and OGT are both often used for oral mucositis.

# 4. Bowel Obstruction/Constipation

In cancer patients after laparotomy and intestinal manipulation, gastrointestinal motility decreases, gastrointestinal transit delays, and intra-abdominal adhesion occurs. Adhesion may cause mechanical bowel obstruction and abdominal pain, resulting in prolonged hospitalization and greater health care utilization in postoperative cancer patients and survivors. In Japan, daikenchuto (DKT) is the most commonly used for prevention and treatment of postoperative bowel obstruction and gastrointestinal disorders. DKT is considered as a safe drug with only a rare incidence of minor side effects [23].

Morphine is one of the most effective anti-nociceptive agents used in pain management of terminal cancer patients. However, it induces severe constipation, causing an obvious reduction in quality of life (QOL) [24]. It is reported that about 60% of patients who take morphine-containing drugs suffer from severe constipation. Other side effects are nausea and vomiting (around 40%), impairment of consciousness (less than 20%) and dysuria (less than 3%). Magnesium oxide or sennoside-containing drugs are typically administered for treatment of constipation, but it is difficult to control the dose of these drugs, and these therapies often become intolerable to the patients. DKT relieves morphine-induced delay of gastrointestinal transit without affecting the anti-nociceptive effects of morphine. Furthermore, DKT causes moderate contraction of morphine-treated longitudinal muscle of ileum and relaxation of morphine-induced contractions of the circular muscle of ileum. These effects of DKT provide a pharmacological basis for recovery from morphine-induced disorder of gastrointestinal transit [25].

DKT is composed of four crude drugs: Zingiberis Siccatum Rhizome, Ginseng Radix, Zanthoxyli Fructus, and Maltosum. The chief ingredient of DKT is Maltosum, which confers a sweet taste and improves the palatability of this formula. DKT warms the intestine and cures abdominal pain, nausea and vomiting. The ''kenchu'' of DKT represents the reconstruction of gastrointestinal tract; therefore DKT can be translated as, ''strong soup for reconstructing gastrointestinal tract.''

The neuronal mechanism of DKT in morphine-induced constipation is partly associated with stimulation of serotonin receptors [26] and vanilloid receptors [27] by components of DKT such as (6)-shogaol and hydroxy-*L*-sanshool. Gastrointestinal transit may be coordinated by relaxation of the circular muscle and constriction of the longitudinal muscle through several neuronal networks including serotonin receptors [26, 28]. The accelerating effects of DKT on the rates of intestinal and colonic transits in morphine-treated mice would result from those of Zanthoxyli Fructus. The effect of hydroxy-*L*-sanshool was significantly inhibited by the capsaicin receptor antagonist, capsazepine [29]. Another DKT component, (6)-shogaol, isolated from Zingiberis Rhizome, acts on gastrointestinal motor neurons and facilitates an intestinal transit [30]. Moreover, it is suggested that (6)-shogaol exhibits a capsaicin-like effect on the terminals of primary afferent nerves containing substance P, causing the initial release of neuropeptides and finally depleting the contents of neuropeptides, by subsequent stimulation of the primary afferents [31].

Several important neurally mediated mechanisms are suggested as mediating the increased effective intestinal motility of DKT. One of these mechanisms of action involves the release of calcitonin gene-related peptide (CGRP), a neuropeptide produced by the sensory neurons of the gut. CGRP is the most powerful vasoactive substance and increases mucosal blood flow [32]. Serum calcitonin gene-related peptide level elevates after administration of DKT [33]. Therefore, CGRP in gut function may reveal diverse actions of DKT in the prevention of intestinal adhesions resulting from inflammation.

CGRP binds to the calcitonin receptor-like receptor (CRLR). The former receptor turns into the CRLR through binding of receptor activity modifying protein 1 (RAMP1), a specific type of modulating membrane protein from the family of RAM proteins. The CRLR family can function as a CGRP receptor or as an adrenomedullin (ADM) receptor depending on the modifying membrane proteins; binding of RAMP2 and/or RAMP3 converts the receptor to the ADM receptor. ADM belongs to the same peptide family as CGRP and has potent vasodilatory effects in the microvascular system. The major difference between CGRP and ADM is that the latter is not produced by neuronal cells, but rather by epithelial, smooth muscle cells, and other non-neuronal tissues. One of the characteristics of the small intestines is the production of ADM from the intestinal epithelial cells. ADM also has anti-inflammatory and powerful anti-cytokine effects and especially inhibits TNF$\alpha$.

The effect of DKT on blood flow in the rat gut with direct intra-intestinal administration of DKT was associated with the release of CGRP from the sensory nerve terminals of the mucosa, stimulating the expression and subsequent interaction of CGRP receptor and modifying proteins (CRLR and RAMP1), and thereby causing an immediate increase in colonic blood flow. This increase in intestinal blood flow, however, was not observed with oral administration of DKT, which suggested that the actions of DKT were mediated locally rather than systemically [34].

Distal gastrectomy (DG) and pylorus-preserving gastrectomy (PPG) have been employed for gastric cancer. PPG is reported to be superior to DG in regard to postoperative quality of life. However, some patients with PPG still suffer from gastric stasis. Rikkunshito (RKT) improves gastric emptying and postoperative symptoms of patients who have undergone a PPG [35].

In Kampo medicine, there are two popular formulas for constipation in cancer patients. Shokenchuto (SHKT) is in the same group as DKT. SHKT means ''small soup for reconstructing gastrointestinal tract''. The ingredients of SHKT are Ginger Rhizome, Maltosum, Zizyphi Fructus, Cinnamoni Cortex, Glycyrrhiza Radix, and Peony Radix. This is a popular formula for treating abdominal pain due to cold. It is indicated for those who are in a generally weak and debilitated disposition associated with the loss of essence such that the patient looks pale, is easily exhausted, or feels cold but sweats easily.

Mashiningan (MNG) is composed of Paeoniae Radix, Rhubarb Rhizome, Aurantii Fructus Immaturus Armeniacae Semen, Cannabis Semen and Magnoliae Cortex. MNG is a variation of shojokito that purges heat accumulation and relieves moderate constipation. The chief herb, Cannabis Semen, is rich in oil that moistens the intestine and facilitates bowel movement.

# 5. Neuropathy

Neuropathy is one of the major reasons that limit treatment tolerability, often necessitating treatment delay or cessation. Neuropathic symptoms may persist for a long time. All platinum analogs are potentially neurotoxic. Oxaliplatin is especially associated with a unique spectrum of neurologic symptoms. Severe oxaliplatin-induced neuropathy, such as sensory ataxia or functional impairment, occurs in 10–20% of patients receiving a higher cumulative dose [36, 37].

The Kampo medicine, goshajinkigan (GJG), is composed of 10 crude drugs: Rehmanniae Radix, Achyranthis Radix, Corni Fructus, Dioscoreae Radix, Plantaginis Semens, Alismatis

Rhizoma, Hoelen, Moutan Cortex, Cinnamomi Cortex, and Aconiti Tuber. It is traditionally used for the treatment of lower back pain, leg pain, difficulty of urination, or knee-joint deformities. It suggested that GJG improved vibration sensation in patients with diabetic neuropathy [38]. GJG is also reported to improve taxanes-induced neuropathy [39]. In a retrospective study, GJG was effective for peripheral neurotoxicity of oxaliplatin in patients with advanced or recurrent colorectal cancer [40]. GJG safely reduced the incidence of severe neuropathy by mFOLFOX6 regimen without any adverse influence on the response rate to mFOLFOX6. It is useful in preventing oxaliplatin-induced neuropathy in patients with non-resectable or recurrent colorectal cancer. Moreover, GJG did not have an influence on tumor response to mFOLFOX6 therapy [41].

GJG may alleviate peripheral neuropathy by several mechanisms [42–44]. The first is that GJG promotes the release of dynorphin, and thus improves numbness/pallesthesia via the opiate system. The second is that GJG promotes nitric oxide production, and thus improves the circulation and blood supply to the nerves. Additionally, oxaliplatin acts on IB4-positive C-fiber nociceptors to induce an oxidative stress-dependent acute painful peripheral neuropathy [45], and GJG reduces transmitter proteins and sensory receptors associated with C-fiber activation [46].

This effect may be one of the mechanisms of GJG that prevents oxaliplatin-induced neuropathy.

## 6. Vasomotor Symptoms Associated with Cancer Therapy

Vasomotor symptoms associated with cancer therapies are increasingly common problems for breast cancer survivors given the increasing use of ovarian suppression with anti-estradiol (E2) agents, adjuvant chemotherapy in premenopausal women, and aromatase inhibitors in postmenopausal women. Estrogen receptor (ER) positive breast cancers are with additional risks; approximately 60% of breast cancers are ER-positive [47]. In general, hormone replacement therapy (HRT) effectively treats estrogen-deficiency symptoms, but it is probably associated with an increase in breast cancer risk, especially with prolonged use. Thus, it is still difficult to manage estrogen-deficiency symptoms in breast cancer survivors with HRT. In Japan, for vasomotor symptoms of menopause, traditional herbal medicines (Kampo) have been widely used in primary health care. It is possible that Kampo medicines may also be beneficial for breast cancer survivors with estrogen deficiency symptoms. Some clinical use of Kampo medicines for breast cancer survivors has already been reported.

Nyoshinsan (NSS) is indicated for menopausal symptoms such as hot flashes and transient feelings of anxiety. Yet chemicals that possess E2-like activity have not been reported in NSS. NSS is composed of 12 crude drugs: Cyperi Rhizoma, Cnidii Rhizoma, Atractylodis Lanceae Rhizoma, Angelicae Radix, Cinamomi Cortex, Ginseng radix, Arecae Semen, Coptitis Rhizoma, Glycyrrhizae Radix, Carophyllis Flos, and Saussureae Radix. Although NSS contains various chemical substances, neither an elevation in the serum level of E2 nor a decrease in the serum level of FSH is observed. Therefore, the action of NSS may not be based on estrogenic behavior [8].

Unkeito (UKT) is another alternative for menopausal symptoms. UKT is composed of 12 crude drugs; Ophiopogonis Tuber, Pinelliae Tuber, Angelicae Radix, Glycyrrhizae Radix, Cinnamoni Cortex, Paeoniae Radix, Cnidii Rhizoma, Ginseng Radix, Moutan Radix, Evodiae Fructus, Zingiberis Rhizoma, and Asini Gelatum. UKT is used for dysmenorrhea, amenorrhea, or menopausal syndrome. Eight weeks of treatment with UKT enhanced the secretion of follicle stimulating hormone (FSH), luteinizing hormone (LH) and estradiol levels in hyper- (robust) and hypo- (asthenia) functioning patients with first and second grade amenorrhea during a 12-week follow-up. No significant difference was observed in the rate of change of these hormones between hyper- and hypo-functioning patients. It suggests that UKT could be used safely for cancer patients with menopausal symptoms.

## 7. General Fatigue

General fatigue is a common problem in cancer patients. The most important factors contributing to cancer-related fatigue are anemia, pain, emotional distress, sleep disturbance, and poor nutrition resulting from cancer therapy. Cancer-related fatigue is particularly prevalent with multimodality or dose-intense treatment protocols, and in patients with metastatic disease. In Western medicine, management of cancer-related fatigue involves specific treatment for potentially reversible causes (i.e., treating anemia or metabolic or endocrine abnormalities, as well as managing pain, insomnia, depression, or anxiety) and symptomatic measures. Nonspecific symptomatic treatment measures include education, counseling, and pharmacologic (e.g., psychostimulants) as well as non-pharmacologic (e.g., exercise, yoga, acupuncture) measures. In Kampo medicine, patients with pronounced general fatigue and malaise can be treated with Kampo formulas. In this condition, often considered as loss of vital energy, especially Ginseng Radix and Astragali Radix formulations "jingizai" are said to be effective. These formulas include hochuekkito (HET), jyuzentaihoto (JTT), or ninjin'yoeito (NYT), and are useful for cancer patients.

HET is composed of ten crude drugs: Astragali Radix, Atractylodis Lanceae Rhizoma, Ginseng Radix, Angelicae Radix, Bupleuri Radix, Zizyphi Fructus, Aurantii Nobilis Pericarpium, Glycyrrhizae Radix, Cimicifugae Rhizoma, and Zingiberis Rhizoma.

HET is distinguished from other jingizais by containing Bupleuri Radix, which relieves physical and psychological stress. One-week preoperative treatment with HET was effective for improving pre- and postoperative nutritional status and immune function in patients scheduled to undergo laparotomy for large intestine carcinoma in randomized controlled trial using sealed envelopes for allocation (RCT-envelope). Mean prealbumin level was higher in the HET group from the day before surgery to 7 days after surgery. IL-6 was lower in the HET group on postoperative day 1. It was suggested that preoperative treatment with HET is useful for early recovery from surgery for colorectal carcinoma [49]. It is also reported that HET during chemotherapy for lung cancer relieves and improves mood and general malaise [50, 51].

JTT is composed of 10 crude drugs: Astragali Radix, Cinnamoni Cortex, Rehmanniae Radix, Paeoniae Radix, Cnidii Rhizoma, Atractylodis Lanceae Rhizoma, Angelicae Radix, Ginseng Radix, Hoelen, and Glycyrrhizae Radix. NYT is composed of very similar components to JTT. NYT is consist of 12 crude drugs: Rehmanniae Radix, Paeoniae Radix,

Atractylodis Lanceae Rhizoma, Hoelen, Astragali Radix, Ginseng Radix, Cinnamoni Cortex, Angelicae Radix, Polygalae Radix, Schisandrae Fructus, and Glycyrrhizae Radix. JTT significantly prolonged survival rate for advanced breast cancer patients when the JTT group was stratified by Kampo diagnosis [52]. NYT is effective for patients with psychological fatigue and insomnia. The combination of NYT and JTT is effective for reducing myelosuppression and nephrotoxicity associated with chemotherapy [53]. These effects would alleviate general fatigue.

## Conclusion

In this chapter, we introduce some formulas mainly with recent clinical and basic researches in Kampo supportive therapy for cancer patients. It is certain that the effort to clarify the mechanism of Kampo formulas, but it is important to understand that the concept of Kampo medicine is to understand and improve the general condition of patients. There are many things to learn from the method of Kampo examination. The integration of western medicine and Kampo medicine would make new progress in cancer supportive therapy.

## References

[1] Kusunoki H, Haruma K, Hata J, Ishii M, Kamada T, Yamashita N, et al. Efficacy of Rikkunshito, a traditional Japanese medicine (Kampo), in treating functional dyspepsia. *Intern Med.* 2010; 49 (20): 2195-202.

[2] Arai M, Matsumura T, Yoshikawa M, Imazeki F, Yokosuka O. [Analysis of the Rikkunshito efficacy on patients with functional dyspepsia]. *Nihon Yakurigaku Zasshi.* 2011;137(1):18-21.

[3] Tschop M, Smiley DL, Heiman ML. Ghrelin induces adiposity in rodents. *Nature,* 2000; 40(7)908–913.

[4] Takeda H, Sadakane C, Hattori T, Katsurada T, Ohkawara T, Nagai K, et al. Rikkunshito, an herbal medicine, suppresses cisplatin-induced anorexia in rats via 5-HT2 receptor antagonism. *Gastroenterology.* 2008; 134(7):2004-13.

[5] Fujitsuka N, Asakawa A, Hayashi M, Sameshima M, Amitani H, Kojima S, et al. Selective serotonin reuptake inhibitors modify physiological gastrointestinal motor activities via 5-HT2c receptor and acyl ghrelin. *Biol Psychiatry.* 2009; 65(9): 748-59.

[6] Takeda H, Muto S, Hattori T, Sadakane C, Tsuchiya K, Katsurada T, et al. Rikkunshito ameliorates the aging-associated decrease in ghrelin receptor reactivity via phosphodiesterase III inhibition. *Endocrinology.* 2010; 151(1):244-52.

[7] Hattori T. Rikkunshito and ghrelin. *Int J Pept.* 2010; 2010.

[8] Oikawa T, Ito G, Hoshino T, Koyama H, Hanawa T. Hangekobokuto (Banxia-houpo-tang), a Kampo Medicine that Treats Functional Dyspepsia. *Evid Based Complement Alternat Med.* 2009;6(3):375-8.

[9] Hecht JR. Gastrointestinal toxicity of irinotecan. Oncology. 1998; 12(8 Suppl 6):72–78.

[10] Masuda N, Fukuoka M, Kudoh S, Kusunoki Y, Matsui K, Takifuji N, et al. Phase I and pharmacologic study of irinotecan in combination with cisplatin for advanced lung cancer. *Br J Cancer.* 1993;68(4):777-82.

[11] Kaneda N, Nagata H, Furuta T, Yokokura T. Metabolism and pharmacokinetics of the camptothecin analogue CPT-11 in the mouse. *Cancer Res.* 1990;50(6):1715-20.

[12] Takasuna K, Kasai Y, Kitano Y, Mori K, Kobayashi R, Hagiwara T, et al. Protective effects of kampo medicines and baicalin against intestinal toxicity of a new anticancer camptothecin derivative, irinotecan hydrochloride (CPT-11), in rats. *Jpn J Cancer Res.* 1995;86(10):978-84.(Japanese)

[13] Sakata Y, Suzuki H, Kamataki T. [Preventive effect of TJ-14, a kampo (Chinese herb) medicine, on diarrhea induced by irinotecan hydrochloride (CPT-11)]. *Gan To Kagaku Ryoho.* 1994;21(8):1241-4.

[14] Mori K, Kondo T, Kamiyama Y, Kano Y, Tominaga K. Preventive effect of Kampo medicine (Hangeshashin-to) against irinotecan-induced diarrhea in advanced non-small-cell lung cancer. *Cancer Chemother Pharmacol.* 2003; 51(5):403-6.

[15] Narita M, Nagai E, Hagiwara H, Aburada M, Yokoi T, Kamataki T. Inhibition of beta-glucuronidase by natural glucuronides of kampo medicines using glucuronide of SN-38 (7-ethyl-10-hydroxycamptothecin) as a substrate. *Xenobiotica.* 1993; 23(1):5-10.

[16] Napenas JJ, Shetty KV, Streckfus CF. Oral mucositis: review of pathogenesis, diagnosis, prevention, and management. *Gen Dent.* 2007; 55(4):335-344.

[17] Lalla RV, Pilbeam CC, Walsh SJ, Sonis ST, Keefe DM, Peterson DE. Role of the cyclooxygenase pathway in chemotherapy-induced oral mucositis: a pilot study. *Support Care Cancer.* 2009.

[18] Kase Y, Hayakawa T, Ishige A, et al. The effects of Hange-shashin-to on the content of prostaglandin E2 and water absorption in the large intestine of rats. *Biol Pharm Bull* : 20(9):954-957,1997.

[19] Kase Y, Hayakawa T, Ishige A, Aburada M, Komatsu Y. The effects of Hange-shashin-to on the content of prostaglandin E2 and water absorption in the large intestine of rats. *Biol Pharm Bull.* 1997; 20(9):954-7.

[20] Samosorn S, Tanwirat B, Muhamad N, Casadei G, Tomkiewicz D, Lewis K, et al. Antibacterial activity of berberine-NorA pump inhibitor hybrids with a methylene ether linking group. *Bioorg Med Chem.* 2009;17(11):3866-72.

[21] Grycova L, Dostal J, Marek R. Quaternary protoberberine alkaloids. *Phytochemistry.* 2007; 68(2):150-175.

[22] Kono T, Satomi M, Chisato N, Ebisawa Y, Suno M, Asama T, et al. Topical Application of Hangeshashinto (TJ-14) in the Treatment of Chemotherapy-Induced Oral Mucositis. *World J Oncol.* 2010: 1, 6, 232-235.

[23] Itoh T, Yamakawa J, Mai M, Yamaguchi N, Kanda T. The effect of the herbal medicine dai-kenchu-to on post-operative ileus. *J Int Med Res.* 2002;30(4):428-32.

[24] Mancini I and Bruera E: Constipation in advanced cancer patients. *Support Care Cancer.* 1998; 6, 356 – 364.

[25] Nakamura T, Sakai A, Isogami I, Noda K, Ueno K, Yano S. Abatement of morphine-induced slowing in gastrointestinal transit by Dai-kenchu-to, a traditional Japanese herbal medicine. *Jpn J Pharmacol.* 2002;88(2):217-21.

[26] Prins NH, Akkermans LM, Lefebvre RA, Schuurkes JA. 5-HT(4) receptors on cholinergic nerves involved in contractility of canine and human large intestine longitudinal muscle. *Br J Pharmacol.* 2000;131(5):927-32.

[27] Shibata C, Sasaki I, Naito H, Ueno T and Matsuno S: The herbal medicine Dai-Kenchu Tou stimulates upper gut motility through cholinergic and 5-hydroxy-tryptamine 3 receptors in conscious dogs. *Surgery.* 1999; 126, 918 -924.

[28] Shibata C, Sasaki I, Naito H, Tsuchiya T, Takahashi M, Ohtani N, et al. Intragastric capsaicin stimulates colonic motility via a neural reflex in conscious dogs. *Gastroenterology.* 1995; 109(4):1197-205.

[29] Satoh K, Hashimoto K, Hayakawa T, Ishige A, Kaneko M, Ogihara S, et al. Mechanism of atropine-resistant contraction induced by Dai-kenchu-to in guinea pig ileum. *Jpn J Pharmacol.* 2001;86(1):32-7.

[30] Yamahara J, Huang QR, Li YH, Xu L, Fujimura H. Gastrointestinal motility enhancing effect of ginger and its active constituents. *Chem Pharm Bull (*Tokyo). 1990;38(2):430-1.

[31] Onogi T, Minami M, Kuraishi Y, Satoh M. Capsaicin-like effect of (6)-shogaol on substance P-containing primary afferents of rats: a possible mechanism of its analgesic action. *Neuropharmacology.* 1992;31(11):1165-9.

[32] Katsoulis S., Conlon J. M., Calcitonin gene-related peptides relax guinea pig and rat gastric smooth muscle. *Eur. J. Pharmacol.* 1989; 162, 129-134.

[33] Sato Y, Katagiri F, Inoue S, Itoh H, Takeyama M. Dai-kenchu-to raises levels of calcitonin gene-related peptide and substance P in human plasma. *Biol Pharm Bull.* 2004;27(11):1875-7.

[34] Kono T, Kanematsu T, Kitajima M. Exodus of Kampo, traditional Japanese medicine, from the complementary and alternative medicines: is it time yet? *Surgery.* 2009;146(5):837-40.

[35] Takahashi T, Endo S, Nakajima K, Souma Y, Nishida T. Effect of rikkunshito, a chinese herbal medicine, on stasis in patients after pylorus-preserving gastrectomy. *World J Surg.* 2009;33(2):296-302.

[36] Krishnan AV, Goldstein D, Friedlander M, Kiernan MC. Oxaliplatin-induced neurotoxicity and the development of neuropathy. *Muscle Nerve.* 2005;32(1):51-60.

[37] Land SR, Kopec JA, Cecchini RS, Ganz PA, Wieand HS, Colangelo LH, et al. Neurotoxicity from oxaliplatin combined with weekly bolus fluorouracil and leucovorin as surgical adjuvant chemotherapy for stage II and III colon cancer: NSABP C-07. *J Clin Oncol.* 2007;25(16):2205-11.

[38] Uno T, Ohsawa I, Tokudome M, Sato Y. Effects of Goshajinkigan on insulin resistance in patients with type 2 diabetes. *Diabetes Res Clin Pract.* 2005;69(2):129-35.

[39] Yamamoto T, Murai T, Ueda M, Katsuura M, Oishi M, Miwa Y, et al. [Clinical features of paclitaxel-induced peripheral neuropathy and role of Gosya-jinki-gan]. *Gan To Kagaku Ryoho.* 2009;36(1):89-92.

[40] Kono T, Mamiya N, Chisato N, Ebisawa Y, Yamazaki H, Watari J, et al. *Efficacy of Goshajinkigan for Peripheral Neurotoxicity of Oxaliplatin in Patients with Advanced or Recurrent Colorectal Cancer.* Evid Based Complement Alternat Med. 2009.

[41] Nishioka M, Shimada M, Kurita N, Iwata T, Morimoto S, Yoshikawa K, et al. The Kampo medicine, Goshajinkigan, prevents neuropathy in patients treated by FOLFOX regimen. *Int J Clin Oncol.* 2011;16(4):322-7.

[42] Yamada K, Suzuki E, Nakaki T, Watanabe S, Kanba S. Aconiti tuber increases plasma nitrite and nitrate levels in humans. *J Ethnopharmacol.* 2005;96(1-2):165-9.

[43] Gotoh A, Goto K, Sengoku A, Shirakawa T, Akao Y, Fujisawa M, et al. Inhibition mechanism of Gosha-jinki-gan on the micturition reflex in rats. *J Pharmacol Sci.* 2004;96(2):115-23.

[44] Hu X, Sato J, Oshida Y, Xu M, Bajotto G, Sato Y. Effect of Gosha-jinki-gan (Chinese herbal medicine: Niu-Che-Sen-Qi-Wan) on insulin resistance in streptozotocin-induced diabetic rats. *Diabetes Res Clin Pract.* 2003;59(2):103-11.

[45] Joseph EK, Chen X, Bogen O, Levine JD. Oxaliplatin acts on IB4-positive nociceptors to induce an oxidative stress-dependent acute painful peripheral neuropathy. *J Pain.* 2008;9(5):463-72.

[46] Imamura T, Ishizuka O, Aizawa N, Zhong C, Ogawa T, Nakayama T, et al. Gosha-jinki-gan reduces transmitter proteins and sensory receptors associated with C fiber activation induced by acetic acid in rat urinary bladder. *Neurourol Urodyn.* 2008;27(8):832-7.

[47] Kroman N, Jensen MB, Wohlfahrt J, Mouridsen HT, Andersen PK, Melbye M. Factors influencing the effect of age on prognosis in breast cancer: population based study. *BMJ.* 2000;320(7233):474-8.

[48] Kogure T, Ito K, Sato H, Ito T, Oku Y, Horiguchi J, et al. Efficacy of Nyoshinsan/TJ-67, a traditional herbal medicine, for menopausal symtoms following surgery and adjuvant chemotherapy for premenopausal breast cancer. *Int J Clin Oncol.* 2008;13(2):185-9.

[49] Nishimura G. Evaluation of clinical efficacy of hochuekkito in improving nutritional/immune status in patients with surgery for large intestine carcinoma*. *Progress in Medicine.* 2009; 29: 84-85.(Japanese)

[50] Inui H, Yamagata T, Minakata Y, et al. Prevention of side effects during lung cancer chemotherapy by Hochuekki-to. *Kampo to Saishin-chiryo.* 1993; 2: 56–60. (Japanese)

[51] Mori K, Kondo T, Kamiyama Y, Kano Y, Tominaga K. Preventive effect of Kampo medicine (Hangeshashin-to) against irinotecan-induced diarrhea in advanced non-small-cell lung cancer. *Cancer Chemother Pharmacol.* 2003; 51(5):403-6.(Japanese with English abstract).

[52] Adachi I. Supporting therapy with Shi Quan Da Bu Tang in advanced breast cancer patients. *Biomedical Research.* 1990 ; 11 suppl: 25–31.

[53] Hasegawa K. Clinical usefulness of Kampo medicines (Ninjin-yoei-to, Juzen-taiho-to) for side effects in gynecologic cancer chemotherapy – Effects on reducing side effects by CDDP in CAP therapy. *J. Trad. Med.* 1994; 11, 181-187. (Japanese with English abstract)

In: Traditional Medicine: New Research
Editor: Yoshiharu Motoo
ISBN: 978-1-62257-448-3


*Chapter 2*

# NEXIA as a Promising Non-toxic Cancer Therapeutic Agent in Various Types of Cancer

***Won Cheol Choi***
Kyung Hee University Hospital of Oriental Medicine, Korea

## History

NEXIA is a non-toxic cancer therapeutic agent for use in various types of cancer in East-Asian countries, with a history of 1800 years in CHINA and 800 years in KOREA in its original form (Lacquer Tree) according to the Medical Classics.

What is NEXIA?

- NEXIA is allergen-removed *Rhus verniciflua Stokes* (Lacquer Tree) extract developed by Dr. Choi, Won Cheol
- Korea has the first and unique knowhow in making this drug for cancer among East-Asian countries
- *Non-Toxic* (The leader of US Food and Drug Administration Oncology said "I wish all cancer drugs were non-toxic.")
- Can be combined with over 60 western Chemotherapeutic agents

*About Academician and Professor Choi*

- Academician of RAMS (Russian Academy of Medical Science) as a foreign member
- Professor of Kyung Hee University Hospital of Oriental Medicine
- PhD in Science in Oriental Medicine
- PhD in Pharmaceutical Science
- Number 1 Doctor in treating advanced cancer rated by the Korean Association of Cancer Survivors
- Number 1 Doctor of the Future elected by 1,500 opinion leaders of Korea

- Number 1 Doctor Alive elected by 1,500 opinion leaders of Korea

*Achievements*

- Ongoing Phase II Clinical Trial for approval as a new drug in Korea
- Ongoing collaboration with the U.S. National Cancer Institute
- Introduced in many magazines, journals, television news, and newspapers in Korea and Reuter's news

*Publication*

- Over 100 papers in peer-reviewed domestic and international journals since 2006:
- Among these, one paper presented two cases, renal cell carcinoma with clinically or pathologically diagnosed multiple metastases, and demonstrated complete remissions (completely cured from advanced cancer) with monotherapy of NEXIA, first in the World
- Over 80 successful case series published in "NEXIA Review (Volume 1 and 2)"

*Patent*

Korea: 20 pending & 5 issued patents
Foreign: 13 pending & 2 issued patents

*Value*

As we learned from Taxol, discovered and isolated from the bark of the Pacific yew tree, ,the Value of NEXIA would run into astronomical financial figures according to a U.S. National Cancer Institute program at the Research Triangle Institute in 1967.

# Why NEXIA as an Oncology Drug?

## Oncology Drug Development Process and Costs

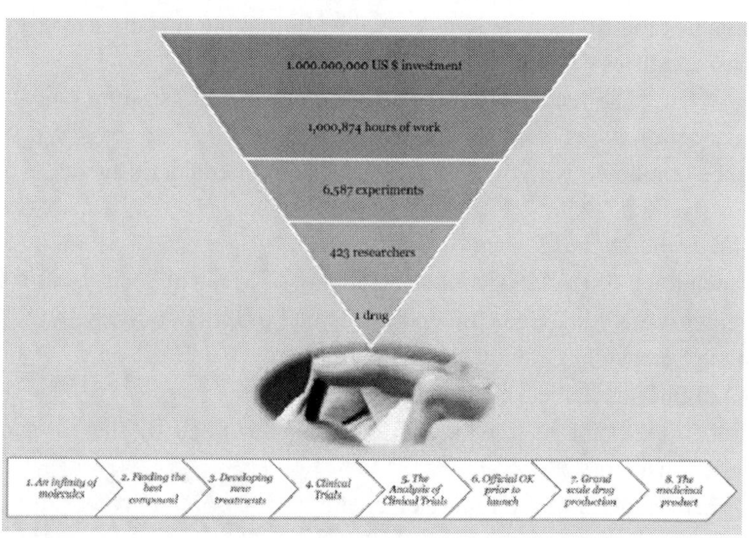

It is a risky and expensive business: With net cost of more than $800 Million ($1,200 Million for an oncology drug) and investing for 15 years, 1 out of 10,000 screened can be approved as a new drug (probability of success = 0.01%)

## Success Stories from the Natural products

• Taxol (Paclitaxel): the bark of the Pacific yew

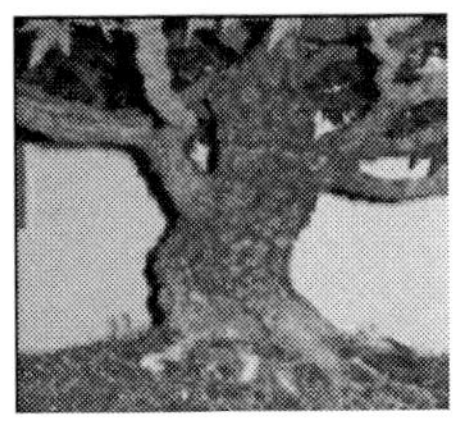

Taxol, the world's best-selling anti-cancer drug, is a natural product found in the bark of Taxus brevifolia (the Pacific yew) and a chemical substance that was discovered and brought to the point of commercial production in the public sector.

• Tamiflu (Oseltamivir Phosphate): *Anisi stellati Fructus*

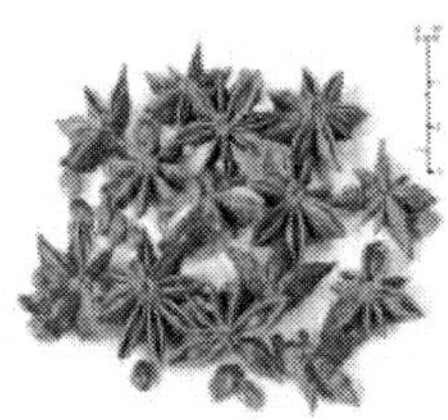

Shikimic acid extracted from the pods (which wraps the seeds) of star anise (*Anisi stellati Fructus*) is the starting material of Tamiflu. Tamiflu is an antiviral drug that slows the spread of the influenza (flu) virus. It has been used to treat and prevent Influenzavirus A and Influenzavirus B infection in over 50 million people since 1999.

**Possibility of NEXIA as a New Anti-Cancer Drug**

- Non-cytotoxic (Non-Toxic) from the natural product
- Since NEXIA is in Phase IIb, it has already been invested for >10 years with necessary costs, and the probability of success is >>30~50% rather than 0.01%
- NEXIA is targeting maintenance therapy after the first line of therapy for non-small cell lung cancer and it can be combined with chemotherapeutic agents available today (on going PhaseII Trial)

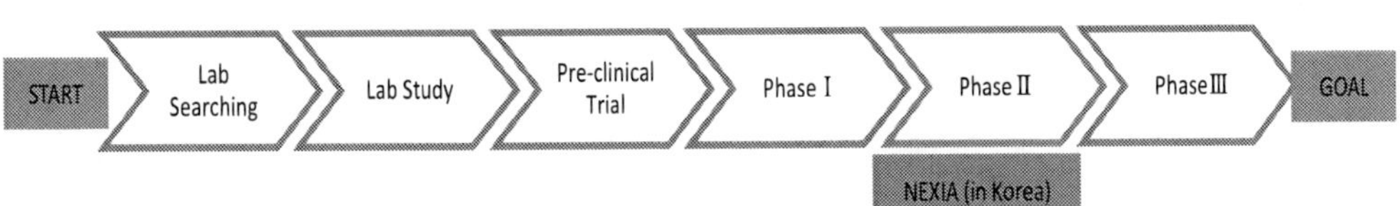

## Anti-cancer Natural Product Derivative

**ABSTRACT**

*Rhus verniciflua* Stokes *(RVS)* of the Anacardiaceae family commonly known as the lacquer tree was a traditional herbal medicine for various stomach diseases including cancer in Korea and China. Owing to a property of breaking up blood stasis and purging hardness based on traditional medicine theory, it could be a drug against malignant tumor. Recently flavonoids from RVS have also been experimentally proven to have apoptotic activities in human cancer cell lines. Therefore, we manufactured a standard extract from RVS (**AZINX75**) for the purpose of prolonging survival, and improving the quality of life in cancer patients with only palliative therapy available.

**GRAPHIC ABSTRACT**

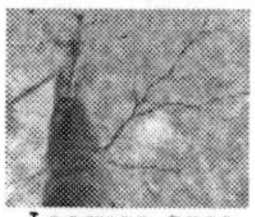

Lacquer tree

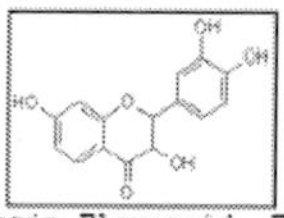

Fustin Flavonoid, Fisetin

**MECHANISM OF ACTION**

AZINX75 was experimentally proved to have anti-angiogenic activities by inhibiting the vascular endothelial growth factor (VEGF) and was recently shown to have an inhibitory effect on matrix metalloproteinase-2 (MMP-2) and MMP-9 activities in a human fibrosarcoma cell line.

**QUALITY CONTROL**

A component analysis method using high performance liquid chromatography showed that the AZINX75 contained fustin, fisetin, sulfuretin, and butein, among others. The quality of the AZINX75 was tested and controlled according to the quality standards of the Korea Food & Drug Administration and our hospital's standards (fustin > 13.0%, fisetin > 2.0%, urushiol not detected). Daily oral administration with 1350mg (1 capsule containing 450 mg three times a day) of AZINX75 was prescribed.

**TOXICOLOGY**

AZINX75 administered orally is well tolerated with no obvious side effects such as weight loss. There were no reported drug-drug interaction between AZINX75 and concurrent chemotherapy agents

**COMPETITION**

Compared to conventional chemotherapy agent, AZINX75 has no serious side effects. It mitigates adverse effects of conventional chemotherapy treatment, and it is easily administered as long-term treatment. It has immune-stimulatory effects and can be administer in combination with existing synthetic drug.AZINX75 is a supplemental treatment and would not replace primary chemotherapy agent, so it would be an uncomplicated decision for physicians.

**PATENTS**

Korea:20 pending & 5 issued patents
Foreign: 13 pending & 2 issued patents

***NCI collaboration study**

AZINX75 effect on Endothelial Cell tube formation

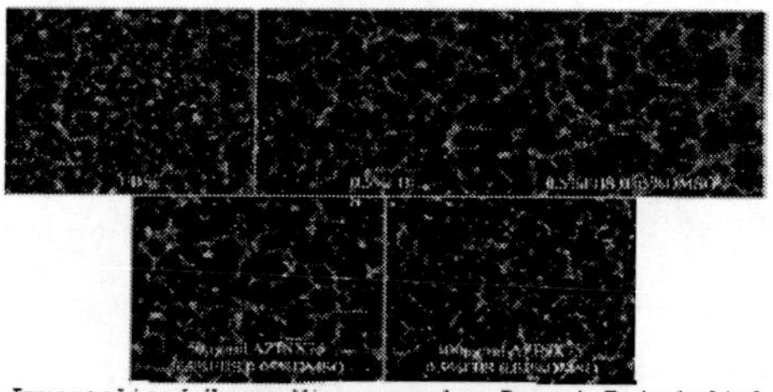

Immortalized Human Microvascular Dermal Endothelial Cell Line (HMEC-1) 28,000 Cells/Well + AZINX75 [ug/ml] for 3hrs

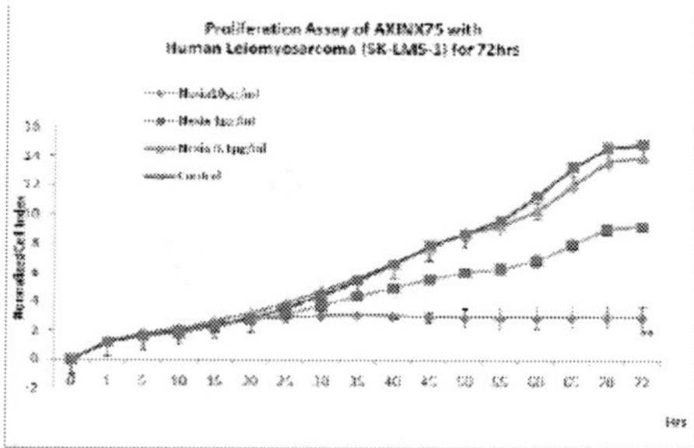


**81% Inhibitory Effect of Proliferation**

US-NCI Collaboration **Electric Cell-substrate Impedance Sensing (ECIS)**

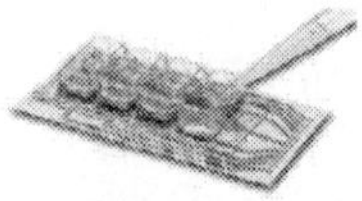

(Roche Has an Equivalent System Know As ACEA)

In: Traditional Medicine: New Research
Editor: Yoshiharu Motoo
ISBN: 978-1-62257-448-3


*Chapter 3*

# Creating an Appropriate Modern Herbal Formula for the Adjuvant Treatment of Cancer

*G. G. L. Yue, C. B. S. Lau and P. C. Leung*
Institute of Chinese Medicine, The Chinese University of Hong Kong,
Shatin, New Territories, Hong Kong

## Introduction

Caner is a pathological condition. Removal of the cancer is a necessity in the treatment process. However, removal has reached its limitations as the cancer could be too extensive, or, in spite of the removal, still recur . When the pathological process is not stopped, no matter how effective the cancer removal is, the formation of cancer is going to be repeated. Cancer treatment has therefore gone beyond the stage of cancer removal and other approaches such as controlling the blood supply, initiating apoptosis, and regulating the responsible genes. The treatment approach needs to be modified from a single target, eliminative direction towards a multiple target, holistic direction. Modern medicine still lacks a perfect understanding of the causative factors of cancer formation, hence it follows a multi-target holistic approach. As new systems of cancer treatment are not yet mature, using Chinese medicine as an adjuvant therapy could be an innovative and practical investment to bring about better results of cancer control.

## Chinese Medicine and Cancer

Putting classical Chinese Medicine principles into modern understanding, the practicing herbalist of today would administer his/her treatment regime according to his/her observations of various syndromes. Before chemotherapy and before surgical treatment, he/she would start strengthening treatment for the maintenance of "Qi", that is internal balance. During chemotherapy, he/she would use herbs to strengthen the digestion. After chemotherapy and/or surgery, he/she would support lung functions and use blood-strengthening herbs, as well as a means to facilitate kidney clearance in an attempt to detoxicate.

## Experience at our Laboratory

In the laboratory, based on the standard needs of modern cancer research, we have developed research platforms to study the direct cytotoxicity, immunomodulation, and anti-angiogenesis of Chinese medicine (CM) as shown in Figure 1. In the following paragraphs, we will describe some basic work accomplished under the different platforms.

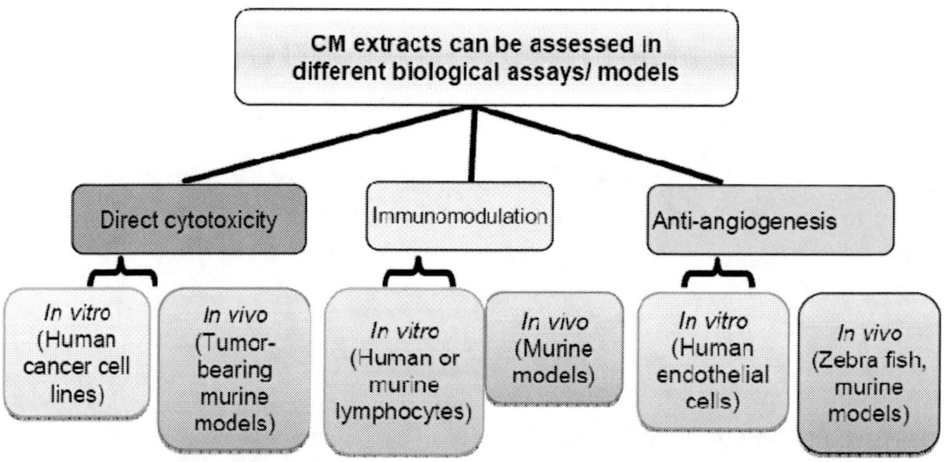


Figure 1. Research platforms for anti-cancer Chinese medicines (CM).

Although many different Chinese herbal medicines and their combinations have been reported to be effective against cancer, both in the laboratory and clinically, we want to limit our study to the least number of herbs which presumably would cover the area of direct cytotoxicity, anti-angiogenesis, and immunomodulation. Based on our early screening results of *in vitro* direct cytotoxic, immunomodulatory, and anti-angiogenic activities, the hot water and/or ethanolic extracts from five Chinese medicinal herbs, namely, *Scutellaria baicalensis* (黃芩), *Ganoderma lucidum* (靈芝), *Hedyotis (Oldenlandia) diffusa* (白花蛇舌草), *Andrographis paniculata* (穿心蓮), and *Acanthopanax senticosus* (刺五加) have been selected to form an innovative and complementary formulation. This formulation was subjected to evaluation of its efficacies in the following assays.

### I. Platform on Direct Cytotoxicity

Diagrammatically, *in vitro* and *in vivo* experiments are performed accordingly (Figure 2). Important findings include the following:

a. The formulation significantly inhibited proliferation of various human cancer cells, such as breast cancer (MCF-7, MDA-MB-231), liver cancer (HepG2, R-HepG2), and uterine sarcoma (MES-SA, MES-SA/Dx5), in a dose-dependent manner. The $IC_{50}$ values ranged from 66.7 to 208.1 μg/ml. The multi drug-resistant cell line R-HepG2 was derived from HepG2 in our university.
b. The formulation induced cell cycle arrest at G2/M phase of R-HepG2 cells, which was detected by flow cytometry.
c. The formulation induced R-HepG2 cells underwent apoptosis, which was confirmed by annexin-V & propidium iodide staining, and DNA fragmentation assay.
d. The expression of pro-apoptotic proteins, Bax and Bad, as well as PARP (poly ADP ribose polymerase) cleavage were induced by formulation treatment in R-HepG2 cells.
e. The formulation could significantly inhibit the growth of MCF-7 xenografts in nude mice.

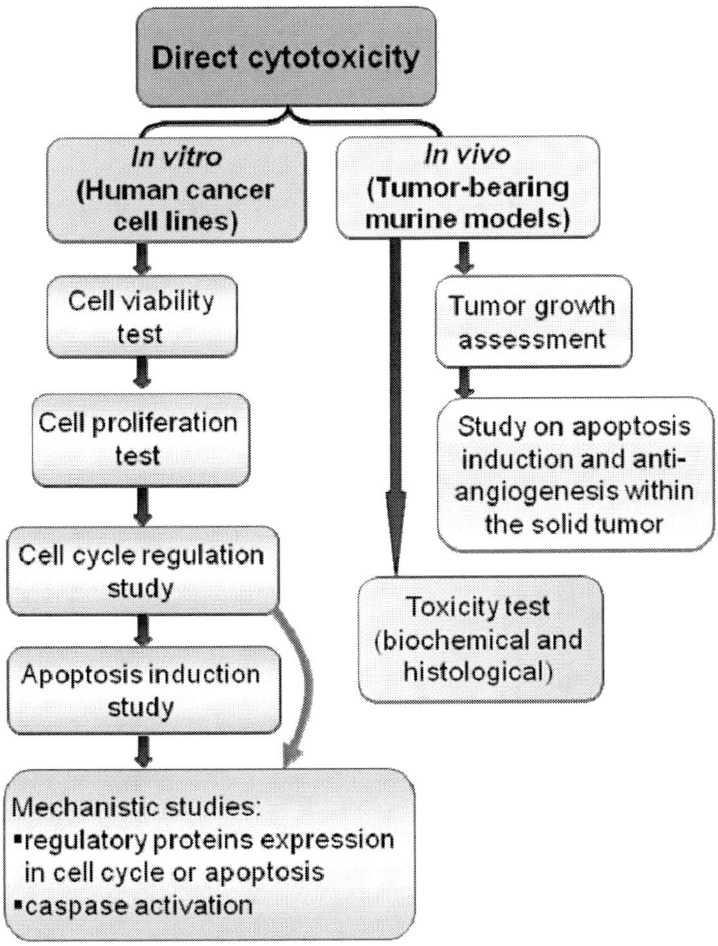


Figure 2. Study on direct cytotoxicity.

## II. Platform on Immunomodulation Effects which Should Be Responsible for the Tested Animals' Indirect Defense against Cancer Invasion (Figure 3)

Important findings include the following:

a. Formulation could enhance the proliferative response and TNF-α production of PHA-stimulated human peripheral blood mononuclear cells.
b. *Ganoderma lucidum*, one of the compositions of the formulation, has been shown to enhance the proliferation and cytokine production of mouse spleen lymphocytes from tumor-bearing mice.

### III. Platform on Anti-Angiogenesis

Both *in vitro* cultures and *in vivo* animal models will suffice for this study (Figure 4). Important findings include the following:

a. The formulation significantly inhibited proliferation of human umbilical vein endothelial cells (HUVEC) in a dose-dependent manner.
b. The formulation could inhibit the formation of inter-segmental vessels of zebra fish embryos.

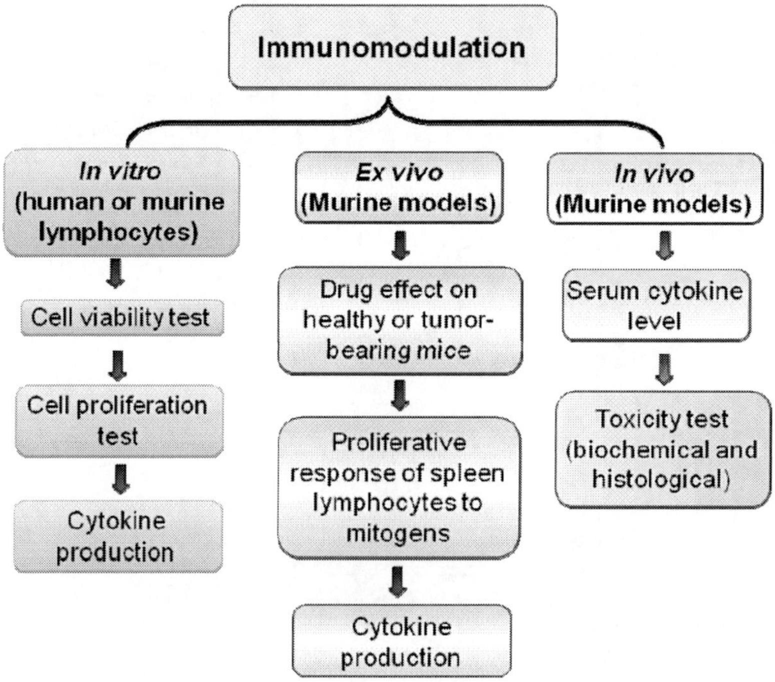


Figure 3. Study on immunomodulation.

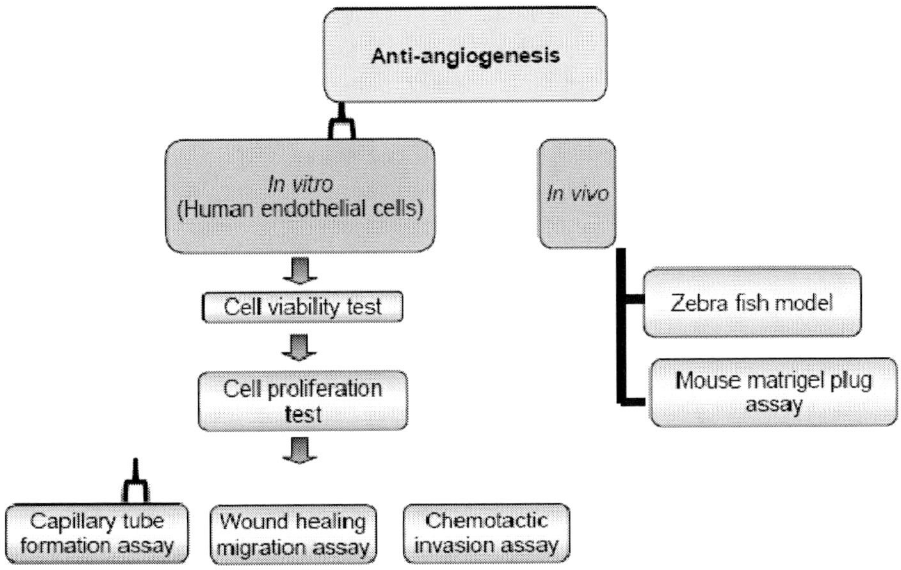


Figure 4. Study on anti-angiogenesis.

Apart from the above-mentioned platforms, the study of anti-metastatic Chinese herbal medicine was added in our research recently. The *in vitro* anti-invasive and anti-migration assays of cancer cells as well as the *in vivo* tumor-bearing animal models will be adequate for this study. The mouse breast cancer (4T1) metastasis model was newly established. The intratibial breast cancer model, which is in collaboration with Prof. Andreas Evdokiou, University of Adelaide, Australia, has been established and verified using conventional western drugs. The anti-metastatic effects of our formulation will be evaluated in these models.

## Experience on Clinical Applications

While active comprehensive *in vitro* and *in vivo* studies are conducted to verify the multiple efficacy targets of the anticancer herbal cocktail, the ultimate aim is to offer it to cancer patients as an adjunctive treatment supplement.

In the Chinese community in Hong Kong, over 90% of cancer patients are receiving supplementary treatments of various natures in an attempt to gain better chances of cancer control and survival (Wong *et al.*, 1993). It is therefore justified to explore the effectiveness of the adjuvant use of the popular herbs through clinical trials. Such efforts should not be viewed as a proper endorsement of popular beliefs. But rather, they are practical, responsible plans of clinical study, if well designed according to the modern concepts of good clinical practice, and could have a lot to offer in the holistic care of cancer treatment. After all, developing an innovative drug is expensive and time-consuming. The use of herbal supplements could be readily administered and safety is not difficult to ensure.

Of all the possible pathways of action offered by different herbs, since their active components and chemistry are still unknown, the most logical selection would be those that aim at holistic support through nutritional or immunological modulations. Innovative new pharmaceuticals offer specific, immediate effects. Holistic support offers non-specific, slow influences that could be defined as supplementary, palliative, or preventive.

A reasonable aim of cancer treatment is not only to remove the tumor mass and the harmful cells, but also to stop the dynamic process that has led to the development of the cancer. The logical expectation is: the holistic support works through complicated, yet unknown indirect pathways, whereby the cancer development process is kept at bay. In the following paragraphs, examples of clinical trials using herbal preparations as adjuvants will be given.

## A Clinical Trial Using Herbal Preparation as Supplements to Chemotherapy for Cancer

A Phase II, randomized, placebo-controlled trial using herbal preparations was conducted at the Prince of Wales Hospital of Hong Kong in 2002-2004, whereby 60+60 patients suffering from advanced cancer of the breast or colon were being treated with cytotoxic chemotherapy. The use of herbal preparations as supplementary support to control pain and other symptoms, tumor size, and survival was checked. A qualified, experienced Chinese medicine expert served as the partner of the oncologist in charge. The expert was responsible for the prescription of the herbal preparations given according to the symptom complexes and their individualized indications. The results of this study indicated that symptom control over pain, appetite, and diarrhea were improved more with the herbal medicine group compared with the placebo group. The most remarkable improvement was observed with the control of nausea. The important parameters of survival, tumor size, and chemotherapy-induced hematological toxicity were not improved in both groups.

This randomized controlled trial was carefully planned to objectively measure the efficacy of herbal supplements in attempts to make chemotherapy more comfortable. Thousands of cancer patients have been relying on the support from traditional Chinese medicine healers who prescribe individualized treatment. This form of individualized treatment was fully respected in the trial. The results might have supported the popular supplementary use of herbal medicine because it did no harm and was alleviating symptoms like nausea. However, the results failed to improve survival and other vital parameters like cytotoxic complications affecting the haematological state (Mok *et al.*, 2007).

## A Clinical Trial Using a Herbal Formula as a Supplement to Radiotherapy for Cancer Patients

The second trial was conducted in the same hospital on nasopharyngeal cancer patients receiving radiotherapy, which was the standard curative treatment for this cancer, common for the male population of South China. It was designed as a small pilot, randomized, placebo-control and double-blinded trial. Apart from general fatigue, the head and neck symptoms related to irradiation were well-known and included local skin irritations, muscle tightness and spasms, mouth stiffness, loss of taste, loss of salivation, dry eyes, etc.

For this study, a uniform herbal formula consisting of two herbs was used and the principle of generalization was observed rather than individualization of treatment. This preparation contained a fungal component, *Coriolus*, which had the reputation of immuno-boosting property. For this reason, the immunological state of the 20 + 20 clients was assessed before and after four months of treatment.

Results of the pilot study revealed that fatigue was significantly relieved in the treatment group compared with the placebo ($p \leq 0.05$), but the general trend of decline in the quality of life score in both groups after irradiation showed no difference between the two groups. In the immunological assessment, T-lymphocyte suppression was obvious in both groups, but the decline was significantly less in the herbal supplement group (Bao *et al.*, 2006).

The objectives for the use of herbal supplements in this study were not confined to the control of symptoms arising from the radiotherapy. Instead, possible positive effects of the herbal preparation in the promotion of immunological defense were explored. Moreover, this cancer is unique in that it possesses a serological marker, the DNA of Epstein-Barr Virus (EBV-DNA), which offers a direct indication of cancer activity. A significant decline indicates a positive control of cancer growth. After radiotherapy, EBV-DNA dropped dramatically. The herbal study tried to look for possible supplementary effects of the *Coriolus* preparation, which might initiate further drops of EBV-DNA. No difference, however, was seen between the herbal and control groups, both of which showed limited changes of the DNA. This observation might indicate that the *Coriolus* preparation did not work through a direct control of the cancer growth, but rather indirectly via the immuno-supportive pathway.

## A Clinical Trial Using Herbal Preparation as a Palliative Agent in the Treatment of Multiple Bone Metastases

This was a clinical trial performed in the same hospital in Hong Kong on 46 + 46 patients known to be suffering from multiple bone metastases arising from various types of cancer. It was a randomized, comparative trial using a herbal formula and a bisphosphonate. The assessments included Bone Mineral Density (BMD), control of secondaries, biochemical bone markers, quality of life, and adverse effects.

The design was based on observations on the use of bisphosphonates for bone secondaries. Bisphosphonates suppress the bone resorption initiated by osteoclasts without affecting the osteoblasts. The newer bisphosphonate preparations were first for bone metastasis when they were found to be effective in the control of pain arising from bone destruction. Later, it was observed that bisphosphonate also lessened the destruction of bone, hence it might even prevent more secondary deposits. It was therefore deduced that if there were herbal agents which supported bone mineral density, the same agents should have protective effects on bone metastases like bisphosphonates. A herbal preparation active for the support of osteoporosis was therefore compared with a bisphosphonate (clondronate), and the parameters of assessment followed those of BMD studies closely (Wu, 2006).

A total of 46 + 46 patients were recruited randomly into the clondronate and herbal groups. Six months of respective treatment was given, followed by six months of further assessment.

The study was not totally successful because too many (45%) recruited patients died before the completion of treatment. Analyzing the fully treated patients, the herbal group showed some trend of superiority over the bisphosponate group in pain control and the average quality of life scores.

As some modern drugs, non-specific for cancer treatment, have started to be used in cancer patients to achieve secondary benefits, such as the control of angiogenesis and the relief of bone pain, many herbal preparations could be studied and developed for similar effects in an attempt to look for practical solutions for symptom control in cancer patients.

## A Clinical Trial Using Herbal Preparation as a Preventive Agent for Immuno-Support

Many herbal items are popular among the general public in the Chinese community for use as health promotion agents. These are particularly popular among the elderly, the frail, and weak after illnesses, survivors of serious accidents, and those bothered by different forms of derangement. Apart from the large choices of food rarities, well known energizers and life-supporting herbs include the ginsengs, *Cordyceps*, *Ganoderma*, and other fungi.

A large scale clinical trial using healthy volunteers was designed in 2002 to examine the immunomodulating effects of a simple preparation consisting of a fungus, *Coriolus*, and another herb. It was a randomized, placebo-controlled, cross-over trial. A group of 50 volunteers given the herbal preparation was tested against 50 others who received placebos. Four months of consumption were required for each group, followed by a cross-over for another four months.

The results showed very convincing immuno-boostering effects of the herbal preparation on all immunological parameters - T-helper cells, T-suppressor cells, T- helper/T-suppressor ratio, and B-lymphocytes levels were all increased. Quality of life also showed significant improvement when the volunteers were maintained on the herbal preparation (Wong *et al.*, 2005).

## Conclusion

Removal of the cancer is a necessity in the treatment process. Removal has been achieved through surgery, radiotherapy, or chemotherapy. However, removal has reached its limitations as the cancer could, in the first place, be too extensive, or, in spite of the removal, still recur, which happens too frequently.

Cancer is a pathological process in which the cells either grow too much or too rapidly, or the normal programmed process of cell death (apoptosis) is not functioning properly. When the pathological process is not stopped, no matter how effective the cancer removal is, the formation of cancer is going to be repeated (van de Greef, 2003).

Cancers spread indiscrimatorily or recur in spite of apparently effective treatments because, presumably, the etiology of the cancer is either unknown or is not removed. The etiological factors exist either on the molecular or genomic levels. Systems biology has confirmed the complex problems, and scientists in this field have actively engaged in new problem solving efforts. One difficulty is that cancer etiology involves not one, but many factors, hence the usual single target aim of the cure probably does not work. On the contrary, the multiple target approach should have greater promise. In this context, traditional Chinese Medicine, still short of thorough scientific explanations but emphasizes a multiple target approach and protection of internal harmony, should have a lot to offer.

Cancer treatment has therefore gone beyond the stage of cancer removal and other approaches aiming at the causations, such as controlling the blood supply, initiating apoptosis, and regulating the responsible genes . The treatment approach needs to be modified from a single target, eliminative direction to a multiple target, holistic direction. Chinese medicine has followed a multi-target holistic approach. As new systems of cancer treatment are not yet mature, using Chinese medicine as an adjuvant therapy could be an innovative and practical investment to bring about better results of cancer control.

Our earlier experience using either single or multiple herbs as supplementary, preventive, and palliative adjuvant therapies which yielded reasonable results have encouraged us to persue a more proactive approach of developing an innovative herbal formula to be used as adjuvant cancer treatment. Our laboratory experiments of the five selected herbs have yielded very positive results on apoptosis, anti-angiogenesis, and immunological support. In the near future, we are ready to design a proper clinical application.

## References


[1] Wong JW, Wong SL, Donnan S. Traditional Chinese Medicine and Western Medicine in Hong Kong. *J. Hong Kong Med A* 1993; 45: 278-84.

[2] Mok SK, Yeo W, Johnson PJ *et al.* A double-blind placebo-controlled randomized study of Chinese herbal medicine as complementary therapy for reduction of chemotherapy-induced toxicity. *Annals of Oncology* 2007; 18:768-74.

[3] Bao YX, Wong CK, Leung SF *et al.* Clinical studies of immunomodulatory activities of Yunzhi-Danshen in patients with nasopharyngeal carcinoma. *The Journal of Alternative and Complementary Medicine* 2006; 12(8): 771-6.

[4] Wu K. Clinical observation and pharmacological study of the efficacy of a Chinese Medicine Formula on malignant tumor bone metastasis. *PhD thesis,* Graduate School The Chinese University of Hong Kong, 2006.

[5] Wong CK, Bao YX, Wong EL. Immunomodulatory activities of Yunzhi and Danshen in post-treatment breast cancer patients. *Am J Chinese Med* 2005; 33: 381-95.

[6] Jan van de Greef. The role of analytical science in medical systems biology. *Current Opinion in Clinical Biology* 2003; 8: 944-54.

In: Traditional Medicine: New Research
Editor: Yoshiharu Motoo
ISBN: 978-1-62257-448-3


Chapter 4

# Suggestions for Changing Some Future Research Intentions and Directions in the Field of Integrative Medicine in Cancer Care: From a TCM Clinician and Theorist's Perspective

*Ofer Baranovitch*
Ph.D; L.Ac, Israel

## Traditional Medicine Concepts Could not Have been Understood Better than Today Is it a Paradox?

Traditional medicine such as Chinese, other East Asian medical theories, and other sources of world antique wisdom regarding mind and body health, such as the writing of the Israelite civilization, and the Hebrew language itself, may contribute some major new ideas that may be found as a breakthrough in the quest for a better understanding of the principles of the balances that preserve Human health, longevity, and good shape. Such ideas may shed more light on the principles of loosing those balances and thus allowing development of illnesses.

Traditional medicine diagnostics and working tools in cancer care are falling, most of the time, way behind modern medicine practices. While modern medicine has been developing science and technology side by side, traditional medicine, while preceding the modern era, did not develop the same way. The ability to identify a single active ingredient and understand its pharmacological structure and its biological routes and influence, and reproduce it artificially again and again in such a concentration that it will be a very potent, accurate, and effective form of medicine, is one of the trademarks of modern medicine and its technologies and knowledge. We can accurately identify the active ingredient, ginsenoides in a Ginseng root, but we do not know how or if it does assist with immune modulation, or with

Zheng Qi tonification, and rarely explains the biology behind those terms. Even though traditional medicine suffers from an extreme technologies, and microscopic knowledge deficiencies, this weakness does not have to be applied to its theoretical principles and macroscopic knowledge. Those principles originated in an early mass of knowledge that was further validated through means of investigation, interpretation, experimentation, and further development all along Human medical history. Traditional medical theory offers us the skills of observing unarmed, in a macroscopic eye, the reflections of the "larger world" on our "small Human world" thus allowing us with a macroscopic recognition of the above super-harmonization/balancing – systems. Our possible ability to further recognize the routes of information transference in our bodies, which is needed to conserve balance, will allow us to construct new integrative theoretical models. Our new hypothesis will be followed by research methods constructed to fit it specifically. Paradoxically, this scientific and technological era that features fantastic microscopic and telescopic observation capabilities can validate the axiom that traditional medicine was built upon. It is easier today for one's imagination to grasp the vast, undiscovered, physical zone and to only speculate the infinite number of waves, and other particles passing through it, building up within it, establishing Cosmic and Human communication route systems.

## The Ocean of Void and the Yuan Qi

The traditional concept of Qi is well understood today. Every existing entity and subject is made from Qi particles. Every thing is made from small electrical charges: 'positive' and 'negative' ones i.e, Yin and Yang. The illusive world of forms hides infinite spaces within them. It is like an ocean yet to be discovered. It is like the sun, for which one needs to travel millions of miles to reach it. So many possibilities of movement, containment, and discharge mechanisms exist within that ocean and sprout from it. The infinite Qi interactions between the cosmic and the Human, within the great void.

*How much do we really know about those spaces,and what is that is circulating in it? Who is responsible for each space cleaning and performance? What are the laws and reasons of narrowing of that void? How is a disease being formed? We do know some of the answers already, but how many of them still elude us?*

We can assume that any existing form of being is the sum of its electrical components and that their composition builds it, and as a consequence is composed of the sum of the vacant spaces within it. Each form of being has a will to be, and to be present, in time and space. That will is the very did of creation, the seal of the infinite shapeless Creator, it is the Original, the Yuan. The Original Qi in our bodies is present as a source for any electrical components' will to form structures, by binding to other components using binding knowledge carried on through time ever since the dawn of man and other forms of existence. The Original Qi circulates through the spaces and within the form's nano-void; controlling, adjusting, balancing, and allowing the togetherness that is needed to exist.

## The San Jiao as a Phenomena

The San Jiao's Yuan circulation system offers us an excellent example for how Traditional Chinese Medicine (TCM), in this case, describes a phenomena, which is hard to grasp, even macroscopically. This phenomena is being presented through the genius idea of a San Jiao meridian, a description of its internal and external path, mainly by drawing a straight line running from below the belly button to the center of the chest, pointing at three different main stations along that line: lower, middle, and upper ones. Those stations represents the San Jiao subdivisions, an additional macroscopic understanding of the changing internal climate and its influences on it.

Even though the San Jiao is named after an organ (Fu organ), there is no evidence that such an organ exists, but rather offers us a different concept which defines a specific Qi system, i.e an intelligent authority that may or may not include an 'organ'. The San Jiao allows the circulating Yuan to reach its infinite destinations, thus its purposes, serving the Kidney intelligence authority storing the Yuan.

Where is the location of the Kidney? Some of the traditional descriptions tell us that its territory is at the lower abdomen, named traditionally as the Dan Tian , or the Cinnabar Field, while others extend the presence of that entity to the brain, to bones and bone marrow, to the Kidney organ and to the adrenal gland, to the lower back and knees, etc. What is the connections between all of those Kidneys? The answer in this case is easy: the Kidney's intelligence authority is the sum of all. One can influence that intelligence system and manipulate it using its meridian by applying medical techniques such as acupressure, acupuncture, shiatsu, etc. This is a great idea which grants us access to a multi lock safe. Even though we are far from being exact while manipulating it, we can influence it as a whole.

The Kidneys store fear. Whaoo!! Is this real or just a metaphor? Do fearful memories of one's ancestors influence his/her Kidneys? how?

Well, Jing and Yuan Qi, in the form of gens, being the heart of every cell, are actually a memory storing device that allows inherited and maybe an on-going acquired Kidney intelligence to be presented in every cell in our bodies.

The Yuan being circulating via the San Jiao spaces to and from every cell is the tool that keeps Kidneys together. One whole made from infinite cells, just like the infinite stars circulating in space in a perfect order, the "larger world" and the "smaller world" governed by the Creator of all, a oneness present in and through spaces by the Yuan Qi. While recognizing the Dan Tian , located at the middle of the lower abdomen, the place and zone where the Kidney's Qi is being gathered, we learn that Qi is present in every unit, but at the same time gains power and intelligence from a major Qi field.

## Drawing a Meridian

The simple drawing of the meridians i.e, Jing Luo, on the body, offers the observer a detailed location of all major Qi fields. Each one of those major Qi fields is actually the sum of the infinite Qi events, influenced by their root Qi field and influencing it, constructing its power and intelligence and obeying it, transforming all kinds of received information thus allowing a gathering of fragments of power, knowledge, etc. When examining the geometry of the meridians of one in relation to the others, a relationship between major Qi fields can be seen, suggesting cooperation, coordination, communication, and sharing of certain activities, responsibilities, and certain Qi dynamics.

Asking huge questions such as: *why does an oncogen give abnormal orders to a cell's core i.e, nucleus? What is the overall system's intention while doing so? Its will?* Yes, we can block its communication routes with the cell's core, and we can slow that "mal" communication down, using certain genius biological blockers, *but why does the system behave like that?*

Understanding some of the ideas behind this meridian system may offers us with some new hypothesis and direct our research into new horizons.

## The Shao Yin and its "Treasures"

The Kidneys and Heart meridians are known to be the Shao Yin mega system i.e, the controlling pivot of it all, mind and body. The collective Shen which resides in the Heart's intelligence system is the total of spiritual, emotional, and awareness present in every atom, molecule, cell, and tissue of the body. The traditional Heart's Qi field includes the brain which is considered to be an "extra organ" thus, the brain's infrastructure and activities are part of Shao Yin, i.e an intelligence and Qi power system shared by Heart and Kidneys. Shao Yin communicates, absorbing and sending information by different means such as the San Jiao and Pericardium Qi fields and pathway systems , and/or modern titled endocrine, neurological, and immune systems, etc. Traditionally, Yuan Qi, Shen, and Jing are considered to be the Emperor's "treasures" i.e the divine tools needed to allow Shao Yin with the means needed in order to allow it to rule life, just like the "Emperor of heaven" rules heaven and earth, the Human Emperor rules mind and body. "Physical", and "non-physical" pathologies must have been derived from a reduction in Qi power, effectiveness of Qi communication pathways , and the levels of establishment and presence of Yuan, Jing, and Shen in every system's components, as isolated as it could be.

*How can we better tonify Qi? How can we assist a deteriorating intelligence in the major Qi fields ensuring that Qi remains potent, Yuan vigorously circulates and is present, and Shen would be more aware and capable with better handling awareness?*

Traditional medicine has its techniques directed in enhancing Qi capabilities; *are they enough?* The answer is simply no.

*Do we invest enough in integrating these ideas into modern research?* The answer is once again no.

The Jing, the basic stone and cement of every composition of structures, carries the Creator knowledge and reflects it. Jing is the living memory, the sum of all memories, being the "blue print" of the Qi's skeleton, and the right sequence of the amino-acids. Even the earth remembers, wood remembers, and a bird remembers without being aware of the way it roams between autumn and spring. Individuals remember loved ones who have left him/her, hurt and carry this memory over a lifetime, curved in his/her Shen and Jing deep in one's blood, one's bone marrow, and one's Heart.

*Can we find out the depth of that hurt? Can we define its location? Can we understand eventually how that forgotten incidence developed into such a level being able to affect Qi and Yuan potency and thus allowing some "isolated cells" to form an isolated tumor? Can we estimate the pressure of this accumulative stress that such a memory, deeply buried for years, creates on the bone marrow finally resulting in leukemic crisis or forming a Multiple myeloma?*

## Tao, Immunity, and the Mutation of Cell's DNA

An effective immune system depends on its ability to identify and eliminate foreign, penetrators, proteins, and cells. Some self cells, surviving immune screenings, had been "kidnapped", mutating and developing autonomic agendas, detached from the general will of the entire system. Observing the latter's behavior may lead to a simple conclusion that this frightening pathology was generated by an idiopathic accident. Is it?

This is reminiscent of the Taoist monks that were ordered to get crazy while indentifying that their surrounding societal norms represent madness, or any violation of Tao, thus keeping sanity, obeying the laws of Tao, which has no name or shape; composed of true being.

Traditional medicine describes an effective immunity as the total power of Wei and Ying i.e, defensive and nutritive Qi mechanisms. Master Zhang Zhong Jing went even further by constructing the famous *Gui Zhi Tang* formula designed to enhance failing immune response by balancing Wei and Ying. Improving their communication will increase the effectiveness of the immune response, just like modern concepts of the acquired and adaptive levels of the immune system. Traditional medicine relates to the extremely important relationships between the internal and the external in almost any theoretical model describing Humans. Wei and Ying is a prominent example of this .

The way an individual grasps his/her position in time and space is crucial and is being reflected in all of his/her existing dimensions; "physical" and " non physical". Me and my family, Me and my people, Me and myself, Me and my Tao, etc. *Can we really know and understand which are the exact effective pharmacological ingredients found in the Paeonia root or in the Cinnamon twig that improves Wei and Ying balance? Do we want to know? Are we clever and modest enough to assume that traditional wisdom may lead to the formation of new attitudes in research?*

Well I think we should. An integrative medicine does not mean solely working together using different disciplines of medicine in order to enhance treatment, but also integrating theories for the sake of finding more and new ways to prevent, handle, and even cure diseases by a better understanding of their etiologies and pathologies. This is the sole reason for writing this chapter. I would like to call for the attention of scientists and researchers who might find the notion of this chapter close to their hearts, looking for ideas without any discrepancy. I prefer to share some of the Classic principles that I have further developed along the twenty years of my theoretical and clinical work, as to increase the chances that some of them will reach the novel goal of finding new solutions for all kinds of diseases people are suffering from. This chapter does not aim at teaching Traditional Chinese Medicine, nor does it suggest ideas that can be found in Chinese medicine only. I usually integrate some Israelite Classical ideas in my theoretical and clinical work. Human knowledge with regards to health should be integrated with no discrepancy.

# The Holy Temple in Jerusalem and Camouflage Phlegm

The Bible differentiates groups of some diseases from others. A cluster of skin and skin tumor diseases were treated by the priests serving in the Temple through the performance of a set of "mystical" ceremonies. The priests had to wear special "spiritually defending" clothes while in the Temple, serving in any ceremony included being the mediators in some sacrifice ceremonies. By mentioning a cluster of diseases and not others, and by suggesting their treatment should be in the Temple and not anywhere else, and that their treatment will be conducted by the priests and not by any other kind of medicine men, the Bible advises and teaches us that some of the etiologies to certain ills are rooted in the moral dimension. Wrong doing to ourselves or to others, objectively or subjectively, may affect the Qi and damage its clarity by means of dampness and phlegm. Such a turbidity forms an obstructive climate that may initiate immune response and reduction in immune clarity, i.e the immune ability to well identify, leading to its over activity, allergic reactions, autoimmunity, and reduced immunity.

One might produce damp/phlegm as a means of concealing undesired emotions and memories etc, being unaware of course to his/her did. We may fight chronic rhinitis, crohn's or mioma, without paying attention to the reasons that formed the phlegm to begin with. The presence of an excessive phlegm narrows the spaces needed for the circulation of Yuan, Shen, and Jing. Once an ongoing self induced phlegm process had been initiated, the transformation to a serious disease could and should be prevented, depending on a professional ability, based on new technology, to clearly identify that process.

# Self induced Phlegm and the Formation of Tumors

The following was discovered in clinic: using a specially designed questionnaire, specific pulse reading, and tongue observations, a large grope of ill women diagnosed with *ovarian* and *right breast cancers* indicated some extreme difficulties in their relationships with one or more important feminine figure. The location of those diseases at those particular organs, both actually located on the Ren (Conception vessel) meridian, i.e Ren intelligence and memory system, led to the idea that the Ren is actually an intelligence system that reflects the sum of all engagements with dominant feminine figures such as the grandmother, mother, daughter, etc. The Ren remembers, and stores many of the above engagements concealed and unaware. Within the depth of it, an ongoing work is being done to solve and discharge all kinds of unresolved issues and emotions such as guilt. For different reasons some women can not deal, while being aware, and even while being unaware to certain levels, with such issues. In the beginning of the clinical treatment sessions, some of them denied the very existence of such an issue. This type of denying behavior actually discloses their abusive productions of self induced phlegm as a masking mechanism for those stressful and toxic emotions. This sometimes lifelong masking mechanism involves the constant production of phlegm in all forms: damp/phlegm, "non substantial" spiritual phlegm, and more. Eventually, the abuse of that tool, originally made to give them time to continue with their ordinary and routine daily survival , put aside difficult things to later be resolved, and discharge had led to the formation of isolating groups of cells, forming a mass, separating themselves from the whole , using phlegm as a means to define their new entity. We should look for ways to better identify the processes of the formation of this kind of phlegm, treats its roots , and find a better technique to clear it, while convincing the system overall to stop production. We do use herbs and acupuncture to resolve phlegm, but usually we mark phlegm as our target to be eliminated. The practitioner should keep in mind that the patient has chosen, even if it is an unconscious type of decision making, to produce and use phlegm for its needs. So, instead of working with the patient, one might work against his/her phlegm. The clinical reality shows that the work is insufficient. A better and more effective treatment and treatment strategy needs to be found. Maybe our attitude in treating cancers overall, and in an advanced stages in particular, is too limited; killing the cell is not enough most of the time. We may need to change the way we think. Instead of just killing that cell or blocking its supply and other routes of communication, find a way to allow the cell to belong again to the whole by convincing it that change is possible and true. Then, Shao Yin governing Yuan Qi and Shen will gain the entire kingdom's respect again, so isolation will be no longer needed.

One may ask, why are the numbers of the above mentioned diseases increasing in our days? Are those so called "Ren issues" new? The answer is no.

But, society has changed, women's position in the family has changed, careers and the diminishing concept of motherhood status has its pressures and sanctity, etc. In accordance with the "Double Hit" theory, the spiritual and emotional difficulties mentioned above, involving unresolved and toxic issues with one or more feminine figures might be the straw and work should be done to eliminate that straw.

A single digit percentage reduction in the Ren's load might retain a "single hit" situation, dangerous but not malignant.

*Do we have an effective spiritual-physical method to reach an ailment? Can we understand the principles practiced in the Temple at Jerusalem? Can we learn anything from that tradition, identifying some of the above mentioned diseases, pathologies and etiologies, offering solutions and treatments?* One needs to better understand the reason in order to initiate a search and navigation for a new mode of solutions.

## Tears and Resins

Crying is a great tool to overcome the toxicity of depressed emotions. Tears are part of the Liver's intelligence system, a master of discharging techniques, power, and means. Tears act just like a spring reaching the surface while originating from the deep . Tears release an accumulative stress saturated with toxic Qi. Tears can overcome the clouds of masking buried emotions, assisting clarity. While looking at injured trees, the resin they secrete can be identified as tears. Can we use different kinds of resin such as Mo Yao (Myrrha), Ru Xiang (Olibanum), Hu Po (Succinum), etc., as a means of breaking the veils of phlegm, thus allowing a better communication in between different levels of consciousness, assisting the Yuan Qi with increasing unity and reducing isolation. Furthermore, reduction in phlegm load will actually improve the modulation of certain mechanisms within the immune system, such as the ability to better identify self and non self, friend and enemy, performed by natural killer cells and other pointing cells.

*Does Zhong jing's harmonizing method of Wei and Ying to improve their mutual communication lead to the same modulation effect?* Let us invest more and truly understand that idea and find the biological logic to explain it. Let us find new and modern techniques to better express this idea in clinic.

*Is strengthening clarity, or Qi power and Qi circulation, reflected in the ability of certain genes within a cell's nucleus to perform better? Fixing wrong sequences in protein chains, or inducing normal apoptosis, and more?*

## Incense, Sense of Smelling, and Evils Revealing

At the Israelite Temples, a special daily incense was burned. The prescriptions of the substances mixed to produce that incense are Biblical. A high percentage of that mixture was made from tree resins such as the Mo Yao (Myrrha) and Ru Xiang (Olibanum) mentioned before.

*Does a healing process initiate by smelling their burning smoke? Does the process of inhaling that Qi in the form of smoke, and within the Holy environment of the Temple, allow a safe and open environment for our "internal evils" to reveal themselves? Such evils as fear, abandonment , emptiness, and more? Does forcing them to the surface through the fog that has been hiding them ease the stress within?*

Reducing the stress from the "Blood Level", and from the Shao Yin zone within that level where Shen resides should be considered a true physical pressure reduction. This kind of pressure build up can explain different types of internal "accidents" in every "Blood Level" component such as: Chong's intelligence system, Jing-bone marrow, Shen-central nervous system, Yuan/Jing-DNA, etc. *Can we use the sense of smell as a part of a future healing protocol?*

## Searching for the Biology of Tao

Traditional medicine theory is being constructed on an axiom which considers the linkage between human Tao, Shen, Yuan, and "physical" health, as the skeleton of one's very being. If we can allow ourselves to seriously check the possible logical assumption that Human life has a definite purpose, and that this purpose is the main cause for existing , we will be able to broaden the "cause and effect" way of analyzing and diagnose making. Accepting the validity of it, with some doubts which are normal, can open new horizons in seeking restoration of health for some complicated diseases such as cancer.

What kind of natural vehicles does Tao use in order to navigate us through life to fulfill our purpose for living? Traditional medicine has recognized, within the realm of Shen i.e, our spiritual, emotional, cognitive, and behavioral capacity, an autonomic entity named Hun. The Hun has been described in the Classics as an integral residence of the Liver intelligence system, which allows one to live according to his/her Tao.

By cleansing the Liver while crying, we free our Hun from the weight of unresolved issues, thus enables us to restore our vision of ourselves in time and in space, and strengthens our sense of being on the right track toward fulfillment. Just like those Taoist monks that I have mentioned earlier, when the Hun realize that some living principles such as moral, family relations, dream fulfillment, and others, are out of "normal" track, it has to resist this "abnormality".

*Isn't it a wonderful thing to be able to strengthen the Hun's capacity to enforce change by needling the Hun Men( Urinnary Bladder 47) acu-point, for example? What other biological means does our body use in order to initiate change in a "perfect Status quo", which is necessary in the process of initiating recovery, regaining a new, fresh, and more accurate balance, in all realms of being?*

Remember that the individual needs to convince the monks i.e, the "isolated" cells, with his/her sincerity, so that they can start to feel and be belong again to the whole, back to their roots, intelligent, true, and respectful.

## Wind and the Ability to Make a Change

Traditional medicine uses the nature of wind to explain certain changes in the dynamics of Qi, Jing, and Shen. Dr. He a collegue from Guan An Men hospital in Beijing uses the term wind in order to explain the metastatic nature of some cells. According to Dr. He, the intention of those cells and the development of their intelligence, as presented in the process of preparing future sites for their new colonies, had taken place long before cancer was diagnosed.

I found in my clinical work that one can issue a superficial Wei/Immune crisis which involves different kinds of "external wind" battling with his/her Wei Qi, in order to pacify internal Ying and blood level issues . Maybe that assumption can explains Dr. He's tendency to use wind expelling herbs such as Gui zhi (Ramulus cinammomi Cassiae), Gao ben (Rhizoma Ligustici), and Bo he (Herba Mentha) while treating cancer. It is better to fight on the castle walls than fighting from door to door inside the palace. It is better to make all kinds of changes, thus restoring clarity to the Tao's navigation system, moving us unified once again toward our next station in life, than to ignore that inner need to discharge, organize, and restore proper Qi, Jing, and Shen circulation to and from every and each cell. An external moderate crisis using an external wind is a much better option than a severe internal crisis i.e., an" internal wind".

*Is it possible that we invite some kind of friendly viruses in order to quarrel with our immune system and accelerate all kinds of psychological, neuro -endocrine, and immune system communication mechanisms aimed in reset? If some of the viruses are considered to be friendly, is it possible that those viruses are a form of wind serves Tao's mysterious ways actually? Can we identify means of communication between different systems within ourselves and viruses? Can we train them, use their help, and initiate some controlled, easy to moderate crisis in order to be able to prevent severe ones? What does a visit of Epstein Barr Virus in a system mean; is it an immune failure? Could it be a fake failure, actually challenging the entire system, forcing it to slow down, and acknowledge its false drive?*

# The Earth Envelopes, Order, Chaos, and Wind

Dr. Oz Argash, a colleague at the Rabin Medical Center's Integrative Medicine Unit, Israel, and a friend who recently passed away, was using the term chaos to describe the prerequisite condition that sometimes invites and encourages the eruption of cancerous diseases. Working with children diagnosed with cancer for a long time, Dr. Argash had realized that stormy winds have been shuttering and cracking their world such as their parents' divorce "which is a terrible thing" he repeatedly said. Chaotic situations in one's life may produce pressure on the Earth element. This element, as part of the Five element/ Wu Xing model, defines the center power of our being, which is anti-chaotic by nature. Chaos causes the positive spaces within Earth to be no longer regulated, thus an internal wind is being formed.

The term "Great Envelopes of the Spleen and Stomach" i.e, The Earth Envelopes (EE), defines a unique cooperative mechanism which originates in the Heart, the master of contraction and relaxation, to construct the intelligence system of the middle Jiao. The EE are actually the sum of two dynamic opposing vectors constructing the Earth together. The EE mechanisms form an "empty" zone in between them, while contracting and relaxing toward the other named the Inter Envelopes Gap (IEG). The Spleen envelope wraps around the Stomach envelope, while the latter resists that surrounding and maintains a multi purpose void/emptiness. The IEG formed by the latter two correspond to the Qi level in the Four Levels model and to the Shao Yang stage in the Six Stages model. The IEG reflects a balanced communication between Wei and Ying, which is the balance between our "inner" and "outer" selves, our mutual desire to reach out and reach within, and the wisdom of our Wei and Ying to resist and to permit wind formation, and to reign wild and domestic wind within the illusive stability and oneness of Earth. Master Zhong jing' formula, named *Xiao Jian Zhong Tang* i.e, Minor Construct the Middle decoction, a modified *Gui Zhi Tang* formula, presents Zhong jing mastering of the Wei and Ying co-factors, directing and regulating order verse disorder, and normality versus abnormality. Controlling the IEG means controlling Qi power, Qi circulation, and Qi intelligence to use wind when necessary in order to calm chaos and sometimes provoking it to allow the process of change.

*Can we design a chip that can estimate the effectiveness of the IEG, diagnosing the EE status, and assist with their regulation when needed, thus boosting Zheng/True Qi i.e, Yuan Qi? Does the enforcement of Yuan Qi reduce gene aneuploidy, regaining DNA stability, and allowing adequate gene expression?*

*Is it possible to learn the way that the Shang Han Lun herbs Bai Shao(Radix Paeonia alba), and Gui Zhi (Ramulus Cinnammomi cassia) maintain middle Qi harmony, just by defining their known active ingredients? Thereby forcing it to be part of what we can conceive and judging it through those eyes only?*

The central Qi path has been described as a midline meridian that runs from top to bottom through our chest and abdomen. Along that Qi path, some major Qi reservoir acu-points are located, such as Qi Hai (Ren 6), Guan Yuan (Ren 4), Zhong Wan (Ren 12), and Shan Zhong (Ren 17). This Qi path is actually a reflection and a macroscopic overlook at the total of Qi being gathered, empowered, and circulates at and from the IEG. The masters of Traditional medicine that had drawn the San Jiao pathway within the latter Qi path had proposed the idea that the San Jiao, a Shao Yang entity, has a central role in maintaining the effective proximity between the EE, often distancing one from the other.

The diminishing will of the Spleen envelope to astringe itself toward the Stomach envelope often reflects one's attempt to distance itself from the Stomach envelope which is loaded with all kinds of external "substantial" and "non substantial" elements, thus leaving them out, away from the "inner self". The Stomach envelope reflects one's desire to be involved with his/her surroundings. An over whelmed Stomach envelope, being excessively filled with the "external", tends to "shut down" and over contract inwardly, narrowing, in order to reduce further exposure.

That mutual distancing causes reduction in IEG total effectiveness. This is actually a major crack at the heart of the Earth. The Shao Yang (San Jiao plus Gall Bladder Qi fields) acts to ensure sufficient communication between exterior and interior by definition. The San Jiao uses the Yuan Qi force, which originates and is stored in the Kidneys, to keep "mother earth" united, while the Gall Bladder, through activating of the Dai (Girdle vessel), an extra ordinary intelligence system that forms a giant envelope itself, enveloping the Spleen envelope, forcing it and assisting it to get back closer to the Stomach envelope.

## The Separation Process of the Envelopes Mechanism and Colon Cancer

I have noticed in clinic that patients diagnosed with Adeno carcinoma of the Colon, do present a long history of cracked Earth, distancing EE, and weakened Shao Yang components. The Colon meridian is the only meridian that crosses the mid- line of the body. It crosses it while reaching the nose to the opposite nostril. By crossing the mid-line, the Colon meridian presents a special role of the Colon intelligence system: keeping the central Qi field, the IEG, vital. The Colon Qi system joins the Shao Yang Qi system, and both work to maintain the structure of Earth and its functional oneness. When the other compensation mechanisms are no longer capable of sharing their Qi power, the Colon is being called to the flag. I have also noticed that some of these patients were generating phlegm in order to camouflage all sort of things they could not cope with. The phlegm, "substantial" and "non substantial", enters the IEG at the Earth envelopes system, and at the "Sleeve" mechanism envelopes system. The IEG is the reflection and the sum of all the spaces i.e, the nano-spaces, that separate the inner world from the outer world. This kind of separation is natural and functional, and is being formed in substantial structures such as the intestinal wall, the interneurons synapse, and in the "non-substantial" realm of awareness: the conscious, sub-conscious, and unconscious realm of existence. While the envelopes move away from each other they conceal hard to cope with data and hides difficult and complex emotions. Phlegm is produced in order to assist with this task. This phlegm accumulates in the nano-spaces, being part of the total IEG in both envelope systems, as described above. While this process of Wei and Ying separation is proceeding, the normal compensation reflex of the Shao Yang is being issued, trying to reduce the level of distancing/separation, defending the Zheng Qi/Yuan Qi.

Colonic polyps and/or tumors can be the substantial reflection of the Colonic effort "to keep it together", and overcome the obstacles made by the process of self produced phlegm, masking the clarity of Qi, Jing, and Shen, in the IEG being in fact the "Central Qi Field", where Qi prospers, gains its power, its intelligence, and its circulation potential.

*Is it possible that the above scenario could be the another straw that breaks the camel's back ? Negatively contributing to a parallel process of mutativity/gene aneuploidy under toxic pressure made by the presence of pesticides left over in the Colon's tissue, for example ?*

We can use traditional medicine to reduce the pathological processes that affect Earth wholeness, such as the distancing/separating EE, preventing chaos and the over use of the compensation mechanism, tonifying Shao Yang' components, and Colon Qi as a consequence.

We can reduce phlegm production and induce a more dynamic shifting of matter between levels of consciousness. But our traditional tools are often not sufficient. When talking about cancer, the level of pathology's complexity, which involves an extreme damage to the Yuan, Jing, and Shen, leaves this author, a practitioner of traditional medicine, often frustrated.

*We have a good base of theory, but we often lack the ability to use that theory as a research hypothesis, free from the need to be appreciated and accepted by certain academic systems. So, most of the research today on traditional medicine is merely a poor attempt to prove that traditional medicine works. We know it works, but we also know that we need to squeeze more out of it. Integrated ideas that lead to an integrative research might find new techniques to better understand, treat, and cure some cancers. This should be our goal.*

## Planning a New Medical Device Programmed to Diagnose and Treat the Reduction in Inter Envelope Gaps' Qi Output

The structure of Earth can give a fake impression of one which is solid, stable and safe , built upon a long term and confident routine on the one hand, while on the other, its true fragility allows, with flexibility, to better withstand earthquakes and sometimes even inviting them to happen. While I observe the symmetry of the meridian pathways on the abdomen, those of the Spleen, Stomach, Gall Bladder, and on the abdominal midline, the San Jiao and the Ren, I can only imagine the myriad microscopic different sites of the entire system that are being presented by those meridians and the composition of relationships and communications that are known to be taking place in between them. Furthermore, I can influence those myriad microscopic sites in a macroscopic fashion simply by applying an acupuncture to some elected acu-points demonstrating a logic of point selection such as: Needling Da Heng (Spleen 15), and Tian Shu (Stomach 25) (one toward the other will positively affect the IEG). This is an example of how an acupuncture might work: by "convincing" the whole system's intelligence to allow the distancing EE to reduce their "inward" reflex and to get closer to each other again. Tian Shu, being the Mu(Alarm) point of the Colon intelligence system, will also send a signal that actually reflects the improvement in the IEG condition. Such a signal will free the Colon from compensating for the distancing EE, so it can focus its Qi power and intelligence on other important tasks.

Da Heng, posted at a crucial Qi junction, just like Tian Shu, will send a similar signal that reflects the improvement in the IEG condition. Such a signal will free the Gall Bladder and the Dai intelligence system from being over worked as a compensation system for the EE, regardless of their other tasks, and lets them rest and gain their strength once more.

Furthermore, Da Heng as part of the Yin Wei's extraordinary intelligence system (Yin Linking vessel), and part of the Yin Wei within the Sleeve mechanism , will improve the physical/emotional flooding mechanism of that system and thus will reduce the levels of concealment, an increase in the chances for a lesser camouflage to be produced, and a more exact Tao navigation to be taking place.

*We might be able to invent some new devices that will prove to be more potent than acupuncture techniques alone, but the rational for such inventions may emerge from the inspiring theoretical base and clinical experience of acupuncture. Such a device will be intelligent enough to use the right communication signal system and communication routes. While being considered friendly by the hosting body, it can penetrate the codes and the enigmas of the different security systems and gain cooperation.*

## The Colon, Reign of Wind

The Colon intelligence system presents a unique capability to cross the midline of our body from side to side. The midline is a route for the Ren, Du, San Jiao, Pericardium/Xin Bao, Kidneys, and Chong meridian, and overall it should be considered a Central Qi Field for the entire system, being the sum of all inter-envelope gaps, of all Qi level aspects, where ever they exist. The ability of crossing the midline may offer the idea that the Colon holds a unique and strategic position in regard to the central Qi field/IEG overall, and that from it, the Colon allows or denies the entrance of winds into the IEG and out of it.

When needed, the total and the integrated intelligence system of our mind and body/Jing and Qi and Shen/Ying and Wei, issues an invited and friendly crisis. A crisis as such is needed for different kinds of tasks to be taking place, such as: training some of the immune systems components by inviting friendly wind to imitate war games, destroying malignant cells, and promoting the discharge of toxic wastes, "physical" and "non-physical" , through initiating fever and sweat. As mentioned before in this chapter, an external wind reaching one's borders and entering his/her superficial spaces is often the "cure" for a much more complex and dangerous internal wind.

The Colon is part of the Metal element in the Five Element/Wu Xing Traditional medical theoretical and clinical model. A harmonized Metal should be capable of letting go of past fixations, thus preparing the vacant spaces needed for a re-vital Qi to re-circulate in it, "announcing" the promise of a better tomorrow. The "invited" wind is actually the help our body needs in order to accelerate the process of change, just like different friendly bacteria are needed for the acceleration of some chemical processes being part of our normal intestinal flora.

By needling the acu-point, He Gu (Colon 4), one can initiate a sequence of events issued by the Colonic Qi system, allowing the "penetration" of an External Wind and the provoking of the Inner Wind which resides in the internal zones, exposed for identification and elimination, by means of flooding and sweating. Never getting sick is therefore not a wholely positive thing . A limited crisis is needed in order to prevent a non-limited one, and the acceptance of its importance as such, gratefully, is important in constructing the immune system's confidence. Sometimes friends can turn out to be enemies. A simple invited wind may turn out to be violent and not cooperative , masking its true nature, or igniting a chain of errors leading to a severe complexity.

The fact that the path of the Colon meridian crosses the midline around the nose of all other possible options may symbolize the importance of fragrance based communication between the external messengers of Tao, in the form of an external wind, and the different kinds of internal intelligence systems such as the immune system, Hun and Shen, San Jiao and the Colon, and more. As mentioned before, the Biblical prescription of the daily use of incense in the Temple had included materials made from different kinds of tree resin, awakening the Yuan, allowing its prevalence again through the mist.

*Is it possible that a certain type of fragrance may induce healing processes, being actually the mediator, just like a wind, between the laws of the Creator and one's inner knowledge of it, hidden and masked in a chaotic and toxic environment awaiting the discharge which is needed to gain clarity? Can we identify the signals which are used in that process? Can we simulate such a process in a lab observing this hidden form of communication? Do certain dogs smell some form of cancer? Can we imitate that capability using certain technology?*

## The Gall Bladder's Intelligence System, Lymphoma, and Leukemia

The Gall Bladder(GB) intelligence system has to perform multi-dimensional tasks. As San Jiao's (SJ) partner in the Shao Yang system, the GB assists with keeping a correct and a functional climate in the different Jiaos. The GB and the SJ form the Yang Wei extraordinary intelligence mechanism. The Yang Wei is responsible for discharging the Ying zone (Ying Level) and eliminating the excess dampness and heat that tends to accumulate within it. By doing so, the Yang Wei allows drainage from the inner Blood zone (Blood Level).

The drainage of the Blood zone is crucial for the maintenance of a clear inner void that is needed for a stable and well functioning Shao Yin different components such as the modern concept of DNA, and the similar traditional concept of Shen and Jing. Thus, reduction in overall functioning capabilities of the GB Qi will cause the accumulation of different kinds of internal excesses termed traditionally as damp heat, damp phlegm, and blood heat, which are the "physical" reflections of unresolved emotions, and untreated memories, buried and forgotten, lacking the power to be unconsciously discussed and solved, flooded, and discharged. The above excesses will reduce the total free space and voids needed for proper circulation, communication, and power building of a valid and potent Qi. A persistent damp heat environment tends to form phlegm. This climatic kind of phlegm accelerates the build up of damages being formed by a self produced phlegm.

I have noticed that many of the patients diagnosed with Lymphomas or Leukemia clinically present the macroclimate which is described traditionally as Ying toxic fire and Ying damp heat. I relate to the lymphatic system as a Ying zone system and as a Ying portion of the immune system, and to the bone marrow as part of the Blood zone. The GB Qi is responsible for keeping an internal proper climate through its crucial involvement in climatic maintenance systems such as the Dai, Yang Wei, and San Jiao. However, the burden on that busy system reduces its functioning capabilities. We are living in an era that put a lot of emphasis on the GB's intelligence system. Decision making, initiative, and assertiveness are all traditional GB functions. I would add that its major role is in the Sleeve Envelopes' mechanism , which describes the GB as a mediator between different levels of consciousness. In that mechanism, the GB role is to allow the flooding process of hidden memories/emotions from all kinds of hidden spaces in our brain and body into a more superficial level of consciousness, thus allowing the natural problem solving mechanism to disengage their explosiveness. One's ability to resolve things has to go through different routes of disclosure, such as the dreaming process and imaginative and artistic expression. Dr Zhang Pei Yu, a colleague and a friend from the oncology department in the Guan An Men hospital in Beijing, often uses the *Huang Lian Wen Dan Tang* and *Shu Gan Wan* formulas in order to regain as much GB Qi as possible for the complex battle with cancer. By addressing the GB, Dr Zhang tries to clear the pivot, paving the way for a whole Jue Yin, Shao Yin, and Ying and Blood level cleansing, and for an improved Yuan circulation known as the Fu Zheng strategy.

## The Gall Bladder and the Accumulation of Guilt

The GB might be a major system that gets saturated with guilt. My Ph.D thesis and the appendix of my book: Stages, Levels, Envelopes dealt with an attempt to prove the mind-body connection between guilt and the traditional description of some intelligence system i.e, meridians and organs.

In the Israelite Temples, the guilty could resolve their guilt through the offering of a guilt sacriffice. Excessive guilt might have been transferred from the one that was offering the sacriffice to some body parts of the sacriffied animal. Those parts that were thought to be saturated with toxic guilt were burned on the altar, while the non-toxic parts were eaten by the priests serving in the Temple. Prolonged clinical observations, interviews, and patients filling out questionnaires, including a follow up questionnaire, led to the conclusion that the GB's intelligence system, as TCM described it, is the most important system where guilt tends to be collected , and reductions in its entire performance capabilities influence other zones, and other intelligence systems that are usually influenced from reduced GB functioning, as was described above. The research also made clear that guilt is transferable from one person to another. In Traditional Israelite society, guilt seemed to also be a collective issue. We are all responsible for each other, and we all share the society's total toxicity.

*Do we pay attention to those traditional understandings of Human psych/spirituality? Can we use that knowledge while treating cancer? Is it possible that some patients are the carriers of our society's contagious guilt and other spiritual toxicities? Is it possible that practitioners who are offering a spiritual cleansing as a means to survive cancer or to get cured from it put themselves in danger?*

It was discovered in clinic that using Jing Men (GB 25) acu-point, and a cluster of extra (A-shi) points, located under the inferior and posterior border of the rib cage named the "guilt belt", while using an acupuncture dispersal technique proved to reduce the accumulation of excessive guilt in the GB and other systems such as the Kidneys, improves all kinds of GB Qi capabilities. The physical location of the latter cluster of acu-points presents the past-future symmetry as it is reflected in our trunk aligment and balance. While the lower parts of our trunk get loaded with unresolved issues, our forehead points to future possibilities, so needling an acu-point such as Shen Ting (GV 24) might put more pressure on the dilemma's solving center of our entire being, and it might convince it to issue a conceptual and strategic change. We need to find better ways to communicate with our inner intelligence and to talk to it, convince it, and prove to it that our new intentions are sincere, to better engage with Tao, and to be a better listener of the Yuan's true voice within ourselves and around us.

## The Rakia and the Cell's Membrane

The Hebrew language offers many clues in regard to Human health. The word Rakia - רקיע is a synonym of the word Shamaim- Sky – שמים. The Bible describes the existence of the Rakia dividing the water above the sky from the water below it. The word Rakia is constructed from the Hebrew root RKA-רקע, which means to be hammered out, just like the earth was hammered out from the sea. One's Gall Bladder's nature and intelligence has a role in influencing its bile's capability to engage fat molecules thus enabling the construction of well formed cholesterol, and other lipid based constructing materials.

A cell membrane, while being constructed from lipids, is in fact a microscopic Rakia of oil that separates the water within the cell from the water outside it. This uniqueness of the Rakia which reflects a divine idea repeats itself over and over, in macroscopic and microscopic levels of existence of our world and body.

The mathematic of the word sky - שמים ( the Hebrew technique of gimatria ) is equal to that of the word שמן which mean oil. This ability to form a form in our waterfylic environment is a chemical/physical/electrical miracle. Our cell membranes are a major battle field in oncology. We try to understand its normal and abnormal behavior , and the signals that are received by it and those issued by it.

We try to influence it through radiation, chemotherapy, and biological weapons. However, are the vast concept of the GB's intelligence system and it's reflection on the cell's membrane considered?

Traditional medicine's ideas such as those that were presented briefly are hopefully attractive enough to inspire those of you that are very close, and those of you who are already here. Thinking clearly about the traditional concepts that were mentioned in this chapter, and learning to better integrate the ideas of the Gall Bladder, the Dai, and the Shao Yang together with the ideas of the Colon, the wind, and the Envelopes into the modern concepts of the Immune system, Psychology and Neurology, and Endocrine fields of thinking and research may offer many different starting points for a new era of integrative research.

## Epilogue

*A few month ago, I was attending a meeting in a hospital between a few members of an integrative medical unit, specializing in oncology, and a director of a famous drug company's research and development department. The director was presenting to us the inconceivable negative ratio between the amount of money invested into developing new medication and to the poor results of that development process. He mentioned a lack of a scientific breakthrough as a possible major barrier along the objective barriers of regulations and biocracy. I suggested investing some of his department's budget into establishing an Integrated Ideas Unit, specialized in translating traditional medical ideas into a more advanced and integrated form of language that will be able to truly express both worlds of ideas regarding the etiology and pathology of cancer and the construction of a more effective way to understand it and cure it. He replied and said, surprisingly , " I believe that you are right, traditional medicine can offer us some breakthrough ideas, but I don't think that science is ready for it... " Is this so?*

# References


Ader R, Felten D, Cohen N. Psychoneuroimmunology. *Brain Behav Immun J.* 1990: 2.

Baranovitch O. *Solomon ships in the sea of China* (in Hebrew). Tel Aviv: Astrolog, 2006.

Baranovitch O. *Chronic Fatigue Syndrom* (in Hebrew). Hotam Cin (Isr J TCM). 2004; 2: 37 – 42.

Baranovitch O. *Stages levels envelopes.* Tel Aviv: Avigdor, 2006.

Baranovitch O. *Phlegm camouflage and defense.* (in Hebrew). Hotam Cin (Isr J TCM). 2007; 5: 33-8.

Baranovitch O. *New clinical approach to patients presenting excess guilt as a major etiology for a complex: psychological and physical pathologies, and some behavioral tendencies: Doctoral dissertation.* Nitra: Constantine the Philosopher University, 2008.

Baranovitch O. An integrating Pilates and Chinese medicine treatment for patients that are suffering from breast cancer, a case report (in Hebrew). *Hotam Cin* (Isr J TCM). 2009; 7: 15-21.

Baranovitch O. The traditional use of Chinese herbs in the molecular Era of herbalism and within the frame of integrative medicine (in Hebrew) *Hotam Cin* (Isr J TCM). 2009; 7: 44-6.

Baranovitch O. The extraordinary vessels Du and Ren and their relation to archetypes in our lives, as they are expressed in disharmonies between right and left (in Hebrew). *Hotam Cin* (Isr J TCM). 2010; 8: 19-26.

Becker S. A handbook of Chinese hematology. Boulder: *Blue Poppy*, 2000.

Ben-Eliyahu S, Page G, Schleifer S. Stress NK cells and cancer. *Brain Behav Immun J.* 2007; 21: 881-7.

Bensky D, Barolet R. *Formulas and strategies.* Seatle: East Land, 1990.

Bensky D, Clavey S, Stoger E. *Chinese herbal medicine materia medica. Seattle:* East Land, 2004.

Caspi O, Baranovitch O. When science meets medical tradition – what is needed for a dialogue on integrative medicine. *J Altern Complement Med.* 2009; 15: 579- 83.

Chiang A, Massague J. Molecular basis of metastasis: *N Engl J Med.* 2008; 359: 2814 – 23.

Goldfarb Y, Ben -Eliyahu S. Surgery as a risk factor for breast cancer recurrence and metastasis. *J Breast Disease.* 2006; 26: 99 – 114.

He Y, Han J. Relationship between the wind and tumor metastasis (in Chinese). *Chin J Basic Med TCM.* 2006; 12: 124- 6.

Lahans T. *Integrating conventional and Chinese medicine in cancer care.* Philadelphia: Churchill Livingston Elsevier, 2007.

Melmed NR. *Mind body and medicine:* Oxford University, 2001.

In: Traditional Medicine: New Research
Editor: Yoshiharu Motoo
ISBN: 978-1-62257-448-3


*Chapter 5*

# Seeking Care from Traditional Healers (*Mor boraan*): Traditional Practices in Southern Thailand

***Dusanee Suwankhong, Pranee Liamputtong*[*] *and Bruce Rumbold***
School of Public Health, La Trobe University, Bundoora, Australia

## Abstract

Traditional healers care for people in their own localities at low cost, and their work can increase access to primary care for people in rural areas in particular. In this chapter, we discuss qualitative ethnographic research using participant observation and in-depth interviews that was carried out with 18 traditional healers and 23 customers. The findings provided in-depth understanding of traditional approaches to consulting and remunerating traditional healers. The options available for remuneration are shown to be an important part of the traditional therapeutic system. The main aims of remuneration are to maintain a close relationship between traditional healers and their patients, and to preserve traditional cultural practices. Remuneration is not solely about payment for treatment, even though in Southern Thailand payment of money rather than payment in kind has become the norm. Although patients seek help for different ailments, the traditional practice in all cases is for payment to be made at the first visit and also after treatment is completed and the patient has been healed. We conclude that, in seeking care from traditional healers, payment is a means of honouring traditional healers and their place in Thai culture, and ensuring that traditional healing remains part of the Thai health care system.

[*] Corresponding author: Professor Pranee Liamputtong, School of Public Health, La Trobe University, Bundoora, Victoria, Australia 3086. Email: Pranee@latrobe.edu.au.

# Introduction

The folk healthcare sector is accepted as one of the healthcare resources most readily available to laypeople in developing countries, particularly when they have little or no access to modern health care. Building upon close rapport between healers and patients, folk healing encourages patients to believe that their illnesses can be managed outside the formal healthcare system. This informal traditional medicine healthcare sector thus not only increases access to care but is also a low cost healthcare option for people in many communities [1, 2]. Because the various strategies for healing aim to cure the root causes of illnesses, an holistic approach [1, 3, 4] is taken, and treatment often includes either religious ceremonies or spiritual rites alongside the primary treatment method, so as to better serve the total health needs of the patient [5, 6]. Treatment involves not only religious ceremonies or spiritual rites but also remuneration; payment and cultural gestures that honour the healers.

The folk healing system in most developing nations costs customers little, and payment options are flexible. Customers can choose their mode of payment, which can be monetary or other types of gifts. These flexible options allow customers to pay for the treatment based on what they can afford [7]. Customers usually do not incur significant travelling expenses when visiting traditional healers because the services are available in their own or nearby communities. In contrast, accessing modern health services can entail not only considerable financial expenditure for consultation fees and pharmaceutical costs, but also expenditure in terms of time and costs of travel [2, 8]. The process of receiving treatment from traditional healers is usually less complicated. It only requires that customers bring traditional objects at the first visit. This is a symbolic gesture to show honour to the master, or teacher, of the traditional healer being consulted, and can influence whether the treatment will have a successful outcome [9].

Traditional payment practices are one aspect of providing customers with holistic health care. Traditional healers are usually not concerned with collecting large amounts of income [10]. Rather, seeking help from indigenous practitioners is a traditional custom, which is often not associated with payment. Remuneration strengthens the positive relationship between healers and their patients. Apart from the customary fee, patients may provide additional non-monetary forms of payment after they have been healed, depending on the practice of each community [11]. When visiting healers in other communities, even when those healers do not request additional payment, visitors will always express gratitude and honour the healer when they are healed. Traditional practitioners prefer to preserve the traditional practices for remunerating and honouring healers. They practise traditional medicine (TM) because of an interest in the profession, the desire to help people and the wish to preserve TM for future generations [12, 13].

We turn now to discuss the traditional practices of seeking out and remunerating traditional healers in southern Thailand, a geographical area with unique social and cultural characteristics. These traditional practices keep service costs low and increase access to care for people in rural communities.

## The Setting

The study was conducted in Phatthalung province in the South-Eastern region of Thailand, approximately 850 kilometres from Bangkok [14]. Phatthalung is the 10th largest area in this region. Phatthalung today is divided into 11 districts with a population of about 500,800. The majority are Thai Buddhists, although approximately 11 per cent of the population adheres to the Islamic faith. Each district has its own distinctive features in terms of geography, natural resources, historical sites, local products and businesses [15, 16].

*Phatthalung is now fast developing into a modern society. It has an increasing number of modern supermarkets, department stores, shopping centres, local markets and other facilities to support a comfortable lifestyle. Most of the policy makers, government organisations and businesses are located in the cities. The socioeconomic status of citizens ranges from high to low across both modern and traditional lifestyles. Phatthalung has both private and public healthcare facilities at the provincial, district and subdistrict level, thus affording easy access to services and variety of choice [16].*

Thung Tong community (fictitious name), located in Phatthalung province, was chosen as the study site because of the large number of traditional healers living there. Of the 260 traditional healers across the province, 103 practise their craft in this community. They use different healing methods for complaints or illnesses such as muscle and ligament disorders, malaria, peptic ulcers, hypertension, common colds, pregnancy care, dysmenorrhoea, abdominal pain, diabetes, rashes, bone dysfunctions, snake bites, haemorrhoids, pale skin and spiritual unease [17]. One reason for the large number of traditional healers in this community could be a lack of access to formal healthcare for, although a primary health care centre at the village level provides people with modern health services [16], this community is about 20 kilometres from the community hospital and approximately 35 kilometres from the provincial hospital.

## Methodology

Ethnography is a suitable method for observing the traditional practices of customers seeking help from traditional healers. Ethnographic research allows the use of a mixture of methods and sources of data for triangulation purposes [18-20]. The methods employed in our study included participant observation, unstructured in-depth interviews and unobtrusive observation.

Participant observation involved sharing the daily lives and activities of traditional healers and their customers; watching what they were doing and listening to their interpretations of the world was critical for understanding the phenomena under study [21, 22]. The first author was granted permission to visit the healers' homes at any time, so that observing their practice and asking questions became a routine part of her activity [23]. Unstructured interviews were conducted in the local Thai language. Open questions were asked, which encouraged the participants, be they traditional healers or customers, to offer their views freely [24, 25]. All the conversations took place at participants' homes at a time that was convenient to them. The participants were given an information sheet, informed consent form and a withdrawal form prior to an interview. Their permission was sought for the researcher to tape-record the interview and take photos. A first conversation with each traditional healer took about one hour and the first author was allowed to visit at other times for further discussions.

A purposive sampling method was used to choose the key informants who met the study criteria and who could provide rich data relevant to the study. The traditional healers were selected based on the forms of healing they used and their current practice of their craft. Customers with a variety of illnesses who asked for help from traditional healers were invited to be participants. A snowball sampling technique was used to expand the number of key informants. This approach was adopted until little new data emerged [26].

All participants were asked for their permission to tape-record the interviews and to take their photographs. The recordings were transcribed for data analysis. The transcription was done in the Thai language in order to preserve its subtle meanings, as recommended in cross-cultural research [23]. The in-depth data were analysed thematically [26]. In presenting the participants' verbatim responses, we have used fictitious names to preserve the confidentiality.

Ethics approvals were granted by the La Trobe University Human Ethics Committee and the Ethics Committee for Research in Human Subjects in the Fields of Thai Traditional and Alternative Medicine, Department for Development of Thai Traditional and Alternative Medicine (DTAM), Ministry of Public Health (MoPH), Thailand. Formal informed consent was given by each individual participant, as was permission for taking photographs.

## Results

The findings were that remuneration of traditional healers in this region was carried out at two points; when customers first asked for treatment or help, and in a further ceremony once they had recovered.

## Traditional Practice Prior to Receiving Treatment

Honouring traditional healers is an inherent aspect of the traditional healing system that has been maintained from generation to generation. People seeking help from traditional healers understand that they have to prepare ceremonial materials before they go for treatment. All customers are expected to contribute to the ceremony called *wai kru* (showing respect to ancestors of traditional healers) before they can enter into the process of healing. This traditional practice of presenting ceremonial materials is to show respect and to inform the traditional healers' *kru mor* (ancestor spirits) of one's needs. With help from their *kru mor*, traditional healers are able to determine the customers' health problems or needs and provide the appropriate treatment or support to help their patients recover. *Pee* (older sister) Wasana, a middle aged woman, remarked:

> We all automatically know what we have to prepare when seeking help of *mor baan* (traditional healer); betel leaves, betel nuts from our backyard, incense sticks and some

coins. This has always been our practice. We believe that *wai cru* ceremony can increase healing capacity. We can achieve full recovery, if we just follow this traditional practice.

The common symbolic items used for the ceremony are areca nut, betel leaf with mineral lime paste, flowers, candles, incense sticks and a monetary fee. The traditional fee is fairly flexible and can be, for example, 3 baht (0.10 USD), 9 baht (0.30 USD), 10 baht (0.33 USD), 20 baht (0.66 USD) or 50 baht (1.67 USD). This fee is a customary practice, and customers who seek help from the traditional healers automatically pay it. All the materials are put together in an appropriate receptacle and presented to the traditional healer at the first visit.

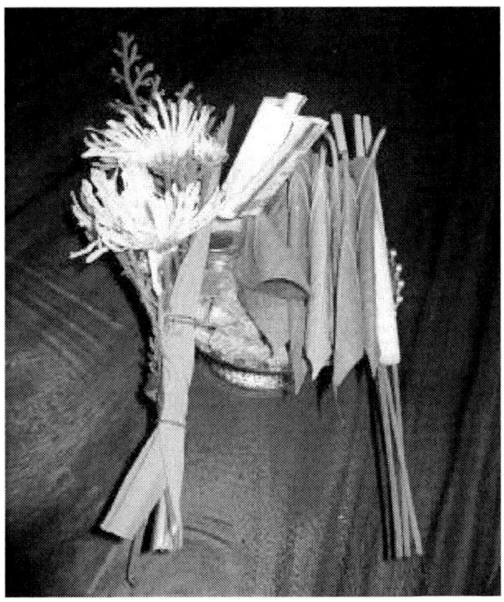

Photograph 1. The symbolic items for seeking help of traditional healers.

Customers hand these symbolic items to the healer according to the established rules. For example, the customer should hand the tail part of the betel leaf to the traditional healer because this shows true respect. The belief is that the customer will recover fully if the gesture of respect is sincere. Customers who present the healer with the head part of the betel leaf may not heal completely as they would be deemed not to have shown true respect. (We observe that the head part of betel leaf is fairly hard, so it may represent a harsh person or someone without gentle characteristics, while the tail is soft, symbolising that the presenter is a gentle person.) Customers have to learn how to adhere to the proper ceremonial procedure if they want to heal permanently, be cured, of their illnesses.

The majority of customers provide the symbolic items shown above when seeking help from traditional healers. However, different illnesses and health problems may require other symbols to enhance full recovery. For example, the treatment and healing of *tor nuea*[1] disorder requires people to provide extra items. This disease involves the growth of the eye membrane which, if left untreated, may develop into a tumour. Meat is needed as part of the

[1] It is an eye disorder involving the growth of medial conjunctiva to form a thickset mass on the cornea. *Tor nuea* or pteryguim mostly grows in triangular shape from the nasal side of the sclera. Sunlight, ultraviolet, dust, wind, or dry air contribute to this eye problem.

treatment to stall the growth of the eye membrane. Patients with this disease thus not only have to prepare the ceremonial items shown above but also to bring some kind of meat to the traditional healer. *Paa* (aunty) Somwang said:

> If seek *mor baan* for healing *tor nuea*, [we] have to bring some meat too, otherwise we will not *haei* (healing). *Mor* (healer) leaves meat on coconut shield and covers my eye and cuts the meat 3 times. I [have to] come to *mor baan*'s house for the same process 3 days in the evening. [I] then always find relief after that.

## Honouring the Healers when Recovered

Customers can choose their own way of honouring traditional healers. Providing *kaa raad* (the traditional fee) is a common practice to show honour when individual patients have recovered. This practice of honouring healers is not compulsory, but customers are encouraged to do so because it increases the chances of them becoming fully healed, and it sustains the traditional healing trade. Although customers generally pay a fee commensurate with what they can afford, this also is not compulsory, as the original philosophy of the traditional healing profession is to alleviate suffering irrespective of remuneration. We found that customers in this community honour and remunerate their traditional healers in three traditional ways: paying only the customary fee, paying the customary fee and giving gifts, and paying the customary fee and performing the *wai kru* ceremony. Some customers prefer to pay the traditional healer after each visit while others remunerate the healers only after they have recovered.

Monetary payment is one option for honouring traditional healers. A fee is not formally set but varies according to what customers can offer. The customers will sometimes make an additional payment if they are satisfied with the treatment. If a patient does not have much money, the healer may provide treatment without asking for any payment. If patients are not completely healed, or if their condition does not improve significantly, payment is deemed unnecessary. Payment, if the customer chooses, may be made at each visit. *Taa* (grandfather) Larb, a bonesetter, understands his customers. He stated:

> When they are healed, they will give me *kaa raad.* It depends on them how much they can provide...if someone is poor, they have insufficient money. Some have been healed but they never turn up to honour the healers.

A number of customers pay traditional healers the customary fee and also present them with a gift. This is done on an important day or a special Thai festival such as the New Year Festival, the Thai traditional New Year celebration or *Songkran* Festival or religious ceremonies related to Thai Buddhist culture. We observed customers giving their favourite traditional healers fabric and necessities for everyday living. Bathing materials and shirts are popular gifts for male healers. Female healers are often provided with sarongs or round necked sleeveless blouses. Another popular present is food or dessert. People will visit traditional healers' homes with these presents to honour them.

The *Wai kru* ceremony is a unique traditional practice for honouring traditional healers and is the acknowledgement preferred by most traditional healers. The *Wai kru* ceremony takes place at the healer's house on a Buddhist Holy Day. The appropriate time for starting the ceremony is between eight and nine in the morning. Soon after the ceremony, the healer will take food to the temple. This ritual provides traditional healers and their customers with a chance to honour the healers' forebears and previous traditional healers, as the ancestors are believed to have had considerable influence on the effectiveness of the treatment. Customers, therefore, should show *ka tun yu* (gratitude) to these spirits.

To observe the *wai kru* rites, healed customers or relatives have to prepare, in advance, some symbolic items for the ritual. These include areca nut, betel leaf with mineral lime paste, flowers, candles, incense sticks, fresh banana, food in tiffin carriers and a customary fee of an amount similar to that paid at the first treatment session. Fruits and food in particular can be of different types, depending on what the customers can afford or prefer. Customers must also inform the healer in advance of their intention to perform these rites so that traditional healers can prepare themselves for the ceremony. The ceremony starts when the customer arrives at the healer's house. All the symbolic items are arranged before the spirits of deceased healers or *kru ar jarn* (teacher or master of the traditional healers). The traditional healer then commences incantations to inform the spirits of the honouring ceremony. The customer stays beside the traditional healer for approximately 30 minutes until the praying finishes. It is believed that the *wai kru* rites will reward both customers and traditional healers. Customers will never get that illness again; they are healed completely. The good fortune of the traditional healers will increase and the blessing prolongs the viability of their profession.

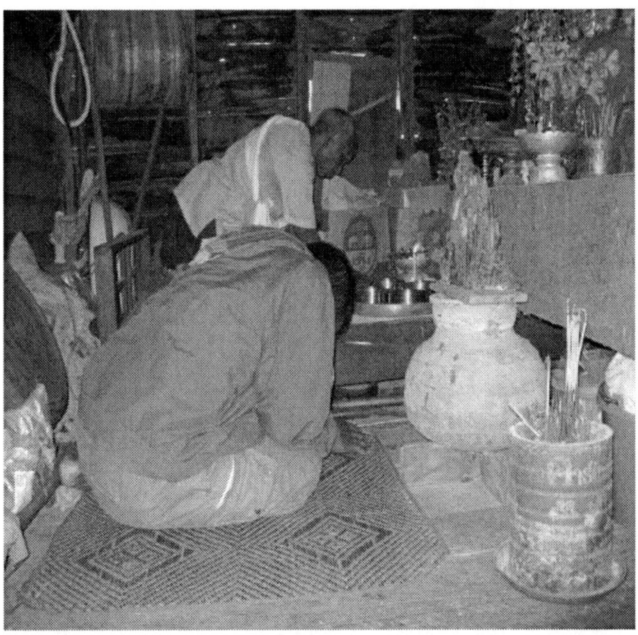

Photograph 2. *Wai kru* ceremony in front of traditional healer's forefather statue.

*Tud raak* (cut the root out) is the final step in the process of traditional healing. This stage is very important as it is believed that, if customers follow the entire healing process until they get *tud raak*, they will recover completely. Traditional healers can be paid to provide this service to their customers. Customers must prepare the symbolic items for *tud raak,* including betel leaf and areca nut. The traditional healers begin the process by praying *katha tud raak* (incantation for cutting root) for a short time, invoking the spirits to bless the customer with a healthy life and good fortune. When they finish praying, the traditional healers roll the betel leaf together with the areca nut and cut it in two. This symbolises that the illness is permanently healed. The healing process is then complete.

There is a traditional belief that, if customers do not offer any payment when they are healed, they may not recover fully, or the illness may return. This belief is a reminder to the customers of the importance of honouring the healers in some way. Nowadays, the payment options have changed with changing social conditions, and customers tend to choose monetary payment above other options. It is not only convenient for them but also recognition that the traditional healers have to make a living as well. This gesture also gives *kum lung jai* (encouragement) to the traditional healers to continue their role in Thai health care.

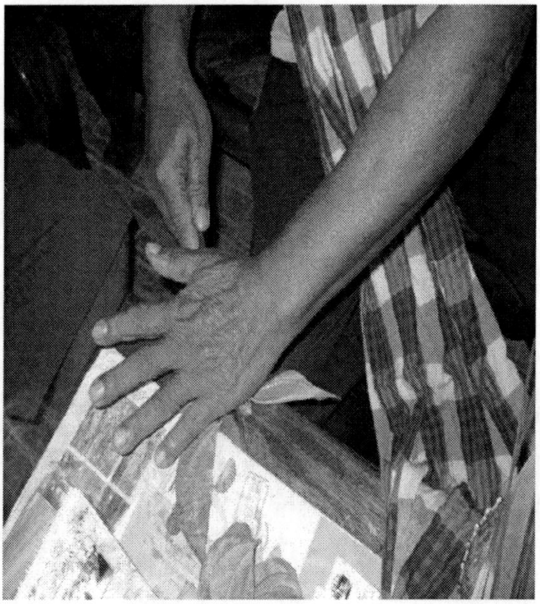

Photograph 3. Chopping the betel leaf and areca nut for *tud raak*.

## Discussion

The remuneration and honouring system in our study has both similarities and differences when compared with those reported for other societies. Costs of treatment in Southern Thailand are generally low, which is not always the case elsewhere. Kale [27] and Nelms and Gorskinote [28] note that the cost of services of traditional healers vary from culture to culture. The amount of the payment is associated with the effectiveness of the treatment. Patients may pay nothing if treatments provide no effective cure. Leonard [29] describes rules of payment among African traditional healers. Initial payments are required, and further payment can be negotiated depending on the effectiveness of the treatment. If the illness is not cured by the treatment, patients are not required to provide any further payment. On the other hand, additional payments need to be made when individuals are completely healed.

Bhatia and colleagues [30] found that Indian patients were charged small amounts of money that varied from 1 to 3 rupees per patient. However, Baskind and Birbeck [31] found different payment options in Zambia, where traditional healers asked for one live goat from their patients and, if patients could not provide the goat, healers refused to provide help.

In Swaziland [11], the payment of a fee is recognised as a traditional custom. It strengthens relationships between healers and patients, but it is not a main concern of the healers. Patients may provide a cow to their healers as a payment after they are healed. In southern Thailand, as we have seen, payment can be of varying amounts [12], although these are usually modest. Hanvattanakul [13] states that traditional healers generally do not ask for big sums of money as payment because people practice TM due to an interest in the profession, the desire to help people and the intention of preserving TM for further generations.

Our findings are similar to those of Whittaker [32], who reported that traditional midwives in Northeastern Thailand received between 100 and 200 Thai baht ($2.50 to $5 USD) from each woman during her pregnancy. One traditional midwife in Whittaker's study said about payment:

> It varies, some people have no money. In the old days people gave me water, rice and cloth in a basket, but now they give money instead. Some of the children I have delivered come at Songkran [Thai New Year] and pour water over my hands and pay respect to me as I am *bun khun* [a person to whom they have a special obligation]. You make a lot of Buddhist merit by helping someone give birth.

Studies in Trinidad and Grenada [33] also show patients having a variety of payment options and reward styles. Clients usually pay the customary fees or provide a gift. Many clients pay as much money as they can afford while others may not make any monetary payment at all.

The majority of customers interviewed in this study pointed out that monetary and time savings were important reasons for them consulting traditional healers. Because healers were local, they did not have to spend long hours travelling to modern hospitals and involving themselves in medical treatment. Traditional healers could get them back to health to resume their livelihoods more quickly. As we have shown, individual customers have various options to remunerate traditional healers, depending on their circumstances. Several studies, such as Applewhite [34], Sawatsing [7] and Cho [5] confirm that patients seek treatment with traditional healers because they are offered care at a lower price compared with treatment in modern facilities. However, this study found that many patients also seek traditional healers outside their communities if they are offered the promise of speedier recovery or if the healers have a good reputation, even if this involves higher expenditure. Expense is not the most important factor for all people in all societies. This is consistent with the findings of Cassidy [35], Sirois and Gick [36], Sringernyuang [37] and Pradubmook and Sringernyuang [38], who state that individuals desire effective healers who will provide them with better prospects for good health, which will in turn allow them to lead their normal lifestyles.

There are, however, risks involved in seeking care from traditional healers. A payment can bring negative results to both patients and healers if the patient fails to follow specific rules related to the payment [9, 29, 39]. This can be illustrated by Oppong's study [39] in Plateau State, Nigeria. Here, patients were charged a fee of 10 Naira ($10 USD), and were sometimes required to provide a chicken as part of the payment. Patients who received treatments from traditional healers but did not pay the full amount would be punished with stomachaches and other health troubles. When they realised their mistake and made the required payments, these problems would go away. Similarly, in Leonard's work [29], it was found that patients were punished with ailments if they did not follow the rules of payment. But a study among Hmong healers living in Australia conducted by Liamputtong Rice [9] found that if payment options were not adhered to by the customers, the traditional healers themselves would suffer the consequences. Patients were expected to pay for treatments by honouring traditional healers and their masters, taking incense sticks tied with red material, gold, banknotes and a few silver coins to the healers. If patients did not provide these forms of remuneration, the traditional healers would become sick.

## Conclusion

Each traditional community has its own system of remunerating its healers. The main purpose is to preserve and reinforce cultural practices. The tradition in southern Thailand is no exception. The remuneration system enhances the relationship between healers and patients through the mutual respect shown to each through the system. Not only that, the remuneration system can through compliance or non-compliance bring either reward or suffering to customers in terms of their health. This cultural belief serves to remind customers to honour traditional healers when they are healed so that what the treatments they have received will remain part of an effective health care system in Thai society.

## Acknowledgments

We are grateful to all traditional healers and customers who have provided us with deep understanding of their remuneration system. We also thank the Faculty of Health and Sports Science, Thaksin University, Thailand and the School of Public Health, La Trobe University, Australia who granted the scholarship to support the first author in carrying out the fieldwork in rural Thailand. We would also like to acknowledge the DTAM, MoPH, Phatthalung Provincial Health Office (PPHO), and all local government organisations and their staff who gave us their invaluable support during the process of our data collection.

## References

[1] Hufford DJ. Folk medicine and health culture in contemporary society. *Primary Care* 1997;24(4):723-41.

[2] Kulsomboon S, Adthasit R. *The status and trend of research in local wisdom for health.* Bangkok: The War Veterans Organization; 2007.

[3] Helman CG. *Culture, health and illness.* 5th ed. London: Hodder Arnold; 2007.

[4] Kleinman A. Patients and healers in the context of culture: An exploration of the borderland between anthropology, medicine, and psychiatry. Berkeley: University of California Press; 1980.

[5] Cho MO. Health care seeking behavior of Korean women with lymphedema. *Nursing and Health Sciences* 2004;6(2):149-59.

[6] Kunstadter P. Do cultural differences make any difference? Choice points in medical systems available in Northwestern Thailand. In: Kleinman A, Kunstadter P, Alexander RE, Gate JL, editors. *Culture and healing in Asian societies: Anthropological, psychiatric and public health studies.* Cambridge: Schenkman Publishing Company; 1978. p. 185-217.

[7] Sawatsing C. *Provision and utilization of traditional health services in rural Thailand.* Bangkok, Thailand: Unpublished master's thesis, Mahidol University; 2003.

[8] Gessler MC, Msuya DE, Nkunya MHH, Schär A, M H, Tanner M. Traditional healers in Tanzania: Sociocultural profile and three short portraits. *Journal of Ethnopharmacology* 1995;48:145-60.

[9] Liamputtong Rice P. Hmong women and reproduction. Westport: Bergin & Garvey; 2000.

[10] Van der Geest S. Is there a role for traditional medicine in basic health services in Africa? A plea for a community perspective. *Tropical Medicine and International Health* 1997;2(9):903-11.

[11] Green EC, Makhubu L. Traditional healers in Swaziland: Toward improved cooperation between the traditional and modern health sectors. *Social Science & Medicine* 1984;18(12):1071-9.

[12] Golomb L. An anthropology of curing in multiethnic Thailand. Urbana: University of Illinois Press; 1985.

[13] Hanvattanakul C. *Using folk wisdom for promoting health during pregnancy: A case study of southern Thai Muslim Women.* Had Yai, Thailand: Unpublished master's thesis, Prince of Songkhla University; 2005.

[14] Thai Cultural Encyclopedia Association. Thai cultural encyclopedia: Southern region volume 11. Bangkok: *Thai Cultural Encyclopedia* Association; 1999.

[15] Phatthalung City Hall. *History of Phatthalung.* Phatthalung2006.

[16] Phatthalung City Hall. *The Phatthalung province 2008.* Phatthalung: Phatthalung City Hall; 2008.

[17] Phatthalung Provincial Health Office. *The list of traditional healers in Phatthalung.* Phatthalung: Phatthalung Provincial Health Office2009.

[18] Gobo G. Doing ethnography. Los Angeles: Sage Publications; 2008.

[19] Madden R. Being ethnographic: A guide to the theory and practice of ethnography. London: Sage Publications; 2010.

[20] O'Reilly K. *Key concepts in ethnography.* Los Angeles: Sage Publications; 2009.

[21] Fetterman DM. *Ethnography: Step by step.* 2nd ed. London: Sage Publications; 2009.

[22] Spradley JP. *Participant Observation.* New York: Holt, Rinehart and Winston; 1980.

[23] Liamputtong P. *Performing qualitative cross-cultural research.* Cambridge: Cambridge University Press; 2010.

[24] Britten N. Qualitative interview in health care research. In: Pope C, Mays N, editors. *Qualitative research in health care.* 2nd ed. London: BMJ Books; 2000. p. 11-9.

[25] Minichiello V, Aroni R, Hays T. *In-depth interviewing: Principles, techniques, analysis.* 3rd ed. Sydney: Pearson Education Australia; 2008.
[26] Liamputtong P. Qualitative research methods. 3rd ed. South Melbourne: Oxford University Press; 2009.
[27] Kale R. Traditional healers in South Africa: A parallel health care system. *British Medical Journal* 1995;310(6988):1182-5.
[28] Nelms LW, Gorski J. The role of the African traditional healer in women's health. *Journal of Transcultural Nursing* 2006;17(2):184-9.
[29] Leonard KL. African traditional healers and outcome-contingent contracts in health care. *Journal of Development Economics* 2003;71(1):1-22.
[30] Bhatia JC, Vir D, Timmappaya A, Chuttani CS. Traditional healers and modern medicine. *Social Science & Medicine* 1975;9(1):15-21.
[31] Baskind R, Birbeck G. Epilepsy care in Zambia: A study of traditional healers. *Epilepsia* 2005;46(7):1121-6.
[32] Whittaker A. The demise of birth attendants in Northeast Thailand: Embodying tradition in modern times. In: Rozario S, Samuel G, editors. *The daughters of Hāritī: Childbirth and female healers in South and Southeast Asia.* London: Routledge; 2002. p. 211-33.
[33] Mischel F. Faith health and medical practice in the Southern Caribbean. *Southwestern Journal of Anthropology* 1959;15(4):407-17.
[34] Applewhite SL. Curanderismo: Demystifying the health beliefs and practices of elderly Mexican Americans. Health & Social Work1995;20(4):247-53.
[35] Cassidy CM. Social science theory and methods in the study of alternative and complementary medicine. *Journal of Alternative & Complementary Medicine* 1995;1(1):19-40.
[36] Sirois FM, Gick ML. An investigation of the health beliefs and motivations of complementary medicine clients. *Social Science & Medicine* 2002;55:1025-37.
[37] Sringanyuang L. Social and cultural dimension of community drug use: Development of knowledge based on theory and research. Nonthaburi: Health Systems Research Institute, Thailand1999.
[38] Pradubmook P, Sringanyuang L. Life situation and self care of diabetic patients. *Health Systems Research Journal* 1994;2(4):272-80.
[39] Oppong ACK. Healers in transition. *Social Science & Medicine* 1989;28(6):605-12.

In: Traditional Medicine: New Research
Editor: Yoshiharu Motoo
ISBN: 978-1-62257-448-3


*Chapter 6*

# Traditional, Complementary and Alternative Medicine (TCAM): A Review of Healing Practices outside the Formal Health Care System

***Pranee Liamputtong, Dusanee Suwankhong and Bruce Rumbold***
School of Public Health, La Trobe University, Bundoora, Victoria, Australia

## Global Utilization of Traditional, Complementary and Alternative Medicine (TCAM)

> Healing and healers are essential to the experience of recovery from sickness or disease. Healers are those who assist in the healing process. Informants indicated that they use informal healers as well as physicians and the formal health care system. Informants described their use of different types of folk healers and compared their experiences with folk healers to their experiences with physicians [1].

This chapter considers the contribution of healing and healers who work outside the formal health care system, with a particular focus upon TCAM. The questions addressed include why TCAM is chosen for health care, who practices TCAM, where TCAM healers find their customers, and whether it is possible for modern medicine to cooperate with TCAM.

Allopathic medicine dominates health care systems worldwide. But facilities providing modern medical care may not be accessible or affordable to all, especially in developing countries [2]. More than two-thirds of the world's population has little or no access to modern health care. Because of this, the World Health Organization (WHO) endorses the use of TCAM as an alternative provider of health care [3, 4], and this option has been included in the national health policies of over 100 countries around the world. Each of these countries develops its own mix of TCAM and modern medicine in attempting to meet the health needs of its people and give them access to care [5].

Over recent decades, public interest in TCAM has increased in both developing and industrialized countries [6, 7]. On average, over half the population in most developed and developing countries use TCAM regularly. About two-thirds of people in Canada, Germany and Chile, more than one-third in China and Colombia, and approximately four-fifths of those living in most African countries use CAM or TCAM [6]. Principal reasons for doing so are the costs of conventional treatment, its side-effects, and its ineffectiveness for certain chronic conditions in particular [8].

TCAM use is also increasing in Asia [9, 10], with estimates that between 70 per cent and 80 per cent of populations in most Southeast Asian countries consult traditional or complementary practitioners. The majority of TCAM patients live in rural and semi-urban regions where access to modern medical care can be difficult. Here, some traditional health care practitioners have found ways of co-operating with modern health care systems, or have become part of a specific TCAM section within modern health care facilities [6]. Some traditional practices are a recognized part of the formal health care systems in many countries, but for the most part these services, once incorporated into the mainstream, are provided by modern health practitioners [3, 6].

TCAM has long been practised in developing countries [4, 6, 11]. Here, it was, until the advent of western medicine, the recognized healthcare system, grounded in the culture and spirit of the country. Leaving aside national variations, the fundamental concept informing TCAM is the need of balance to ensure the healthy functioning of body and mind. All dimensions of the body are interconnected, and individuals should have a balanced relationship with their environment and their society. Disrupting these relationships can cause illness in individuals; however, illness not only affects these individuals but also the well-being of the whole community. Traditional healing, therefore, is not designed simply to cure specific parts of an individual (a limb, an organ), but rather to bring about healing through restoring the balance between the various dimensions of health [6, 12].

## What Is TCAM?

TCAM as a category includes therapeutic practices and techniques considered to be outside the domain of modern medicine [8, 13-16]. TCAM contributes to folk, home and natural remedies and involves the use of plants and herbs, physical manipulation and religious practices, rather than resources developed from scientific investigation [4, 17, 18]. Alternative medicine, complementary medicine, complementary and alternative medicine (CAM) and traditional medicine (TM) are four terms that are used interchangeably within a number of countries [7, 19, 20]. The terminology for, and even the content of, TCAM varies with cultural and geographical differences. Thus, a CAM treatment in a western nation may be a TCAM strategy that has been removed from its indigenous context, or it may be an alternative healing strategy developed within the culture, as is the case with chiropractic and osteopathy in western societies.

TM has been practised by native healers and local people in developing nations for many generations prior to western influence [4, 16, 18, 21]. TM is thus embedded in the indigenous health systems of these countries, providing therapeutic practices based upon local knowledge and traditional beliefs. Healing materials used are local products such as plants and parts of animals. This knowledge and these practices have been handed down through the generations [11].

More recently, other forms of health care have been introduced into these countries [16]. For some, TM remains an alternative to the imported western curative health care system, especially in rural areas [2, 22] and impoverished regions where access and costs create difficulties. For others, the main role of TM now is to complement the imported system so that together a holistic approach that incorporates the interrelated dimensions of health is provided, rather than one that focuses almost exclusively on curing disease. A further attraction of TM is its use natural therapies with potentially fewer side effects than modern medical treatments [22]. Ultimately, it is consumers who decide whether TM is used as complementary or alternative medicine; but that choice may be shaped by a variety of factors, including people's prior experiences of the traditional and mainstream sectors.

## Satisfaction with TCAM

Some people, when they become ill, combine modern and traditional healing methods and may not even be aware of which treatments cure illness [23]. Doing this, however, requires belief in the efficacy of both healing forms [13, 24, 25]. People who use TCAM commonly have strong beliefs about indigenous medicine and are satisfied with its services [26]. Lazar and O'Connor [27] conclude that health beliefs are influential in an individual's decision to use some health care practices rather than others. These health beliefs are formed in a variety of ways.

### Emotional Appeal

CAM has become widely accepted because "patients want to be cured, but they also want to be cared for" (Roe [16]. Patients report that CAM practitioners meet their expectations by treating them as individuals rather than paying attention only to their disease. They seem to prefer the readily-available, uncomplicated single-practitioner strategies of traditional healing. The complex multi-practitioner processes of modern medicine can eliminate the collaborative relationships that these people want to have with their health care providers [16]. Jonas [14] contends that when we are ill, whether with minor or severe conditions, we basically want "a rapid, gentle treatment that cures us or at least can allay out fears and alleviate our suffering".

Patients may have confidence in modern medicine, but may also believe that CAM can help in ways that modern medicine cannot, especially when it comes to the emotional and spiritual dimensions of health [28]. Spencer [20] sees communication problems as illustrating this. Patients worry about their illness because they do not clearly understand their doctors' explanations of the illness and its treatment. They are thus more likely to try the services of local traditional healers they can understand. This problem in communication can also create distrust in the treatments offered by modern doctors.

Individual beliefs and perceptions about health influence the use of CAM. Goldner [29] reported that consumers in San Francisco used CAM because CAM therapies are based on holistic understandings. Their trust in CAM increased once they had positive experience of it. Many preferred using natural products to treat illness in order to reduce their intake of pharmaceuticals. These health beliefs were a good match with CAM principles, but not with modern medicine.

A recent study in Singapore found that patients with cancer used CAM to complement modern treatments because they believed that CAM therapies would increase resistance and improve health in general [30]. This view was also found in young cancer patients, 18 years and over, in the United States [31]. The main reason these patients used CAM was because it increased their hope for recovery.

Cultural beliefs also lead people to trust TM for their health care needs. Many people believe that traditional forms of health care provide effective treatments for particular illnesses [8, 32]. Zhang and Verhoef [32], for example, found that Chinese immigrants believed in the effectiveness of Chinese medicine and not that of modern medicine. They saw TM as providing holistic care and helping with illnesses that require long-term care.

Limits to the capacity of modern medicine to heal seem to lead some people to seek treatment elsewhere. Studies in Thailand showed that patients living with HIV/AIDS used acupuncture because they preferred alternative methods that might more effectively help to reduce negative symptoms [33]. Some traditional methods were used to prevent an illness from getting worse, while others provided pain control when modern medicine failed. This study also found that users of CAM had positive perceptions and beliefs about the capabilities of CAM, while non-users did not. This finding is similar to that of another study of HIV patients in Thailand, which showed that 95 per cent of patients with HIV used more than one type of CAM [34]. The researchers hypothesize that this high prevalence rate may be due to the perception that CAM increases the chance of finding an effective cure.

Patient satisfaction is a key factor in choice of health services. Health care providers thus need to respect the wishes as well as the perceived needs of patients [35]. Many empirical studies show that people use CAM because of dissatisfaction with modern medicine [36-38]. Reasons for this include modern medicine's inability to cure certain conditions, a focus on the disease, lack of adequate holistic care, concern about the possibility of adverse effects from long-term use and lack of interpersonal communication. McGregor and Peay [39], in an Australian study, support these reasons, explaining that patients choose alternative treatments due to a low level of confidence in modern treatments and dissatisfaction with outcomes. Gessler et al. [40] provide further support with findings that dissatisfaction with modern medicine can arise from long waiting times that result in only a short consultation with the doctor. Moreover, patients feel alone and confused when they receive unfriendly explanations about their illness and treatment while visiting the hospital.

Modern medicine may provide less effective treatment than TM, perhaps in part because modern doctors and their patients have different explanations for the causes of illness [40, 41]. Patients bring their hope, beliefs and trust to alternative treatments because they believe that modern medicine offers little chance of recovery in some situations. Folk healing integrates various strategies for managing illness, such as the use of natural products and spiritual ceremonies. These combined practices increase patient beliefs in the treatment and its ability to produce positive outcomes to alleviate illness. Patients may engage in many folk practices to support their well-being. The number of styles of treatment an individual is willing to pursue depends on that individual's intentions and beliefs [41].

Apart from receiving confusing explanations of their illness, patients may not get appropriate treatment due to misunderstandings between clinical managers [42]. Healthy lay people sometimes consult a doctor simply to share the suffering that may be caused by changes in their circumstances and their struggle to make adjustments. Modern medical care often does not meet patients' expectations of support. Doctors will treat diseases by attempting to cure dysfunctional organs, rather than focusing on patients' explanations of their illness that could be more effective for finding a cure. Patients may not follow treatments provided by doctors because they do not understand the medical regimen and they are not sure how the medical treatments can help them with their problems. A failure to engage with patients' understandings and experience of their illness is still a major problem in modern health care [43].

## Physical Appeal

CAM may be used to treat a wide range of health problems [36, 38, 44-46]. In both western and non-western communities, CAM is popular for managing chronic illnesses and relieving symptoms [13, 34, 46-48].

Swartzman and colleagues [48] argue that people in the United States are attracted to CAM treatments for chronic pain conditions because many such treatments can be easily integrated into their health habits and pose a low medical risk. Popular CAM treatments include stretching, relaxation and diet. Individuals are less attracted to treatments that involve modern medical procedures because these tend to be more invasive. Fleming, Rabago, Mundt and Fleming [49] found that patients with lower back pain, headaches and knee pain showed an increased use of CAM to relieve this pain, with treatments including massage, chiropractic, acupuncture, yoga, herbal supplements and prolotherapy. All these treatments were perceived to be helpful. Massage was perceived as the most helpful by 90 per cent of all participants who received it, followed by chiropractic and yoga at 80 per cent and 81 per cent, respectively. Moore [50] suggests that CAM is used by pregnant women in many societies for dietary supplement treatment, alleviation of symptoms and to promote a sense of well-being during pregnancy.

A study by Adler [44] showed that Californian women with breast cancer preferred using CAM over modern medical treatments. About two-thirds of the women already used CAM therapies prior to being diagnosed with breast cancer, and their use increased slightly to 72 per cent after diagnosis. Adler points out that use before and after diagnosis is not significantly different, which could mean that participants use CAM as a regular health care practice. Astin [36] explains that, if a person perceives the benefits of a given therapy, they are more likely to continue to use that treatment. Sirois and Gick [13] conducted a large study of the health beliefs and motivations of CAM users in Canada, finding that individual health awareness was a factor that motivated people to initiate use of CAM, and that this factor also related to continued use.

CAM medicines are intended to increase quality of life mainly among people who have chronic illnesses and severe conditions [51]. Sugimoto and colleagues [51] showed that herbal medicines improved the quality of life for patients living with HIV and AIDS in

Northeastern Thailand. Users of herbal medicines showed greater improvement in overall mental health than non-users did, although physical health outcomes were no different. The greatest improvement in mental health scores was found among patients who were women, widowed, of poor economic status and symptomatic. The researchers hypothesized that these patient groups need support during illness, and expectations of the effectiveness of herbal medicines to cope with illness reduces their social vulnerability. Applewhite [52] reported that elderly Mexican-Americans use traditional herbs because they believe that this treatment can cure some kinds of illness better than modern medical strategies can. Herbs are believed to bring relief for both mild and serious illnesses, and they can help manage headaches and insomnia as well as more serious problems like hypertension and nervous tension.

## Social Appeal

CAM increases individuals' capacity to make healthcare choices. Sirois and Gick [13] found the most frequent reason for choosing CAM over modern medicine was because it increased a person's ability to make their own decisions about health. Sirois and Gick propose that this will influence more individuals to use CAM. Snyder and Lindquist [53] explain that "in complementary therapies the total person is considered: physically, emotionally, mentally, and spiritually. The goal is to create harmony or balance within the person". Mulholland [18] suggests that the advantage TM "holds over modern medicine is its humanity. Each person is treated as an individual". Pawluch, Cain and Gillett [54] state that alternative medicine provides people with the health care of their choice because its philosophy has "an emphasis on individual and personal responsibility over all health care decisions". CAM therapies thus offer patients the opportunity to play an active role in making healthcare choices consistent with their understanding of the world [29].

Patients and modern health care practitioners frequently have different orientations to health and illness, and this can contribute to patients' inability to benefit from modern medicine [23, 26]. CAM maintains an approach that is more focused on culture [2, 55], including people in the decision-making processes of health care instead of requiring them passively to accept the expert decisions of modern physicians [26, 30, 36-38, 53]. A study in Thailand [34], for example, confirmed that patients with HIV/AIDS used CAM because of their cultural orientation; CAM was seen as part of traditional Thai culture. This increasing turn to TCAM is associated with what Furnham and Forey [56] noted: that patients use services that overlap with mainstream health care, as well as choose practitioners that help them achieve their desired health outcomes.

Kelner and Wellman [23] found in their Canadian study that patients turned to alternative medicine because it matched their beliefs that all aspects of health and illness are holistically interconnected and allowed a sense of personal agency in making healthcare choices. McGregor and Peay [39], in an Australian study, found the same. They reported that patients used CAM because it encouraged autonomous decision-making on health care issues.

Social ties influence utilization of CAM as they are an important source of information about CAM methods and techniques. Recommendations from friends and family members can increase patients' beliefs in and utilization of CAM [57]. Arbisi and Panpanich's work [33] found that HIV/AIDS patients in Thailand used CAM both because they received information from friends living with HIV/AIDS and because they had prior experiences with

CAM themselves. Similarly, George et al. [57] found that not only did friends influence patients with chronic illness to consider CAM treatment, but family members, healthcare practitioners and media sources did as well. One study in Singapore [30] reported that patients with cancer gained most of their CAM information from their friends with cancer, although other sources included family members and relatives. CAM information was more rarely provided by health care practitioners, or through seminars or overseas travel. Goldner [29] suggests that word of mouth remains the most successful strategy in promoting the use of CAM.

The services of modern health care professionals can have various disadvantages, some of which have already been noted. Patients report short consultations, an unfriendly atmosphere and long waiting times. In addition, patients are often separated from family members during treatment, most often when advanced technology is being used, and this separation further reduces effective communication. If patients decide to receive modern health care treatment, they are expected to follow all procedures, but treatment can take whole days or even longer to complete [17, 58]. By way of contrast, folk healing techniques are useful for people who want to avoid institutional care, complex technology and the impersonal nature of modern medical treatment [59].

The language used during clinical consultations is another factor creating misunderstanding between doctors and patients. The language of modern doctors differs from that of lay people [42, 60-62]. Helman [63] notes that medical vocabulary includes many technical terms, and clarity is lacking because the language used in consultations is a mixture of general speech and technical terminology. The same terms can mean different things to physicians and to patients. Lay people may also confuse physicians when they use their own terminology to explain their illnesses and health beliefs. Reaching a shared understanding is central to whether or not a patient receives effective treatment.

Economic hardship also influences individual decisions about seeking health care. People on lower incomes may prefer treatment from folk healers because of the lower cost of these services. These individuals tend to ask for help from modern doctors only when they are suffering from a serious illness. People who do not have access to modern medical care, or cannot afford modern medical treatments, initially look to traditional healers for support [64].

## Professional and Legalized TCAM

Regulations to ensure the safety and efficacy of TCAM have been developed in many countries around the world [4, 5]. The purpose of regulation is twofold. First, it is needed to control the harmful possibilities of under-qualified practitioners and unsafe products, so that they do not cause damage to users [5]. Harmful consequences can arise when, for example, patients use medicine with no awareness of its adverse effects, possibly due to the inadequate knowledge of the practitioner who provided it [3, 65]. The second purpose in regulating the field is to increase the possibility of integrating TCAM into formal health care systems [4, 5].

In all industrialized societies regulations apply to the majority of healthcare professions [2, 3, 66, 67]. Practitioners are required to register and are held to specific ethical and legal standards of practice within the health care system. Medical practitioners are licensed to ensure the quality of their knowledge and skills, which allows patients to trust the services they provide [11, 68, 69]. Registration, based on educational qualifications and supervised practice, confers status in the health system [67] for all registered practitioners.

Even when the sort of regulations that apply to mainstream healthcare professions are not applied to CAM practitioners [11, 68, 70], these practitioners nevertheless can be found working to increase the safety and efficacy of their professions [70]. As Shia, Noller and Burford [71], McCabe [66], Kerridge and McPhee [68] and Pal [3] suggest, this trend is likely to be a response to the increasing number of people utilizing CAM and TCAM. Shia and associates [71] also point out that regulation is continuing to develop because the WHO has strongly recommended the evaluation of TM in national policies to ensure its safety and efficacy for users. Many TCAM therapies still lack evidence of their efficacy [65].

Patients play a key role in encouraging TCAM development, for their increasing use of the sector influences national policy-makers to organize and regulate TCAM. In addition to the increasing demand for TCAM, policies promote integration with modern medicine in order to offer people alternative methods of care [6, 29, 72]. This creates new health care opportunities and risks, and safety becomes of significant public importance. Research and evaluation of TCAM is increasing rapidly in the hope of showing the benefits of TCAM products and services [3, 6, 68]. Shein and Maehira [2] assert that providing diverse modalities of TCAM creates more benefits than harm, but that more evaluation is needed to verify TCAM's contribution as a health care resource.

Data from many countries show that, as CAM is increasingly available, there has been a corresponding increase in concern about safety and efficacy [50]. Nagel and colleagues (2004) conducted a three-year longitudinal study in Germany with a group of 305 participants with breast cancer. Three years after being diagnosed, the prevalence of complementary therapy use was at 36 per cent among participants. They further suggested, however, that patients using CAM alongside modern treatments did so because they did not have adequate knowledge about the possible adverse effects of CAM interactions with these treatments.

CAM practitioners do not have the complete trust of the public. Many people assume that they do not have enough scientific knowledge to contribute to health care practice [65]. Armishaw and Grant [8] suggest that CAM therapies might harm patients with acute illness if they lead to delay in seeking modern medical treatment. At the same time, however, they found that CAM therapy offers patients health benefits and had been shown to be safe and effective, whereas modern medicine was ineffective for some conditions.

## Traditional Practitioner of TCAM: Traditional Healers

The contribution of traditional healers as local health care providers [17, 73] is mostly made in rural areas of developing countries, because these areas are less likely to have adequate health care facilitates and resources [17, 24, 40]. Stock [74] notes that their role has appealed to patients since the nineteenth century. Ruff [75], however, contends that their traditional knowledge may no longer pass to younger generations, so that the task of integration with mainstream medicine may be short-lived.

## Great Diversity among Traditional Healers

Different cultures have different names for their traditional healers. For example, traditional midwives in North India and Bangladesh are called *dai* [76] while traditional birth attendants in rural Zimbabwe are labeled as *ngangas* [77]. The spiritual healers in Nepal are identified as *dya: māju* [78]. The shamanic healers among the Hmong community in Australia are commonly known as *txiv neeb* [79]. Traditional healers in the Northern Territory of Australia are *margidjbu* [80].

Characteristics of traditional healers vary throughout the world. Gessler and associates [40] found that, in Tanzania, the majority of traditional healers were elderly, only some were middle-aged (between 30 and 49 years old) and most were male. Their level of education ranged from no formal education to secondary school level. Similarly, in Thailand most practitioners were found to be male [58], most were elderly, 61 to 70 years old, while some others were between 41 to 50 years old. Few individuals who practised TM were younger than 40. The majority of these individuals had obtained some formal education, ranging from primary to secondary school. A few, however, had never received formal education.

Similar characteristics were reported for the Southern Region of Malawi [81], Uganda [82] and Plateau State Nigeria [73]. Most traditional healers were males. In the Southern Region of Malawi, the ages of these healers varied between 34 and 89 years old, and in Uganda, from 20 to 70 years old. In Plateau State Nigeria, the range was from 46 to 70 years old. Although most traditional healers in Uganda had no formal education, most traditional healers in the Southern Region of Malawi and Plateau State Nigeria had obtained some formal education. Oppong [73] also found different ages of entry to the profession. The youngest started training when he was eight years old, whereas the oldest entry was at 34.

There are also specialist areas of healing [24, 83, 84]. Nelms and Gorski [83] report diversity amongst the traditional healers of Africa, where diviners, midwives, herbalists and faith healers are included in the ranks. Similarly, in Southern Thailand, traditional healers are classified in therapeutic and non-therapeutic categories [24]. Therapeutic specialists deal with a broad range of health problems, and include among their number herbalists, masseurs, bone-setters, diviners, midwives and specialists in charms and chronic illness. There is less diversity of traditional healers in Tanzania [40], but even the generalist healers there tend to have one or two specialties [85].

The length of time that traditional healers have been practicing their crafts is difficult to estimate because healers may commence their learning long before they start practising their craft or before becoming independent healers. It is assumed that traditional healers in Tanzania begin their profession when they are mature enough, which is in their late 20s or 30s. The longest reported period of practice as a traditional healer was 50 years, the shortest three years [40]. Bhatia, Vir, Timmappaya and Chuttani [86] found traditional healers in several districts in India had been practising traditional healing for less than two years. Some had been committing for more than 10 years. A study conducted in the southern region of Malawi by Courtright [81] showed that traditional healers in this region have had various lengths of time practicing their crafts, ranging from one to 77 years. In Thailand, most traditional healers have been practicing for about six to 10 years [58].

Training as traditional healer is understood to be an individual's responsibility. Each healer increases his or her healing capabilities in different ways, depending on context and circumstance [24]. Golomb [24] suggests that traditional healers develop their specialties through trial and error, using different methods and various kinds of illness. Not only do they continually practise those methods, but they also read traditional healing texts. It is rare, however, for healers to share their medical knowledge with other traditional healers. Nevertheless, Golumb's findings are inconsistent with findings from another study, which shows that traditional healers develop and gain their skills from experimenting on their own bodies [87]. They monitor an injured part of their bodies, observing the healing process and its duration. This not only increases their knowledge, but also makes them more understanding of clients' suffering when they are ill. Additionally, by doing so, traditional healers gain confidence in their role, which supports them in becoming genuine traditional healers.

Traditional healers tend not to promote themselves and must rely on other ways of becoming known. Their reputations depend upon their healing capabilities, and their image is enhanced if they are able to achieve a high proportion of successful outcomes [24]. The Bureau of Indigenous Thai Medicine [88] supports the idea that traditional healers should not advertise their healing capabilities. Patients whose treatment is effective usually announce this to other people; word of mouth is the normal process that promotes the reputations of traditional healers. Ovuga and colleagues [82] similarly found, in a study in Uganda, that patients learned of the reputations of traditional healers from district hospitals and other traditional healers. Again, word of mouth was the most effective way of promoting traditional healers to the public.

## Pathways to the Traditional Healing Professions

Traditional practitioners are not included in most formal health care systems and their medical knowledge is usually gained outside formal educational systems. Their approach to learning is rooted in tradition and culture [24, 83, 89]. Pathways to traditional healing professions can be varied, and individual healers may combine several pathways on the way to becoming a traditional healer.

Having traditional healers within the family may influence individuals to become traditional healers themselves [24, 82, 84, 90]. The environment familiarizes family members with the profession. They can observe, help, contribute to treatments and ask questions regarding traditional healing practice, so that the learning process becomes part of their family life. The more they attend to cases, the more they gain knowledge, experience and confidence in helping people [90].

In some countries, families select one of their children to become a traditional healer. Children in Nigeria, for example, are trained in traditional healing roles as teenagers. This comprehensive training includes knowledge of the nature of human beings and the use curative plants in clinical practice [91]. Similarly, in Plateau State Nigeria [73], family expectation is a major factor leading a person to become a traditional healer. Traditional healers who enter the profession in this way also encourage the next generation to become traditional healers.

Many enter the profession because of the prompting of ancestral spirits [24, 79, 83]. Golomb [24], in southern Thailand, and Nelms and Gorski [83], in Africa, found that many people became traditional healers because they had been chosen by spirits of practitioner ancestors, who appeared in their dreams, to take on the role. It was also believed that spirits of ancestors keep an eye on these healers' own children to distinguish those who were qualified to be the next generation of healers. Gessler and colleagues [40] reported that, if the spirits' intention was ignored, they could punish them and their family members. Golomb [24] and Nelms and Gorski [83] note that this pathway again demonstrates that traditional professions, knowledge and its practices are preserved within the family and passed down from one generation to the next. This is also the cultural norm among Hmong healers [79], who participate in traditional healing through the influence of shaman spirits.

Individuals who are interested in the traditional healing system and admire traditional healers may be encouraged to take on the role. These people may not have traditional healers within their families, but they seek out healers and learn to practise alongside them [24, 73, 92]. This pathway is also found in Plateau State Nigeria [73] and in Uganda [82], where individuals became healers because they had benefited from treatments provided by traditional healers. Once recovered, these individuals were trained by the traditional healers who had helped them. This is also common among the Hmong [79]. Golomb [24] found others who chose to practise because they wanted to help fellow members and friends. Often, their training was initiated when modern medicine had been unable to provide effective treatment for a family member.

For some, becoming a traditional healer combines more than one of the pathways outlined above: that is, family encouragement, confirmation by ancestor spirits, their own experience of illness, or an interest in healing. Interestingly, one participant from Gessler et al.'s study [40] sought additional knowledge from a university and was able to combine modern and traditional knowledge in his practice.

## Traditional Practices and Service Organization

Traditional healers use indigenous medical knowledge, which is passed down from previous generations and is a local resource for illness management. This knowledge is normally integrated with other knowledge about sacred rites and magic power. Many types of treatment may be needed to control the diverse causes of illness, which include evil spirits, supernatural beings and unseen spirits [24, 93-97]. The literature shows that a majority of healers practice a range of skills, applying these creatively to a variety of illnesses. Only a few are experts who limit their activity to the practice of one particular craft. Overall, a community's healers are likely to be drawn from several categories, with curative, ceremonial and spiritual healers all represented [26, 98].

Golomb [99] reports that traditional healers in southern Thailand earn their reputation from their expertise in a variety of healing modalities, including herbal medicine, psychotherapy and the supernatural. With these, they treat a range of conditions, such as bone fractures, skin diseases, snakebites, infertility and sexual impotence. Traditional healers need to be able to deal with the multiple health problems for which they are consulted, drawing upon a wide knowledge base and demonstrating competence in a number of healing skills. Thus, some healers treat conditions such as stomach aches, headaches, measles, eye disorders and cancer. Others specialize in areas such as psychological disorders and infertility. A similar diversity of healing skills is found in Uganda [82], where most traditional healers can treat people with a variety of illnesses, both physical and mental.

Traditional healers also use a diversity of methods to make a diagnosis, reflecting the fact that an holistic approach requires diagnosis across a number of dimensions of need [83, 99].

Ovuga and associates [82], for example, found that traditional healers in Uganda used history-taking, physical examination, observation and spiritual practices to diagnose mental illness. Observation of abnormal signs was the most widely practised diagnostic method in providing primary treatment for mental disorders. The same skills are used by traditional healers in the southern region of Malawi [81]. Their screening focused on asking patients about the history of their illness, and divination was integrated with this by some traditional healers. Physical examination was used less frequently and only when necessary. Mathole and associates [77] reported that traditional birth attendants in Zimbabwe weighed pregnant women, prescribed herbs, and provided them with protection using spiritual powers. Weighing was an easy way for healers to check that the pregnancy was progressing normally. Spiritual practice supported the mental needs of the pregnant women. Herbs helped to protect them and encourage normal dilatation at full term.

Thus, traditional healers integrate invisible powers with other healing tools to treat the various causes of illness [24, 100-102]. Although each specialist develops his or her preferred combinations, the basic methods are similar, including incantations, the use of holy water and administration of herbs [24, 84, 103]. Some specialists use astrological and numerological charts to select an auspicious time at which to make an accurate diagnosis or provide effective treatment. The magical and spiritual powers invoked lead healers to the appropriate treatment [24]. Similar combinations of healing processes can be found in Plateau State Nigeria, where traditional healers may use both modern medicine and traditional methods for diagnosis and treatment, and a few employ spiritual methods in their practice [73].

The ways in which services are provided vary from place to place. Traditional healers in Tanzania may work part-time or full-time, with part-time workers combining their healing role with their main occupation. This working pattern is normal in Tanzanian society. The majority of younger male healers, however, work full-time. These traditional healers provide both outpatient and inpatient treatment services, with inpatients given access to a place to stay while they are being treated. In some areas, a straw hut is made available; in others a serviced location, similar in style to a hospital, provides all the necessary amenities for living during the patient's stay [40]. Similarly, in the Plateau State Nigeria [73], healers provide hospital-like accommodation. Healers can thus be available to patients 24 hours a day. Some healers provide accommodation only for patients who have travelled a long distance and are not able to return home immediately. In rural Hausaland, Nigeria, traditional healers provide help both at their own home and in their patients' homes [74].

A study from India showed that more than half of traditional healers saw about 50 patients per week [86]. Around 32 per cent of healers in this study had patient loads of up to 150 cases per week, while a small percentage of traditional healers saw more than 150 patients in one week. This is in line with the findings from a study in Tanzania [40], which showed that traditional healers seemed to have quite high patient loads. It was reported that traditional healers who provided services for outpatients had patient loads of up to 200 per week. Oppong [73] found that traditional healers in Plateau State Nigeria saw from 25 to 60 patients daily, with these patients coming from all parts of Nigeria and even neighbouring countries. On the other hand, of course, some traditional healers report seeing just a few patients each week.

Courtright [81] found a much smaller number of patients seeking treatment from traditional healers in a southern region of Malawi. The number varied with the season and the gender of the traditional healer. Male healers treated on average six people a day when it was rainy, while female healers treated five. During the dry season, male healers received four people per day, but female healers only had three. It was also found that patient-load related to a healer's education; literate healers had four times greater patient loads than illiterate healers.

Local healers have their own customary ways of recording patient information. Gessler and colleagues [40] found that traditional healers in Tanzania recorded details that included individual demographic data, diagnosis and medication. This practice is also reported among traditional healers in Plateau State Nigeria [73]. Other traditional healers keep basic data about patients, including names, illnesses and payment information.

## Traditional Healers and their Co-operation with the Health Care system

TM plays an important global role as a complement to modern medicine. Co-operation between traditional and modern healers is accepted as a desirable health care development worldwide, although many issues arise when considering the integration of the two systems [104]. In general, however, such integration should increase benefits to patients because each type of provider has different strengths. Modern doctors cannot assist in all aspects of illness, while traditional healers have more understanding of patients' explanatory models and culture and can better support people in their daily lives. Patients thus do not have to endure chronic suffering and the poor quality of life that this causes [105]. Farge [106] agrees that the co-operation between the modern and traditional models has positive benefits for patients, including improved physical health and shorter healing times. This co-operation not only benefits individuals, but also provides more and better choices to enhance the well-being of communities.

Most of the literature available on the co-operation between traditional healers and modern health care staff relates to African countries. But interest in co-operation is increasing elsewhere. Despite the barriers, there is broad agreement on ways of developing co-operation between these two sectors.

### The Possibility of Co-operation

In South Africa, Freeman and Motsei [107] put forward three options for linking the two models of health care: incorporation, collaboration and total integration. Under the first option, incorporation, traditional healers would become part of the primary health care system. Their functional role would be similar to that of village health workers, and they would be involved in preventing illness and promoting health. They could refer specific cases to specialists if necessary. In the second option, both sectors would collaborate with each other through a mutual referral system to achieve efficient and effective treatment. Under this option, they would have to make agreements as to which illnesses should be treated by which sector. The third, total integration, option combines the healing models. Traditional healers would work as government employees alongside mainstream healthcare practitioners. They point out that patients in their study seemed to prefer this last option because it makes available different explanatory models for illnesses within the one healthcare system. It would increase people's health care choices, and people would have adequate access to care, provided of course that traditional healers continue to practise in their traditional localities and traditional ways. Kale [108] and Van der Geest [109] recommend the second option of collaboration within the primary health care system.

In some societies, selected specialist folk healers are part of the formal healthcare system. Ovuga and colleagues [82] found that Traditional Birth Attendants and bonesetters worked with modern healthcare staff because their healing capabilities were accepted by modern doctors. Courtright [81] reported that traditional healers in the southern region of Malawi created their own collaboration with modern doctors to cure patients with eye disorders because these patients had limited access to modern medical care. The government trained traditional healers to provide basic help for such patients. After receiving care from the healers, the patients were then referred to modern doctors for specific treatment. This collaboration not only benefited the people living in rural areas, but also increased the status of the traditional healers in their communities. Similarly, in Thailand, the Bureau of Indigenous Thai Medicine [110] gave a grant to local provinces to investigate the capabilities of traditional bonesetters. This project encouraged the use of local wisdom as a health care resource, patients with bone fractures had more choices for care, and the health care system benefited by reducing costs. Most importantly, because their practices proved effective, it brought about greater collaboration with modern health staff, especially in the sharing knowledge to provide patients with effective care. A sustainable outcome was that a referral system for bonesetting was developed and implemented.

Co-operation between health care sectors has the potential to increase people's access to care [46]. Nelms and Gorski [83], however, comment that this potential will be difficult to actualize given the many barriers to collaboration, let alone integration. Mistrust of traditional healers' competence and effectiveness on the part of the modern medical community is the largest barrier to establishing collaboration. A remedy for this appears to lie in actual experiences of collaboration. In Africa, traditional healers have contributed to health care delivery for illnesses such as HIV/AIDS and have become accepted as important health care resources connecting local people to formal health care providers. Kale [108] points out that traditional healers face exclusion from the healthcare system in many African nations, including Tanzania [40], because they have no formal registration and there is thus no verification of the standards of treatment they provide. Clearly, further investigation is needed to develop effective strategies for collaboration with the formal health care sector.

In South Africa, Kale [108] suggests that traditional healers should collaborate with modern health care providers because already they play an important role as health care providers for people living in rural areas. These traditional healers could be integrated into the primary level of the nation's formal health care system as a first step, and perhaps eventually into higher levels. (That is, collaboration could lead to integration.) However, there is still a gap between the two sectors, and attempts at integration may irrevocably alter the traditional healers' world, professions and status. It remains unclear if integration is a viable option. Similarly, in Zambia, Baskind and Birbeck [100] contend that even if the national health care sector tries to promote the role of traditional healers, it would face difficulties because the traditional healers have different beliefs and practices, in part because they enter their professions through such different pathways.

When intersectional referrals occur, it is normally traditional healers referring their patients to modern doctors, rather than modern doctors referring patients to traditional healers. Folk healers refer patients if they have failed to cure them, for their principal desire is that the patients should obtain effective treatment. Makundi and associates [111] reported that traditional healers in Tanzania refer patients with severe malaria to other traditional healers or to formal health care centers. In another Tanzanian study [40], it was found that traditional healers refer patients whom they had failed to treat successfully, or whom they felt would be better treated by modern doctors from the start. A small number of traditional healers referred patients to hospitals for diagnosis only. Gessler and colleagues also found that modern health practitioners were critical of traditional healers and their treatments when patients came to the hospital in bad condition having received prior treatment from traditional healers. On the other hand, in the study in Plateau State Nigeria [73], it showed that the hospital providers referred patients with bone fractures to traditional bonesetters after fractures had been confirmed by imaging.

Referral systems can take various forms in Zambia and [82] in Uganda, it was confirmed that traditional healers referred their patients to other traditional healers or to modern doctors when their treatments have failed [82, 100]. A similar practice was also found in Plateau State Nigeria [73]. There, some traditional healers referred patients to a hospital or to other local healers if the conditions were beyond their capability to heal. Some never referred to their traditional healer colleagues, but only to hospitals. In India [86], 90 per cent of traditional healers had referred their patients to other healers or hospitals in the past, but the healers exhibited different referral patterns. Around 37 per cent of traditional healers sent their patients to private practitioners in urban areas and about six per cent directed clients to private practitioners in rural areas. About 12 per cent of traditional healers referred their patients to a primary health centre or other medical centre in a rural area. About one-quarter of traditional healers (26 per cent) referred their patients to hospitals in an urban district. A smaller percentage (22 per cent) showed no consistent pattern of referrals. Some traditional healers referred clients for laboratory tests. The traditional healers who referred patients to the modern health care sector usually had personal contact of some kind with those health facilities.

## What Supports Co-operation?

The literature indicates that links between modern and traditional healers are limited. They are strongest in African countries, though most cooperation there seems to stem from the government sector, which is managed and controlled by modern health practitioners, so that cooperation tends to be on the latters' terms. However, co-operation could contribute to areas such as education, research and policy, and would benefit both traditional healers and modern health practitioners.

The educational system and training programs are basic means for giving practitioners an understanding of principles outside their own professions [66, 109, 112]. Introducing traditional knowledge into medical education could provide modern medical students with knowledge of TM. These practitioners would then have an understanding of both systems. For all health practitioners, this strategy could promote better communication and more positive views of each other, hopefully leading to greater co-operation. Practitioners should have increased levels of understanding of each others' differing principles [112, 113], thus reducing the mistrust that modern health staff have of traditional healers [109, 111].

If TM is to be integrated into the modern medical system, evaluation of its healing practices is required [2]. Evidence of effectiveness would make it easier for the public and modern health care providers alike to accept TM. Research is thus needed to demonstrate whether or not traditional treatments are safe and effective [112, 113]. Given such evidence, the strengths of traditional healing could be incorporated into health care delivery to address some of the weaknesses of modern medicine [71, 112]. Traditional healers would also be informed by the evidence as to the areas in which their practice is effective and of conditions for which immediate referral to mainstream practitioners is required.

Training and registering traditional healers would be a way of increasing their status in the health care system [108, 109]. Meissner [69], however, raises concerns that such training would disrupt traditional pathways into the healing professions. The ideal would be for traditional healers to preserve their indigenous knowledge, not convert it into western knowledge; but both traditional knowledge and healers' professional identities could be put at risk by imposing a western-style education and qualification system.

Although resistance to integration arises from traditional healers themselves, diminishing the possibility for co-operation with modern doctors, healers might still contribute towards the process if they can do so on their own terms, rather than under the direction of outsiders [108]. Kale suggests, in the context of South Africa, that the authority of traditional healers should be encouraged by supporting them in self-regulation and the creation of a registration system based on their own principles. These would be important factors in creating links between the two health systems. Whether or not other nations consider these possibilities, it is clear that the world of the traditional healers should remain reasonably intact, and efforts to incorporate their healing strategies simply as techniques in the conventional medical system should be challenged.

Policy can help direct cooperation between traditional healers and modern health services; but this policy should be consistent [66]. Policy can actively contribute to many areas, including education, training, regulation and the granting of licenses [112]. Policy can play an important role in promoting co-operation between the health sectors provided the focus of policymakers is clearly upon delivering benefits at the population level, not on preserving sectional interests. The interests of both healthcare sectors will need to be given equal attention to reduce confusion during policy formation and implementation. Such an effort could effectively promote the contribution of TM to the mainstream medical sector [66, 112].

## Conclusion

This chapter reviews the literature on healing systems complementary to modern health care, including areas such as the increase of public interest in TCAM, the importance of legalizing TCAM practitioners, the strengths of traditional healers which lead patients to continue seeking their help, patients' perceptions of and experiences with traditional healers, and the co-operation of these healers with the formal health care sector.

TCAM therapies are widely used in developing nations and are co-opted into the CAM systems of industrialized nations. Patients give many reasons for preferring TCAM or CAM over modern medicine, including the most frequently mentioned reason that modern medicine has failed to provide an effective cure, for many chronic conditions in particular. The need to travel long distances to access care, the lack of a holistic approach to care, and the frequent misunderstanding of patients' explanations of their illnesses are other disadvantages of modern health care which cause people to turn to alternative treatments. It is clear that people everywhere are concerned about the broader dimensions of health care, and want to participate more in decisions about their health care rather than deferring them to modern health practitioners. They realize that scientific medicine focuses on high technology and complex treatments, which may not be able to provide them with holistic health care and well-being. People thus seek care from traditional healers, even though modern health care facilities are obviously more advanced in diagnostic and curative techniques.

Traditional healers in developing nations are experiencing increased demand. They are more accessible and affordable, especially for people in rural areas. Importantly, their roles are embedded within local people's belief systems and are integrated into local cultures. The lack of formal qualification of traditional healers makes most modern health care practitioners hesitate to collaborate with them because they do not trust their knowledge and skills, but their patients do not have the same hesitation. National health policies are beginning to recognize the role of traditional healers, developing ways to license them and attempting to integrate their practice into mainstream health care.

Although many countries seem to have similar traditional healing principles, they each build their own systems of traditional health care. Some traditional practices are recognized as coming from specific regions and geographies, and it is difficult to generalize these practices to other regions. TM is used and trusted at the local community level, and can overall provide the population with accessible and affordable health care [4, 15]. Many countries in Southeast Asia have well-formulated national policies regarding TCAM, arising from their commitment to 'Health for All'. Traditional practitioners are a major contributor to this particular mission, and specific organizations and national research councils have thus established policies that promote TM [9].

# References


[1] Zapata J, Shippee-Rice R. The use of folk healing and healers by six Latinos living in New England: A preliminary study. *Journal of Transcultural Nursing*1999;10(2):136-42.

[2] Shein K, Maehira Y. Introduction. In: Bodeker G, Ong CK, Grundy C, Burford G, Shein K, editors. *WHO global atlas of traditional, complementary and alternative medicine.* Kobe: World Health Organization Centre for Health Development; 2005. p. xi-xiv.

[3] Pal SK. Complementary and alternative medicine: An overview. *Current Science* 2002;82(5):518-24.

[4] Kayne SB. Introduction to traditional medicine. In: Kayne SB, editor. *Traditional medicine: A global perspective.* London: Pharmaceutical Press; 2010. p. 1-24.

[5] World Health Organization. *Legal status of traditional medicine and complementary/* alternative medicine: A worldwide review. 2001.

[6] Bodeker G, Kronenberg F, Burford G. Policy and public health perspectives on traditional, complementary and alternative medicine: An overview. In: Bodeker G, Burford G, editors. *Traditional, complementary and alternative medicine: Policy and public health perspectives.* London: Imperial College Press; 2007. p. 9-40.

[7] Lorenc A, Ilan-Clarke Y, Robinson N, Blair M. *How parents choose to use CAM: A systematic review of theoretical models.* BMC Complementary and Alternative Medicine [serial on the Internet]. 2009 [cited 2009 December 16]; 9(9): Available from: http://www.ncbi. nlm.nih.gov/pmc/articles/PMC2680396/pdf/1472-6882-9-9.pdf.

[8] Armishaw J, Grant CC. Use of complementary treatment by those hospitalised with acute illness. *Archives of Disease in* Childhood 1999;81(2):133-7.

[9] Gaitonde BB, Kurup PNV. Regional overview: South-East Asia Region. In: Bodeker G, Ong CK, Grundy C, Burford G, Shein K, editors. *WHO global atlas of traditional, complementary and alternative medicine.* Kobe: World Health Organization Centre for Health Development; 2005. p. 75-82.

[10] Hasan SS, Ahmed SI, Bukhari NI, Loon WCW. Use of complementary and alternative medicine among patients with chronic diseases at outpatient clinics. *Complementary Therapies in Clinical Practice* 2009;15:152-7.

[11] Subcharoen P, Chuthaputti A. Kingdom of Thailand. In: Bodeker G, Ong CK, Grundy C, Burford G, Shein K, editors. *WHO global atlas of traditional, complementary and alternative medicine.* Kobe: World Health Organization Centre for Health Development; 2005. p. 103-6.

[12] Obeyesekere G. Illness, culture, and meaning: Some comments on the nature of traditional medicine. In: Kleinman A, Kunstadter P, Alexander RE, Gate JL, editors. *Culture and healing in Asian societies: Anthropological, psychiatric and public health studies.* Cambridge: Schenkman Publishing Company; 1978. p. 253-63.

[13] Sirois FM, Gick ML. An investigation of the health beliefs and motivations of complementary medicine clients. *Social Science & Medicine* 2002;55:1025-37.

[14] Jonas W. The social dynamics of medical pleuralism, foreword. In: Kelner M, Wellman B, editors. *Complementary and alternative medicine: Challenge and change.* Amsterdam: Harwood Academic; 2000. p. xi-xv.

[15] Fennell D, Liberato ASQ, Zsembik B. Definitions and patterns of CAM use by the lay public. *Complementary Therapies in Medicine* 2009;17(2):71-7.

[16] Roe S. Significance of complementary and alternative medicine in healthcare. In: Herring MA, Roberts MM, editors. *Blackwell complementary and alternative medicine: Fast facts for medical practice Malden:* Blackwell Publishing; 2002. p. 1-8.

[17] Sermsri S. Utilization of traditional and modern health care services in Thailand. In: Quah SR, editor. *The triumph of practicality: Tradition and modernity in health care utilization in selected Asian countries.* Singapore: Institute of Southeast Asian Studies; 1989. p. 160-79.

[18] Mulholland J. Thai traditional medicine: Ancient thought and practice in a Thai context. *Journal of the Siam Society* 1979;67:80-115.

[19] Coulter ID, Willis EM. The rise and rise of complementary and alternative medicine: A sociological perspective. *The Medical Journal of Australia* 2004;180(11):587-9.

[20] Spencer JW. *Essential issues in complementary/ alternative medicine.* In: Spencer JW, Jacobs JJ, editors. Complementary/ alternative medicine: An evidence-based approach St. Louis: Mosby; 1999. p. 3-36.

[21] Mulholland J. *Medicine, magic and evil spirits: Study of a text on Thai traditional paediatrics.* Canberra: Asian Studies Faculty, Australian National University; 1987.

[22] World Health Organization. *WHO traditional medicine strategy 2002-2005.* 2002 [cited 2009 August 15]; Available from: http://whqlibdoc.who.int/hq/2002/ WHO_EDM_ TRM_2002.1.pdf.

[23] Kelner M, Wellman B. Health care and consumer choice: Medical and alternative therapies. *Social Science & Medicine* 1997;45(2):203-12.

[24] Golomb L. An anthropology of curing in multiethnic Thailand. Urbana: University of Illinois Press; 1985.

[25] Naemiratch B. *Who is in control: The diabetic or diabetes? Lived experience of adults living with diabetes in Bangkok.* Queensland, Australia: Unpublished doctoral dissertation, University of Queensland; 2004.

[26] Sugsamran P. *The situation study of traditional health care and healing among the prospective of folk healers in the rural area of Ampur Muang,* Khon Kaen Province. Khon Kaen, Thailand: Unpublished master's thesis, Khon Kaen University; 2006.

[27] Lazar JS, O'Connor BB. Talking with patients about their use of alternative therapies. *Complementary and Alternative Therapies in Primary Care* 1997;24(4):699-714.

[28] Spencer JW. Essential issues in complementary and alternative medicine. In: Spencer JW, Jacobs JJ, editors. *Complementary and alternative medicine: An evidence-based approach.* 2nd ed. St. Louis: Mosby; 2003. p. 2-39.

[29] Goldner M. Consumption as activism: An examination of CAM as part of the consumer movement in health. In: Tovey P, Easthope G, Adams J, editors. *The mainstreaming of complementary and alternative medicine: Studies in social context.* London: Routledge; 2004. p. 11-24.

[30] Shih V, Chiang JYL, Chan A. Complementary and alternative medicine (CAM) usage in Singaporean adult cancer patients. *Annals of Oncology* 2009;20(4):752-7.

[31] Richardson MA, Sanders T, Palmer JL, Greisinger A, Singletary SE. Complementary/ alternative medicine use in a comprehensive cancer center and the implications for oncology. *Journal of Clinical Oncology* 2000;18(13):2505-14.

[32] Zhang J, Verhoef MJ. Illness management strategies among Chinese immigrants living with arthritis. *Social Science & Medicine* 2002;55(10):1795-802.

[33] Arbisi A, Panpanich R. Acupuncture use among people living with HIV/AIDS in Northern Thailand: Motives, barriers, and attitudes. Journal of The Medical Association of Thailand 2008;91 (4):533-41.

[34] Wiwanitkit V. The use of CAM by HIV-positive patients in Thailand. *Complementary Therapies in Medicine* 2003;11:39-41.

[35] Hekkert KD, Cihangir S, Kleefstra SM, Berg Bvd, Kool RB. Patient satisfaction revisited: A multilevel approach. *Social Science & Medicine* 2009;69:68-75.

[36] Astin JA. Why patients use alternative medicine: Results of a national study. *Journal of the American Medical Association* 1998; 279(19):1548-53.

[37] Astin JA. The characteristics of CAM users: A complex picture. In: Kelner M, Wellman B, editors. *Complementary and alternative medicine: Challenge and change.* Amsterdam: Harwood Academic; 2000. p. 101-14.

[38] Vincent C, Furnham A. Why do patients turn to complementary medicine?: An empirical study. *British Journal of Clinical Psychology* 1996;35:37-48.

[39] McGregor KJ, Peay ER. The choice of alternative therapy for health care: Testing some propositions. *Social Science & Medicine* 1996;43(9):1317-27.

[40] Gessler MC, Msuya DE, Nkunya MHH, Schär A, M H, Tanner M. Traditional healers in Tanzania: Sociocultural profile and three short portraits. *Journal of Ethnopharmacology* 1995;48:145-60.

[41] Suarez M, Raffaelli M, O'Leary A. Use of folk healing practice by HIV-infected Hispanics living in the United States. AIDS Care1996;8(6):683-90.

[42] Klessig J. Cross-cultural medicine a decade later: The effect of values and culture on life-support decisions. *The Western Journal of Medicine* 1992;157(3):316-22.

[43] Kleinman A, Eisenberg L, Good B. Culture, illness, and care: Clinical lessons from anthropologic and cross-cultural research. *Annals of Internal Medicine* 1978;88(2):251-8.

[44] Adler SR. Complementary and alternative medicine use among women with breast cancer. *Medical Anthropology Quarterly* 1999;13(2):214-22.

[45] Furnham A, Vincent C. Reasons for using CAM. In: Kelner M, Wellman B, editors. *Complementary and alternative medicine: Challenge and change.* Amsterdam: Harwood Academic; 2000. p. 61-78.

[46] Strozier AL. Introduction. In: Strozíer AL, Carpenter J, editors. *Introductíon to alternatíve and complementary therapíes*. Binghamton: Haworth; 2008. p. 1-7.

[47] Chang Hy, Wallis M, Tiralongo E. Use of complementary and alternative medicine among people living with diabetes: Literature review. *Journal of Advanced Nursing* 2007;58(4):307 - 19.

[48] Swartzman LC, Harshman RA, Burkell J, Lundy ME. What accounts for the appeal of complementary/ alternative medicine, and what makes complementary/ alternative medicine "Alternative"? *Medical Decision Making* 2002;22:431-50.

[49] Fleming S, Rabago DP, Mundt MP, Fleming MF. CAM therapies among primary care patients using opioid therapy for chronic pain. *BMC Complementary and Alternative Medicine* [serial on the Internet]. 2007; 7(15): Available from: http://www.ncbi.nlm.nih.gov/pmc/articles/PMC1885447/pdf/1472-6882-7-15.pdf.

[50] Moore ML. Complementary and alternative therapies. *The Journal of Perinatal Education* 2002;11(1):39-42.

[51] Sugimoto N, Ichikawa M, Siriliang B, Nakahara S, Jimba M, Wakai S. Herbal medicine use and quality of life among people living with HIV/AIDS in northeastern Thailand. *AIDS Care* 2005;17(2):252-62.

[52] Applewhite SL. Curanderismo: Demystifying the health beliefs and practices of elderly Mexican Americans. *Health & Social Work* 1995;20(4):247-53.

[53] Snyder M, Lindquist R. An overview of complementary/ alternative therapies. In: Snyder M, Lindquist R, editors. *Complementary/ alternative therapies in nursing.* 5th ed. New York: Springer Publishing Company; 2006. p. 3-13.

[54] Pawluch D, Cain R, Gillett J. Ideology and *alternative therapy use among people living with HIV/AIDS. Health and Canadian Society* 1994;2(1):63-84.

[55] Niska K, Snyder M. Cultural diversity and complementary therapies. In: Snyder M, Lindquist R, editors. *Complementary/ alternative therapies in nursing.* 5th ed. New York: Springer Publishing Company; 2006. p. 15-23.

[56] Furnham A, Forey J. The attitudes, behaviors and beliefs of patients of conventional vs. complementary (alternative) medicine. *Journal of Clinical Psychology* 1994;50(3):458-69.
[57] George J, Ioannides-Demos LL, Santamaria NM, Kong DCM, Stewart K. Use of complementary and alternative medicines by patients with chronic obstructive pulmonary disease. *The Medical Journal of Australia* 2004;181(5):248-51.
[58] Sawatsing C. *Provision and utilization of traditional health services in rural Thailand.* Bangkok, Thailand: Unpublished master's thesis, Mahidol University; 2003.
[59] Kusinitz M. *Folk medicine.* New York: Chelsea House; 1992.
[60] Spector RE. *Cultural diversity in health and illness.* 7th ed. Upper Saddle River: Pearson Prentice Hall; 2009.
[61] Torsch VL, Ma GX. Cross-cultural comparison of health perceptions, concerns, and coping strategies among Asian and Pacific Islander American Elders. *Qualitative Health Research* 2000;10(4):471-89.
[62] Lewis G. *Knowledge of illness in a Sepik society: A study of the Gnau,* New Guinea. London: Athlone Press; 1975.
[63] Helman CG. *Culture, health and illness.* 5th ed. London: Hodder Arnold; 2007.
[64] Bodeker G, Kronenberg F. A public health agenda for traditional, complementary, and alternative medicine. *American Journal of Public Health* 2002;92(10):1582-91.
[65] Ernst E, Cohen MH, Stone J. Ethical problems arising in evidence based complementary and alternative medicine. *Journal of Medical Ethics* 2004;30:156-9.
[66] McCabe P. Complementary and alternative medicine in Australia: A contemporary overview. *Complementary Therapies in Clinical Practice* 2005;11(1):28-31.
[67] Clarke B, Doel A, Segrott J. No alternative? The regulation and professionalization of complementary and alternative medicine in the United Kingdom. *Health & Place* 2004;10:329-38.
[68] Kerridge IH, McPhee JR. Ethical and legal issues at the interface of complementary and conventional medicine. The Medical Journal of Australia2004;181(3):164-6.
[69] Meissner O. The traditional healer as part of the primary health care team? *South African Medical Journal* 2004;94(11):901-2.
[70] Parkman CA. Regulatory issues in CAM. *The Case Manager* 2004 2004/12//;15(6):26-9.
[71] Shia G, Noller B, Burford G. Safety: Issues and policy. In: Bodeker G, Burford G, editors. *Traditional, complementary and alternative medicine: Policy and public health perspectives* London: Imperial College Press; 2007. p. 83-98.
[72] Jacobs JJ, Pham PTK, Spencer JW. Complementary and alternative medicine in the twenty-first century: Future trends and key focuses. In: Spencer JW, Jacobs JJ, editors. *Complementary and alternative medicine: An evidence-based approach* 2nd ed. St. Louis: Mosby; 2003. p. 543-64.
[73] Oppong ACK. Healers in transition. *Social Science & Medicine* 1989;28(6):605-12.
[74] Stock R. Traditional healers in rural Hausaland. *GeoJournal* 1981;5(4):363-8.
[75] Ruff AM. Medicine -- A boost for old remedies: Once marginalized, traditional Thai medicine is officially back in favour; but critics fear only large companies with financial clout will prevail. *Far Eastern Economic Review* 2000;163(52):100-1.

[76] Samuel G. Introduction: The daughters of Hāritī today. In: Rozario S, Samuel G, editors. *The daughters of Hāritī: Childbirth and female healers in South and Southeast Asia*. London: Routledge; 2002. p. 1-33.

[77] Mathole T, Lindmark G, Ahlberg BM. Competing knowledge claims in the provision of antenatal care: A qualitative study of traditional birth attendants in rural Zimbabwe. *Health for Women International* 2005;26(10):937-56.

[78] Iltis L. Knowing all the gods: Grandmothers, god families and women healers in Nepal. In: Rozario S, Samuel G, editors. *The daughters of Hāritī: Childbirth and female healers in South and Southeast Asia.* London: Routledge; 2002. p. 70-89.

[79] Liamputtong Rice P. *Hmong women and reproduction.* Westport: Bergin & Garvey; 2000.

[80] Soong FS. Role of the *Margidjbu* (traditional healer) in western Arnhem Land. *The Medical Journal of Australia* 1983;1(10):474-7.

[81] Courtright P. Eye care knowledge and practices among Malawian traditional healers and the development of collaborative blindness prevention programmes. *Social Science & Medicine* 1995;41(11):1569-75.

[82] Ovuga E, Boardman J, Oluka EGAO. Traditional healers and mental illness in Uganda. *Psychiatric Bulletin* 1999;23:276-9.

[83] Nelms LW, Gorski J. The role of the African traditional healer in women's health. *Journal of Transcultural Nursing* 2006;17(2):184-9.

[84] Yoddumnern B. *The role of Thai traditional doctors.* Bangkok: Mahidol University; 1974.

[85] Tsey K. Traditional medicine in contemporary Ghana: A public policy analysis. *Social Science & Medicine* 1997;45(7):1065-74.

[86] Bhatia JC, Vir D, Timmappaya A, Chuttani CS. Traditional healers and modern medicine. *Social Science & Medicine* 1975;9(1):15-21.

[87] Kalweit H. Shamans, *healers, and medicine men*. Boston: Shambhala; 1992.

[88] Bureau of Indigenous Thai Medicine. *Thai indigenous medicine: The Thai intellectual property.* Bangkok: Thai Royal; 2003.

[89] White M. Native American healer bridges two worlds. 2003 [cited 2007 March 27]; Available from: http://www.tribalconnections.org/ health_news/features/oct2003html.

[90] Hanvattanakul C. *Using folk wisdom for promoting health during pregnancy: A case study of southern Thai Muslim Women*. Had Yai, Thailand: Unpublished master's thesis, Prince of Songkhla University; 2005.

[91] Adekson MO. *The Yorùbá traditional healers of Nigeria.* New York: Routledge; 2003.

[92] Bureau of Indigenous Thai Medicine. *Case study Thai traditional healer's wisdom (Mor Bunkong Wongsaisin):* The healing for patient with paraquat poisoning. 2003.

[93] Chavunduka GL. Zinatha: The organisation of traditional medicine in Zimbabwe. In: Last M, Chavunduka GL, editors. *The professionalisation of African medicine.* Manchester: Manchester University Press; 1986. p. 29-49.

[94] Easthope G. *Healers and alternative medicine: A sociological examination.* Aldershot: Gower Publication Company; 1986.

[95] Finkler K. Sacred healing and biomedicine compared. *Medical Anthropology* Quarterly 1994;8(2):178-97.

[96] Lopez RA. Use of alternative folk medicine by Mexican American women. *Journal of Immigrant Health* 2005;7(1):23-31.

[97] Staugard F. Traditional health care in Botswana. In: Last M, Chavunduka GL, editors. *The professionalisation of African medicine.* Manchester: Manchester University Press; 1986. p. 51-86.

[98] Watts S. *Disease and medicine in world history*. New York: Routledge; 2003.

[99] Golomb L. The interplay of traditional therapies in south Thailand. *Social Science & Medicine* 1988;27(8):761-8.

[100] Baskind R, Birbeck G. *Epilepsy care in Zambia: A study of traditional healers. Epilepsia* 2005;46(7):1121-6.

[101] Cho MO. Health care seeking behavior of Korean women with lymphedema. *Nursing and Health Sciences* 2004;6(2):149-59.

[102] Kunstadter P. Do cultural differences make any difference? Choice points in medical systems available in Northwestern Thailand. In: Kleinman A, Kunstadter P, Alexander RE, Gate JL, editors. *Culture and healing in Asian societies: Anthropological, psychiatric and public health studies.* Cambridge: Schenkman Publishing Company; 1978. p. 185-217.

[103] Stekelenburg J, Jager BE, Kolk PR, Westen EHMN, Kwaak Avd, Wolffers IN. Health care seeking behaviour and utilisation of traditional healers in Kalabo, Zambia. *Health Policy* 2005;71:67-81.

[104] Mignone J, Bartlett J, O'Neil J, Orchard T. *Best practices in intercultural health: Five case studies in Latin America* 2007: Available from: http://www.ncbi.nlm.nih.gov/pmc/articles/PMC2000867/pdf/ 1746-4269-3-31.pdf.

[105] Ruiz P. Folk healers as associate therapists. *Current Psychiatric Therapies* 1977;16:269-75.

[106] Farge EJ. A review of findings from "three generations" of Chicago health care behavior. *Social Science Quarterly* 1977;58(3):407-11.

[107] Freeman M, Motsei M. Planning health care in South Africa-Is there a role for traditional healers? *Social Science & Medicine* 1992;34(11):1183-90.

[108] Kale R. Traditional healers in South Africa: A parallel health care system. *British Medical Journal* 1995;310(6988):1182-5.

[109] Van der Geest S. Is there a role for traditional medicine in basic health services in Africa? A plea for a community perspective. *Tropical Medicine and International Health* 1997;2(9):903-11.

[110] Bureau of Indigenous Thai Medicine. *Effectiveness of traditional doctors in treating patients with fractures in 9 areas.* 2009.

[111] Makundi EA, Malebo HM, Mhame P, Kitua AY, Warsame M. Role of traditional healers in the management of severe Malaria among children below five years of age: The case of Kilosa and Handeni Districts, Tanzania. *Malaria Journal* 2006;5(1):58-66.

[112] Chi C. Integrating traditional medicine into modern health care systems: Examining the role of Chinese medicine in Taiwan. *Social Science & Medicine* 1994;39(3):307-21.

[113] Pearce TO. Integrating western orthodox and indigenous medicine: Professional interests and attitudes among university-trained Nigerian physicians. *Social Science & Medicine* 1982;16(18):1611-7.

In: Traditional Medicine: New Research
Editor: Yoshiharu Motoo
ISBN: 978-1-62257-448-3


*Chapter 7*

# Efficacy Evaluation of Kampo Medicine in a Mouse Model of Chronic Fatigue Syndrome

***Junichi Yamakawa***
Department of General Medicine,
Kanazawa Medical University, Japan

## Abstract

Modern medicine, which used to be called modern Western medicine, has prevailed in the world and is actively introducing the achievements of modern science, and successfully overcoming many infections in the 20th century. The very simple basic principle of modern Western medicine is that symptoms are treated with counteractive drugs. This principle has culminated in the development of successful treatments for infection. On the other hand, traditional medicines, including Kampo medicine, have been driven out by modern Western medicine because they adhere excessively to tradition and are reluctant to adopt modern technology. In recent years, however, a new tide is rising in the ever shrinking marketplace of traditional medicines. New attempts are being made to introduce traditional medicine into Western medicine and recast traditional medicine as complementary medicine. Among them, Kampo medicine (a unique traditional medicine that continued to evolve after its introduction in Japan) is characterized by clinical efficacy but unknown pharmacological effects as its academic system has taken a classic-oriented attitude for a long time. Thus, the clinical advantages of combinations of Kampo medicine with Western-style medications, for instance, reduction of the latters' adverse effects, need to be determined. In fact, however, Kampo medicines are not readily accepted in daily practice even though they are included in the National Health Insurance (NHI) price list. Much remains uncertain about their pharmacological effects. To be recognized as a potential complementary medicine, for instance, it must be demonstrated that the traditional medicine is useful for treating multifactorial diseases of unknown etiology such as chronic fatigue syndrome (CFS).

The mechanism of development of CFS (also called myalgic encephalomyelitis [ME] and post-viral fatigue syndrome [PVFS]) remains unclear. It is a disease group that is attracting considerable attention. It is characterized by intense fatigue of unknown cause that persists 6 months or more and is usually suspected only after no other diseases are detected by examinations such as computed tomography (CT), magnetic resonance imaging (MRI), and blood tests, and after it has been established that no mental disorder is likely. Nonetheless, nervous system, immune system, endocrine system, etc. abnormalities have been detected. Also, some cases are complicated by mental disorders such as depression or neurosis stemming from the disease itself and/or failure to receive consideration from others. In 1969, CFS was classified by the World Health Organization (WHO) as a central nervous system (CNS) disease on the basis of immunological and neurological findings.

In this paper, the efficacy of the Kampo medicine hochuekkito (補中益気湯; TJ-41; ethical Kampo extract formulation manufactured by Tsumura & Co., Ltd.) to improve exercise capacity in a mouse model of CFS is described. CFS was induced by repeated administration of *Brucella abortus* (BA) antigen over a period of 2 weeks. TJ-41 was orally administered to mice at a dose of 500 mg/kg once daily for 4 weeks starting at 1 week before administration of BA, and the daily running activity was assessed in the treated group comparison with the untreated group. At the time of sacrifice, body weight (BW), spleen weight (SW), SW/BW, and expression level of interleukin-10 (IL-10) mRNA in the spleen were measured in each group. The daily running activity was significantly higher in the TJ-41 group than in the untreated group. Mouse survival during this observation period was monitored. Two mice in the untreated group died 2 days after the second injection of BA, while no mice in the TJ-41 group died. SW and SW/BW were significantly lower in the TJ-41 group than in the untreated group. In the TJ-41 group, splenic expression of IL-10 mRNA was suppressed. These data suggest that hochuekkito can suppress the marked decrease in the running activity after injection of BA.

Secondly, the effects of chronic fatigue syndrome (CFS) on the central nervous system (CNS) are discussed with focus on the literature. Currently, many neuroimaging findings support the hypothesis that patients with CFS have structural and/or functional abnormalities in the brain, and some neurotrophic factors, neurotransmitters, and cytokines have been assessed in order to elucidate the mechanism of abnormal neuropsychiatric findings in CFS. In these situations, the author suggests that the focus of CFS research should be on the CNS.

In addition, brain atrophy and usefulness of hochuekkito in the mouse model of CFS are summarized. The brain-derived neurotrophic factor (BDNF) is related to major symptoms of CFS and neuron apoptosis, but no studies have directly investigated the relationship of CFS, BDNF, and neuron apoptosis. Hence, a modified mouse model of CFS (i.e., CFS induced by six instead of two injections of killed *Brucella abortus* antigen into BALB/c mice) was used to evaluate the effects of TJ-41. The daily running activity, body weight (BW), ratio of cerebrum weight to BW (CW/BW), and expression levels of BDNF and B cell lymphoma-2 (Bcl-2) mRNA in the hippocampus were assessed. The running activity and CW/BW were significantly decreased in the CFS model. Hippocampal expression of BDNF and Bcl-2 mRNA was decreased in CFS model mice and TJ-41-treated mice with no significant difference in expression between the two groups.

The relationship between CFS and brain dysfunction was investigated using the modified model. Although decreased daily running activity may be related to decreased hippocampal expression of BDNF mRNA, hippocampal apoptosis, and brain atrophy, increased daily running activity after TJ-41 activity was not accompanied by neurological recovery of the brain.

Finally, the NK cell activity and neuronal protection were assessed after combined treatment with hochuekkito and interferon-gamma (IFN-γ). The abovementioned modified mouse model of CFS was used to evaluate daily activity and immunological and neurological changes. The running activity and thymus weight were increased in CFS mice in both the TJ-41 monotherapy group and TJ-41/IFN-γ combined treatment group, whereas the thickness of thymic cortex and NK cell activity were increased only in the combined treatment group. Neither group showed significant improvement in hippocampal atrophy or in decreased hippocampal expression of brain-derived neurotrophic factor (BDNF) or Bcl-2 mRNA. These results suggest that TJ-41 combined with IFN-γ can restore daily activity via normalizing host immune responses in the CFS model but not protect neurons.

The relationship between BDNF and CFS pathology, which was studied by the author, has not been previously reported. Moreover, it was shown that the efficacy of the Kampo treatment for CFS, for which there is no established therapy, might be elucidated by analyzing changes in hippocampal expression of the BDNF precursor proBDNF and its promoter III as well as the BDNF receptor TrkB. A broader range of diseases involving BDNF decrease (depression, dementia) might be studied and new therapies for CFS consisting of Kampo medicines and immunotherapeutic agents (such as IFN) might be developed using this approach. In addition, it is suggested that such a therapy may be effective not only for CFS, but also for diseases with a similar brain pathology. Early social rehabilitation of patients with CFS, if achieved, can be expected to have positive economic effects and combined treatment can be expected to be cost-effective because herbal medicines are relatively inexpensive.

## Introduction

Today, we usually visit a hospital and/or a clinic to receive medical care based on Western medicine when we are sick. All nations in the world employ modern Western medicine as authorized medicine. In Japan as well, Western medicine has been used since it replaced conventional Kampo medicine after the Meiji Restoration. Modern medicine, which used to be called modern Western medicine, has prevailed in the world and is actively introducing the achievements of modern science, such as the successful control of many infectious diseases, into standard practice. The basic principle of modern Western medicine is that symptoms are treated with counteractive drugs. This principle has culminated in the development of successful treatments for infection. On the other hand, traditional medicines in the world, including Kampo medicine, have been driven out by modern Western medicine because they adhere excessively to tradition and are reluctant to adopt the principles of modern science. In recent years, however, a new tide is rising in the shrinking marketplace of traditional medicines. New attempts are being made to introduce traditional medicine into Western medicine recast traditional medicine as complementary medicine. Unlike a so-called traditional medicine, Western medicine has incorporated the achievements and concepts of modern science, widening the gap between traditional and Western medicine in this century.

The WHO estimates 65–80% of healthcare provided worldwide is "traditional medical care," emphasizing the importance of traditional medical care (complementary and alternative medicine). According to a survey by Harvard University, 1 in 3 Americans annually receive complementary and alternative treatments, revealing that practitioners of complementary and alternative medicine are more frequently consulted than primary care physicians [1]. In addition, the WHO plans to issue global clinical practice guidelines for traditional medicine [2]. In recent years, standard anticancer therapies in the West have been mostly combination therapies. Western medicine is very effective in the treatment of diseases of known cause such as infection, but has not proved to be as effective against diseases of unknown etiology such as lifestyle-related diseases, exposing the weakness of modern Western medicine. In modern Western medicine, the drugs not only have adverse effects that cause discomfort and anxiety, but also have less effect against chronic diseases such as lifestyle-related diseases. Modern Western medicine is not holistic care that is based on physical examination of systems, but symptomatic treatment dependent on the direct link between laboratory results and clinical action. Indeed, modern Western medicine has successfully overcome many fatal infectious illnesses. However, patients need medical care to not only cure of their pathological symptoms, but also provide psychological well-being, satisfaction, or sense of security (so-called QOL: Quality of Life).

Western medicine provides uniform treatment without considering sex, the patient's constitution, etc., and this practice has been increasing in recent years. For instance, Western medicine (unlike Kampo medicine, which has many remedies for so-called gender-specific symptoms such as female-specific climacteric disturbance, menstrual irregularity, etc.) does not recognize them as illness. Kampo medicine is not standardized, and different prescriptions for the same symptom are available according to the patient's constitution, etc. In addition, the government's harsh criticism of the rising medical cost of technological advancement in modern medicine cannot be ignored.

The current Kampo medicine in Japan has evolved independently from the ancient Chinese medicine brought to Japan long ago. The term "Kampo medicine" means both Chinese traditional medicine and Japanese-style medicine, which are often confused by the public. In fact, Kampo medicine in Japan should be separated from Chinese traditional medicine because there are many differences in healing methods [3,4]. However, the pharmacological effects of Kampo medicine despite its clinical efficacy are largely unknown as its academic system has taken a classic-oriented attitude for a long time. Thus, the clinical advantages of combinations of Kampo medicine with Western-style medications, for instance, reduction of the latters' adverse effects, need to be determined. In fact, Kampo medicines are not readily accepted in daily practice (even though they are included in the NHI price list) because of their uncertain pharmacological effects. Consequently, modern Western medicine will remain the primary form of medical care. Traditional medicine will need to re-evaluate not only its own methods but also those of modern science on which modern Western medicine is based. Therefore, traditional medicine will both remain separated from modern Western medicine and be increasingly recognized as treatment that complements Western medical treatments and compensates for the weaknesses of modern Western medicine. The current challenge may be to clarify the pharmacological effects of Kampo medicine.

To be recognized as effective (i.e., compensating for the weaknesses of modern Western medicine), traditional medicine must be scientifically demonstrated that it is useful in treating multifactorial diseases of unknown etiology such as chronic fatigue syndrome (CFS). The mechanism of CFS development remains unclear, and it is a disease group that is attracting considerable attention. It is characterized by intense fatigue of unknown cause that persists generally 6 months or more. It is also known as myalgic encephalomyelitis (ME) and post-viral fatigue syndrome (PVFS). It is usually suspected only after no other diseases are detected by various examinations including computed tomography (CT), magnetic resonance imaging (MRI), or blood tests, and after mental disorders have been excluded. Nonetheless, abnormalities in the nervous system, immune system, endocrine system, etc. have been detected in CFS, and mental disorders such as depression or neurosis caused by the disease itself and/or by failure to receive consideration from others have been found to complicate CFS. In 1969, CFS was classified by the WHO as a central nervous system (CNS) disease on the basis of immunological and neurological findings. In 1992 and 1993, ME and CFS were consolidated into PVFS, WHO International Classification of Diseases (ICD)-10 G93.3. In 2006, the Centers for Disease Control and Prevention (CDC) reported the results of a large-scale study titled "C3 (CFS Computational Challenge)" involving geneticists, molecular biologists, mathematicians, engineers, etc. that suggested CFS was a physical rather than a mental disease. In addition, a CFS awareness campaign called "Spark" was organized with a budget of 4 million dollars in the US, and the Director of the CDC declared that CFS should be treated as a serious disease. In the US, the disease will be renamed. In 2007, the British government instructed physicians again to treat CFS as a serious illness and issued new guidelines for its management. In Japan, the main criteria proposed by the Health, Labour and Welfare Ministry were intense fatigue severely interfering with daily life and persisting or repeatedly occurring (50% or more of time) for at least 6 months. Diseases listed in the Appendix of the draft criteria were excluded based on medical history, and physical and imaging findings. Minor criteria involved symptoms and physical findings. The symptom criteria are following symptoms that persist or repeatedly occur for at least 6 months. These included slight fever (axillary temperature: 37.2–38.3°C) or chills; sore throat; swollen cervical or axillary lymph nodes; muscular weakness of unknown cause; muscle pain or discomfort; general malaise persisting for 24 hours or more after mild exertion; headache; migratory joint pain with no swelling or redness; and at least one psychoneurotic symptom (photosensitivity, transient scotoma, memory loss, irritability, confusion, reduced thinking, decreased mental concentration, depressed state, sleep disorder [hypersomnia, insomnia]). These minor symptoms associated with the major symptom had to occur within several hours to several days of onset. The physical finding criteria are following findings that had to be confirmed by a physician at least twice within 1 month or more. These included slight fever; non-exudative pharyngitis, and swollen or tender lymph nodes (cervical or axillary). A diagnosis of CFS is made if at least "8 symptom criteria" or at least "6 symptom criteria + 2 physical finding criteria" are met along with the 2 main criteria. "Suspected CFS" is defined as a case meeting the two main criteria and no minor criteria. Among CFS diagnosed cases according to the abovementioned criteria (except for "suspected CFS"), the case with the symptoms following definite infectious diseases is classefied as "post-infection CFS." At present, CFS is diagnosed by ruling out other diseases, raising the demand for biomarkers to facilitate more objective differential diagnosis of CFS. CFS requires that the patient receive physical and mental rest, but many working patients are reluctant to take a leave of absence because of a sense of responsibility, resulting in worsening or lingering symptoms. Currently, it is treated with vitamin C, methycobal (mecobalamin), antidepressants, immunoglobulins, sleeping pills, cognitive behavioral therapy, stepwise behavioral therapy, pacing, etc., but with little effect. With no effective drug available, many patients suffer from the disease for a long period of time.

In this paper, the efficacy of hochuekkito (補中益気湯; a Kampo medicine used to improve exercise capacity in a mouse model of CFS) is described in Chapter 1; the effects of chronic fatigue syndrome on the central nervous system are discussed with a focus on the literature in Chapter 2; brain atrophy and usefulness of hochuekkito in the CFS model are summarized in Chapter 3, and the NK cell activity and neuroprotection are evaluated after treatment with hochuekkito plus interferon-γ in the CFS model in Chapter 4.

The contents of this paper have already been published in the following papers.

i. Wang X.Q., Takahashi T., Zhu S., Moriya J., Saegusa S., Yamakawa J., Kusaka K., Itoh T., Kanda T., *Evid. Based. Complement. Alternat. Med.*, 1, 203-206 (2004).
ii. Chen R., Liang F.X., Moriya J., Yamakawa J., Sumino H., Kanda T., Takahashi T., *Int. J. Med. Red.,* 36, 867-874 (2008).
iii. Chen R., Moriya J., Yamakawa J., Takahashi T., Li Q., Morimoto S., Iwai K., Sumino H., Yamaguchi N., Kanda T., *Neurochem. Res.*, 33, 1759-67 (2008).
iv. Chen R., Moriya J., Luo X., Yamakawa J., Takahashi T., Sasaki K., Yoshizaki F., *Immunopharmacol. Immunotoxicol.,* 12, 1-15 ( 2008). Epab.

# Main Themes

## Chapter 1. Efficacy of Hochuekkito for Improving Exercise Capacity in a Mouse Model of Chronic Fatigue Syndrome

### Part 1. Introduction

Fatigue is one of the most common symptoms in the general population, as shown by a survey [5] in which approximately 50% of respondents reported suffering from fatigue. In addition, another study reported that more than 20% of people who seek medical attention present with fatigue as one of their symptoms [6]. These cases of fatigue are usually transient and self-limiting, and can be explained by pathology [7]. If fatigue cannot be explained, chronic fatigue syndrome (CFS) may be suspected.

CFS is typically characterized by sudden onset of influenza-like illness with the main symptom of severe and persistent fatigue substantially limiting activity. It is hypothesized that CFS may be caused by viral infection that subsequently impairs immune function, but this still remains to be studied. An immunological model of fatigue constructed by intraperitoneal administration of bacterial antigen has been previously reported, but the assessment of wheel running activity in this model showed that the duration of fatigue was short [8]. Ottenweller et al. [9] described the establishment of a mouse model of CFS induced by administration of *Brucella abortus* (BA). In this model, inactivated BA antigen is intravenously administered to mice exercising on a running wheel to induce an acute immune response [9]. Voluntary wheel running activity decreased after administration of BA antigen [9]. It has previously been reported that cytokine gene expression in mouse lymphocytes is affected by administration of BA [10].

In the UK, survey data show that approximately 30% of British people have used some Kampo medicines [11]. Hochuekkito is a Kampo remedy for viral infection, bacterial infection, or postoperative shock. Hochuekkito is reported to increase certain biological activities including the activities of NK cells [12] and macrophages [13] and to inhibit influenza viral infection in mice by enhancing the host immune response [14].

## Part 2. Experimental Materials and Methods

### *Mice and Experimental Conditions*

Female BALB/c mice (8 weeks old) were purchased from Charles River Laboratories Japan, Inc. (Kanagawa, Japan) and individually housed in cages (230 × 100 × 100 mm) each equipped with a running wheel (diameter: 230 mm), wheel turn counter, and water supply (Figure 1). Cages were purchased from Natsume Seisakusho Co., Ltd. (Tokyo, Japan) and mice were maintained on a 10-hour light/14-hour dark cycle under room fluorescent light. During the experimental period, all mice ($n$ = 20) were given solid feed and distilled water every day in a room maintained at a temperature of 24–25°C. For each mouse, the daily running activity was determined at 9 am at intervals of 24 hours and was based on the number of wheel turns.

### *Induction of CFS by Brucella Abortus Antigen*

The fixed killed whole BA ring test (ring precipitin test) antigen (killed bacteria) was obtained from the National Veterinary Services Laboratories, the United States Department of Agriculture. CFS was induced by two tail-vein injections of stock BA antigen solution (0.2 mL per animal) separated by an interval of 2 weeks. In these BA-treated mice, the running activity was decreased 2–3 weeks after administration.

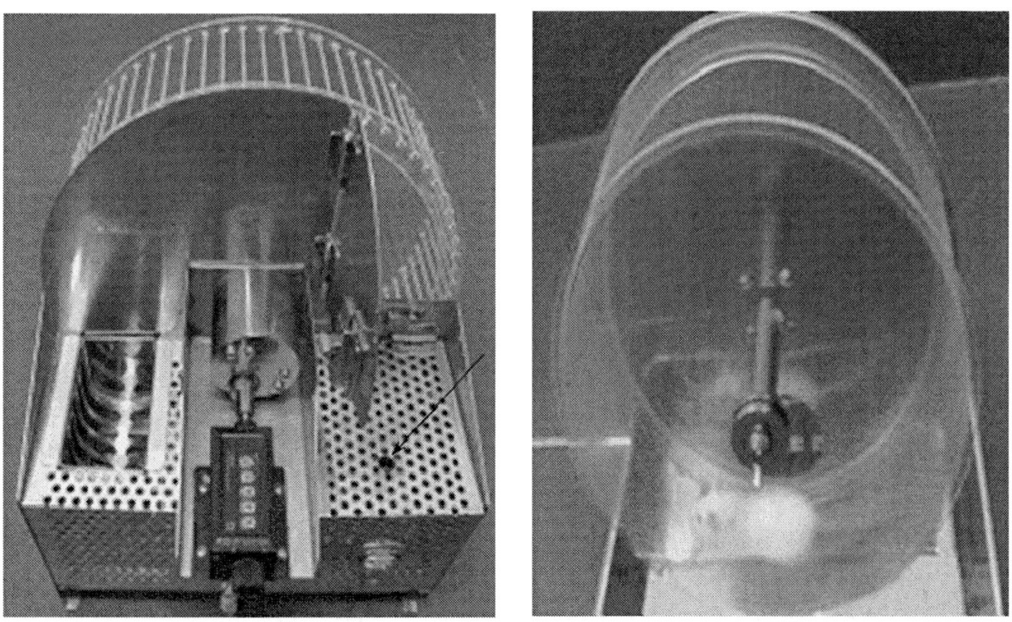

A B

Figure 1. Home cage equipped with a running wheel. A shows the front and B shows the rear of the cage. Food and water were available ad libitum. Mice could enter the running wheel at any time. The counter showed the running wheel activity. The black arrow points to the hole for the water supply.

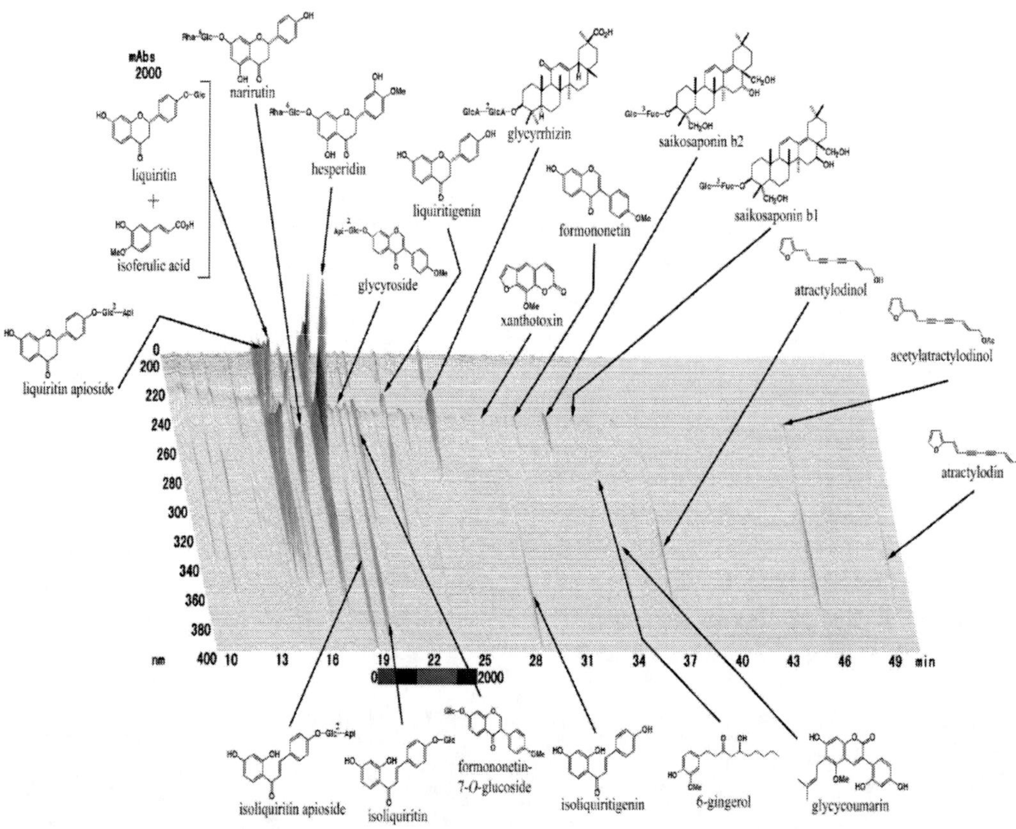


Figure 2. Quantitative assessment of known bioactive compounds in TJ-41 by means of high performance liquid chromatography.

### *Administration of Hochuekkito*

Hochuekkito (補中益気湯) was a ethical Kampo extract formulation (TJ-41) manufactured by Ibaraki Plant, Tsumura & Co., Ltd. It contains Astragalus root (*ogi* [黄耆], *Astragali radix*) (16.7%), Atractylodes lancea rhizome (*sojutsu* [蒼朮], *Atractylodis lanceae rhizoma*) (16.7%), ginseng (*ninjin* [人参], *Ginseng radix*) (16.7%), Japanese Angelica root (*toki*, [当帰], *Angelicae radix*) (12.5%), Bupleurum root (*saiko* [柴胡], *Bupleuri radix*) (8.3%), jujube (*taiso* [大棗],*Zizyphi fructus*) (8.3%), citrus unshiu peel (*chinpi* [陳皮], *Aurantii nobilis pericarpium*) (8.3%), glycyrrhiza (kanzo [甘草], *Glycyrrhizae radix*) (6.3%), Cimicifuga rhizome (shoma [升麻], *Cimicifugae rhizoma*) (4.2%), and ginger (shokyo [生姜], *Zingiberis rhizoma*) (2.0%). The results from analysis of major components by high performance liquid chromatography are shown in Figure 2. This product was dissolved in distilled water and diluted with water to the appropriate concentration. TJ-41 solution was orally administered to mice ($n$ = 10) via a feeding needle inserted into the throat at a dose of 500 mg/kg once daily for 4 weeks starting at 1 week before induction of CFS. This dose was selected based on a report by Kido et al. [15] Animals in the untreated group ($n$ = 10) received physiological saline instead of the study drug.

### *Evaluation Items*

Once the running activity had stabilized 2–3 weeks after the start of feeding, the baseline activity was recorded for 2 weeks. The daily running activity in the TJ-41 group was assessed in comparison with that in the untreated group. Mouse survival was monitored during this observation period. The surviving animals were killed by cervical dislocation 4 weeks after the first injection of BA.

At the time of sacrifice, the ratio of spleen weight (SW) (mg) to body weight (BW) (g) (SW/BW), ratio of thymus weight (TW) (mg) to BW (TW/BW), ratio of heart weight (HW) (mg) to BW (HW/BW), and ratio of lung weight (LW) (mg) to BW (LW/BW) as well as relevant organ weights and body weight were compared between the two groups and assessed. The expression level of interleukin-10 (IL-10) mRNA was determined in each spleen by quantitative real-time reverse transcription-polymerase chain reaction (RT-PCR) [9].

The optimal RT-PCR cycle number was determined for the expression level of IL-10 mRNA. Using the optimal cycle number, glyceraldehyde-3-phosphate dehydrogenase (GAPDH) gene (which was used as endogenous internal reference) and the specific primer were amplified. The expression level of IL-10 mRNA was calculated relative to the expression level in the spleens from normal female BALB/c mice (value = 1).

### *Statistical Analysis*

Analysis was performed using Student's $t$ test. A significance level of $P < 0.05$ was used.

## Part 3. Results

### *Section 1 Running Activity in Mice*

The daily running activity of mice in each group before and after induction of CFS is shown in Figure 3. The daily running activity was not significantly different between the two groups at baseline but significantly higher in the TJ-41 group than in the untreated group after both BA injections (2 weeks after the first injection, 8157.6 ± 3287.6 vs. 5884.3 ± 2977.5; 2 weeks after the second injection, 5584.9 ± 2897.4 vs. 2758.5 ± 2612.1; $P < 0.05$). Two mice in the untreated group died 2 days after the second injection of BA, while no mice in the TJ-41 group died.

### *Section 2. Organ Weights and Expression Level of IL-10 mRNA in the Spleen*

BW, SW, TW, HW, and LW in each group are shown in Table 1. In the TJ-41 group, SW (546 ± 37) was significantly decreased compared with the untreated group (693 ± 107) ($P <$ 0.05), but body weight or weights of other organs were not different between the two groups. At the time of sacrifice, SW/BW was significantly lower in the TJ-41 group (24.2 ± 1.4) than in the untreated group (31.8 ± 6.3) ($P < 0.05$), but TW/BW, HW/BW, or LW/BW was not significantly different between the two groups. The expression level of IL-10 mRNA in the spleen was significantly lower in TJ-41-treated mice ($n = 6$) than in untreated mice ($n = 4$) (5.47 ± 1.81 vs. 11.39 ± 3.99, $P < 0.05$).

## Part 4. Discussion

Wheel running activity is a relatively reliable indicator of severity of CFS. On the other hand, it has been reported that fluffy fur 11 days after injection is an unreliable criterion for distinguishing BA-injected mice from physiological saline-injected mice [10]. In clinical practice, the purpose of CFS treatment is to alleviate symptoms and reduce functional impairment [11]. Therefore, running activity may be a more reliable indicator of the efficacy of TJ-41 than grooming.

**Table 1. Effect of hochuekkito on body weight and weight of organs including spleen, thymus, heart, and lungs at the time of sacrifice**

| | BW (g) | SW (mg) | TW (mg) | HW (mg) | LW (mg) |
|---|---|---|---|---|---|
| Treated mice ($n = 10$) | 22.6 ± 2.3 | 546 ± 37* | 43 ± 12 | 118 ± 19 | 149 ± 11 |
| Untreated mice ($n = 8$) | 21.8 ± 1.1 | 693 ± 107 | 47 ± 25 | 110 ± 22 | 154 ± 21 |

Data are expressed as means ± SD.

Abbreviations: BW, body weight; SW, spleen weight; TW, thymus weight; HW, heart weight; LW, weight of both lungs.

*$P < 0.05$ compared with spleen weight in the untreated mice.

Chao et al. [12] reported spleen enlargement (mg/g body weight) 12 days after inoculation in two mouse models of immune-mediated fatigue (24.1 ± 1.8 in the *Corynebacterium parvum* group and 20.2 ± 1.6 in the *Toxoplasma gondii* group, compared with 5.3 ± 0.2 in the physiological saline group). In the present study, SW/BW was markedly increased after repeated administration of BA, but was significantly decreased in the TJ-41 group, suggesting that the measurement of spleen enlargement may be useful to confirm the improvement from immunostimulation during the treatment.

The author found that splenic expression of IL-10 mRNA was significantly decreased in TJ-41-treated mice compared with untreated mice.

Abnormal gene expression levels of various cytokines (IL-10, IL-4, IL-2, and interferon-$\gamma$) in the spleen have been reported [9, 10]. Since circulating cytokine concentrations may be used in future clinical studies, it may be necessary to measure circulating concentration of the abovementioned cytokines for the assessment of the therapeutic efficacy in this mouse model.

CFS and mental disorders partially overlap and/or simultaneously share important symptoms [7]. The efficacy of hochuekkito and other Kampo medicines for "behavioral despair" and acetic acid-induced writhing in mice have been reported, suggesting that these medicines may have antidepressant and antinociceptive properties [14].

The results of the present study may have implications for the use of hochuekkito in the treatment of psychiatric illness.

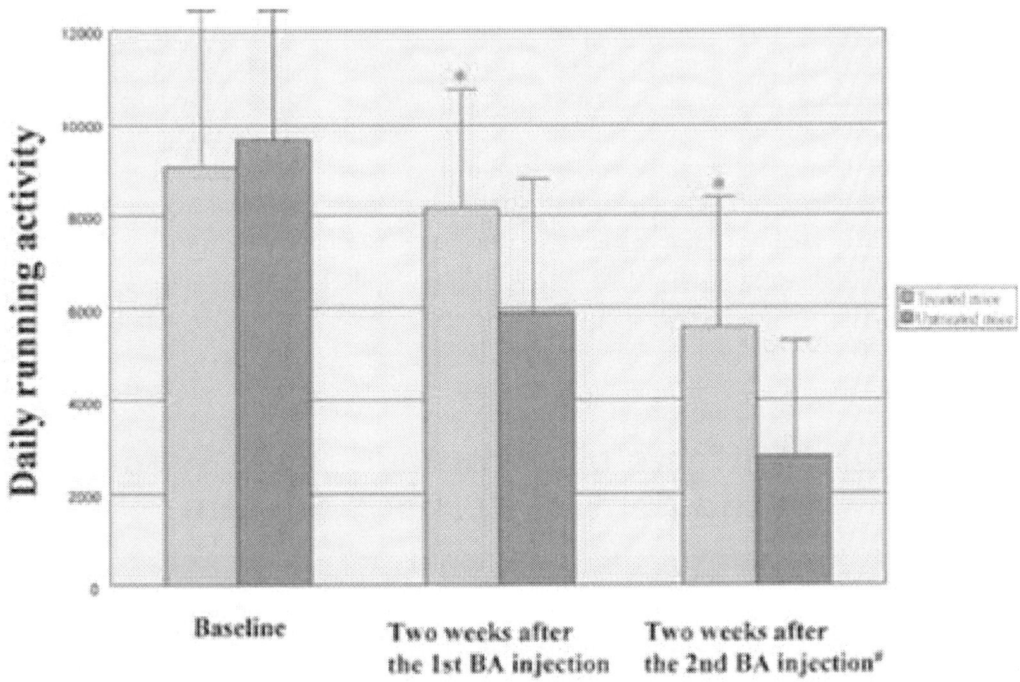


Figure 3. Effect of hochuekkito on the daily running activity in a mouse model of chronic fatigue syndrome.
Data are expressed as means ± SD.
Abbreviations: BA, *Brucella abortus*. Daily running activity was defined as the number of wheel turns per 24 h.
$*P < 0.05$ compared with the daily activity in the untreated mice. † Two mice in the untreated group died 2 days after the second injection of BA, while no mice in the treated group died.

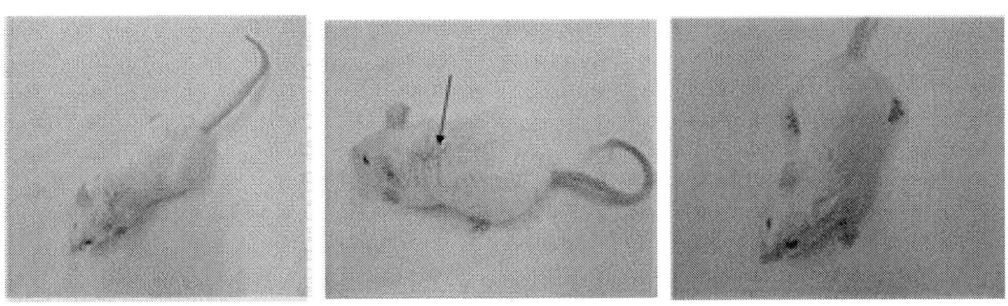

A B C

Figure 4. General appearance of mice in each group before sacrifice.
A was a mouse in the normal control group, which was very active and restless. B was a mouse in the model group, which was slothful and had fluffy fur. C was a mouse treated with TJ-41, which was more nimble than mouse B. The black arrow points to the fluffy fur.

## Part 5. Conclusion

Few studies have demonstrated the efficacy of alternative or complementary therapy including Kampo medicines in patients with CFS [7]. In the mouse model of CFS, the daily running activity was significantly higher and SW/BW at the time of sacrifice was significantly lower in the hochuekkito (500 mg/kg/day)-treated group than in the untreated group. The results of this study suggest that hochuekkito may suppress the marked decrease in the running activity after injection of BA by regulating the host immune response, but the study was not designed to establish the optimal dosage or appropriate timing of hochuekkito treatment. In addition, the efficacy of this product should be evaluated in comparison with that of a positive control of a medication already known to have an effect. It has also been shown that potent antioxidants such as carvedilol (5 mg/kg) and melatonin (5 mg/kg) significantly decrease the duration of immobilization after intraperitoneal administration in the mouse model of CFS [17]. Much remains to be clarified.

# Chapter 2. Effects of Chronic Fatigue Syndrome on the Central Nervous System

## Part 1. Introduction

As defined by the Centers for Disease Control and Prevention, CFS is primarily characterized by fatigue (accompanied by decreased energy) that persists for at least 6 months. Moreover, evidence of an underlying psychiatric or neurological disorder indicates that psychiatric, psychological, or neurological assessments are needed [18]. Accordingly, neuroimaging methods including magnetic resonance imaging (MRI), head single photon emission computerized tomography (SPECT), and positron emission tomography (PET) and radionuclide scanning have been used to assess CFS-related structural and functional abnormalities. [19] Some neurotrophic factors, neurotransmitters, and cytokines have been assessed to elucidate the mechanism of neuropsychiatric abnormalities [20]. In this connection, the author evaluated the effects of CFS on the central nervous system (CNS) and discussed the current approaches used to investigate the neuropathological mechanism of CFS.

## Part 2. Neuroimaging Findings

Available neuroimaging data show not only differences in morphology between chronic fatigue patients and normal controls, but also differences in brain responses to mental fatigue and other complex symptoms of CFS (Table 2).

### *Section 1. Decrease in Cerebral Blood Flow*

In patients with CFS, Ichise et al. [21] and Schwartz et al. [32] determined the cerebral blood flow using SPECT and reported global hypoperfusion. In addition, SPECT showed hypoperfusion in specific regions (anterior cingulate cortex, brainstem, etc.) [22, 26]. Yoshiuchi et al. [30] using xenon-computerized tomography instead of SPECT to determine the absolute cortical blood flow found decreased blood flow in bilateral middle cerebral artery territories. A study in identical twins, however, found no difference in the perfusion between twins with CFS and healthy twins [33].

**Table 2. Neuroimaging findings in patients with CFS**

| Published year | Number of CFS cases | Detection methods | Results in patients with CFS | Reference no. |
|---|---|---|---|---|
| 1992 | 60 | $^{99}$Tcm-HMPAO and SPECT | Lower cortical/cerebellar regional cerebral blood flow ratios, mainly in frontal, temporal, parietal and occipital lobes | [21] |
| 1995 | 67 | $^{99}$Tcm-HMPAO and SPET | Confirmed brain-stem hypoperfusion | [24] |
| 1998 | 18 | $^{18}$FDG-PET | A hypometabolism in right mediofrontal cortex and brainstem | [27] |
| 1999 | 39 | MRI | A larger number of brain abnormalities on $T_2$ weighted images in CFS-No Psych group than in CFS-Psych and HC groups | [33] |
| 2000 | 7 | Proton MRS | ①Reduced concentration of NAA in the right hippocampus; ②No difference in hippocampal volume between patient with CFS and HC | [31] |
| 2003 | 15 | SPECT | less perfusion in the anterior cingulate region | [23] |
| 2004 | 16 | MRI and VBM | Reduced gray-matter volume in the bilateral prefrontal cortex, especially in the right prefrontal cortex | [30] |
| 2005 | 10 | [$^{11}$C]WAY-100635 and PET | A widespread reduction in 5-HT receptor binding potential, especially in the hippocampus | [51] |
| 2005 | 28 | MRI and VBM | Significant reductions in global gray matter volume | [29] |
| 2006 | 25 | Xenon-CT | Reduced absolute cortical blood flow in left and right middle cerebral artery territories | [25] |
| 2007 | 9 | Functional MRI | A greater brain activity in several cortical and subcortical regions such as cerebellar, temporal, cingulate and frontal regions | [32] |

Abbreviations: CFS, chronic fatigue syndrome; CT, computed tomography; $^{18}$FDG, [18F]fluorine-deoxyglucose; HC, healthy controls; MRI, magnetic resonance imaging; MRS, magnetic resonance spectroscopy; NAA, N-acetylaspartate; PET, positron emission tomography; SPECT, single-photon emission computerized tomography; SPET, single-photon emission tomography; $^{99}$Tcm-HMPAO, $^{99}$Tcm-hexamethylpropylene amine oxime; VBM, voxel-based morphometry.

Based on evidence of abnormal cerebral perfusion, cerebral metabolism was studied. Using [$^{18}$F] fluorine-deoxyglucose PET to determine cerebral metabolism, marked hypometabolism was revealed in the right mediofrontal cortex and brainstem in patients with CFS [23]. Taken together with the results of perfusion SPECT studies [22], this finding indicates that hypometabolism in the brainstem is an *in vivo* diagnostic marker of CFS.

### *Section 2. Decrease in Brain Volume*

In patients with CFS compared with normal controls, previous MRI scanning found significant brain volume, white matter, and gray matter abnormalities. Natelson et al. [34] found ventricular or sulcus hypertrophy and increased T2 signal in the white matter in 52 patients with CFS, and de Lange et al. [29] found markedly decreased global gray matter volume in 28 patients with CFS. Likewise, Okada et al. [27] reported decreased gray matter volume in the bilateral prefrontal cortex.

On the other hand, MRI using an unbiased method found no difference in the hippocampal volume between patients with CFS and healthy volunteers, whereas proton magnetic resonance spectroscopy showed significantly reduced N-acetylaspartate concentration (considered as a neuron density marker) in CFS patients [25].

### *Section 3 Neuroimaging Changes Correlated with Symptoms*

The correspondence between brain abnormalities and symptoms of CFS is unknown. It has been reported that decreased gray matter volume is related to decreased physical activity (the central feature of CFS) [29] and that decreased gray matter volume in the right prefrontal cortex is related to severity of fatigue [27]. However, Cook et al. [31] showed that mental fatigue was significantly correlated with brain activity, and fatiguing work was correlated with a greater brain activity in several cortical and subcortical regions (parietal cortex, cingulate cortex, inferior frontal cortex, superior temporal cortex, cerebellum, cerebellar vermis, etc.).

Psychiatric symptoms are another complaint often reported by patients with CFS. CFS without psychiatric problems is associated with decreased cortical blood flow in the right and left middle cerebral artery territories, whereas CFS with psychiatric problems is associated with decreased blood flow only in the left middle cerebral artery territory [30]. In addition, more brain abnormalities were observed on T2 weighted images in CFS patients with no psychiatric symptoms than in healthy controls and CFS patients with psychiatric symptoms. The changes (increases in intensity of mostly small, point-like areas in the subcortical white matter, primarily in the frontal lobe) were observed in CFS patients with no psychiatric symptoms but not in CFS patients with psychiatric symptoms [34].

## Part 3. Pathophysiological Mechanism

### *Section 1. Hypothalamic-Pituitary-Adrenal Axis and Corticosteroids*

In 1981, Poteliakhoff [35] reported an association between chronic fatigue and hypocortisolism for the first time. Since then, many studies have been conducted to verify this finding. The focus of these studies has been on low concentrations of corticosteroids and enhanced feedback in the hypothalamic-pituitary-adrenal (HPA) axis [36]. It is still unclear whether these disorders play a primary or secondary role in the etiology of CFS [38] because there is contrary evidence that HPA axis function in some patients with CFS is decreased [37]. HPA axis dysfunction is still considered to be involved in the development of CFS symptoms although it might be secondary to other factors. More recently, a report by Cleare [38] confirmed the relationship between the HPA axis and CFS.

### *Section 2. Brain-derived Neurotrophic Factor*

In 1982, a German neuroscientist isolated brain-derived neurotrophic factor (BDNF) from the porcine cerebrum [39]. BDNF is widely distributed throughout the CNS (hippocampus, cerebral cortex, basal forebrain, etc.). The author recently found that hippocampal BDNF mRNA expression was decreased in CFS model mice and thus hypothesized that BDNF may play an important role in the development of CFS.

Decreased BDNF levels (especially in the hippocampus) are often associated with major symptoms of CFS. For instance, reduced physical activity is one of the most common symptoms of CFS, and exercise is important to enhance brain health and function. A variable increase in BDNF expression is the main effect of exercise on brain function. In humans, the serum BDNF concentration is transiently increased immediately after brief exercise [40]. In rodents, the BDNF gene and protein expressions in the hippocampus are increased after daily wheel running [41]. Other CFS symptoms (depression, anxiety, etc.) result in decreased hippocampal BDNF mRNA expression [42]. Cognitive dysfunction affects the BDNF level not only in rats but also in a cellular model [43, 44]. Hippocampal BDNF expression is decreased in sleep-deprived rats [45]. In summary, the major symptoms of CFS result in decreased hippocampal BDNF mRNA expression.

Further intensive studies are required to clarify the relationship of hippocampal BDNF with CFS or at least the major symptoms of CFS. BDNF supports the survival and proliferation of many neuron subtypes, and is an important mediator of synaptic, neuronal, and use-dependent plasticity. BDNF signaling is mediated by two different receptors, p75 neurotrophin receptor and TrkB receptor tyrosine kinase. At present, almost all of the synaptic effects of BDNF are known to be mediated by TrkB [46]. Binding of BDNF to TrkB leads to autophosphorylation of the tyrosine residue in the intracellular domain, which, in turn, leads to the activation of one of the following three signaling pathways: mitogen-activated protein kinase (MAPK); phosphatidylinositol 3-kinase (PI-3K), and phospholipase Cγ [47] or N-methyl-D-aspartate (NMDA) receptor [48]. Exercise-induced hippocampal BDNF expression results in increased expression of several important intermediate metabolites in the MAPK, [49] PI-3K/Akt, [50] and NMDA receptor pathways [51]. These pathways are partially involved in sleep disorders, [52] long-term synergy, and depression [53]. Nonetheless, the involvement of BDNF expression in these mechanisms of CFS remains unknown and requires more studies.

### *Section 3. Serotonin System*

Cleare et al. [28] found that the number or affinity of 5-hydroxy-tryptamine 1A (5-HT1A) receptors was decreased in CFS. This important characteristic of CFS is associated with its pathophysiology or with findings secondary to other processes (previous depression, other biological changes, changes in behavior, etc.). In addition, studies of serotonergic neurotransmitters in patients with CFS showed that changes in the serotonergic system in the rostral anterior cingulate cortex play an important role in the pathophysiology of CFS [20]. More specifically, a polymorphic study of serotonin transporter (5-HTT) gene promoter showed that the expression of long allelic variant was significantly increased and transcriptional activity of the long allelic variant was higher than that of the short allelic variant. In addition, treatment with fluvoxamine, a selective 5-HT reuptake inhibitor, resulted in the return to work of approximately one third of CFS patients [54].

In a rat model of polyriboinosinic acid: polyribocytidylic acid (poly I:C)-induced fatigue, 5-HTT was involved in the central mechanism of fatigue, suggesting that the decreased effect of 5-HT on the 5-HT1A receptor may be at least partially involved in poly I:C-induced fatigue [55].

This clinical and experimental evidence showed that loss of serotonergic function is part of the mechanism of CFS. In some neurodegenerative diseases, the change in the function of the serotonin system is also related to changes in the hippocampus, prefrontal cortex, and HPA axis [56]. However, it is unknown whether the serotonin system contributes to those changes in CFS.

### *Section 4. Cytokines*

It has been reported that most patients with CFS have experienced infection [57]. In response to peripheral infection, innate immune cells produce proinflammatory cytokines, which then act on the brain. Constant activation of the peripheral immune system results in immune signaling to the brain and thus increased feelings of fatigue [58]. Since it is well known that cytokines in the brain have various effects on the CNS (activation of the sympathetic nervous system and HPA, impairment of learning and memory, etc. [59]), brain cytokines may play a role in the etiology of CFS.

Natelson et al. [60] detected eleven cytokines in the spinal fluid from patients with CFS and found the following: (i) the granulocyte-macrophage colony stimulating factor level was lower in CFS patients than in healthy controls; (ii) the interleukin (IL)-8 level was higher in CFS patients with sudden onset of influenza-like illness than in those with gradual onset disease or healthy controls, and (iii) the IL-10 level was higher in CFS patients with abnormal spinal fluid than in those with no abnormality or healthy controls.

In a rat model of poly I:C-induced fatigue, brain interferon-α (IFN-α) mRNA expression was significantly increased in the cortex, cerebellum, medial preoptic area, lateral hippocampus, and hypothalamic paraventricular nucleus, whereas expression of IL-6 or tumor necrosis factor α (TNF-α) mRNA was not increased [55]. In this model, an increase in transforming growth factor β was also observed in the cerebrospinal fluid and associated with fever [61].

It has been reported that some cytokines are involved in the development and exacerbation of mood disorder and behavior disorder (depression, anxiety, fatigue, etc.) in CFS. For instance, proinflammatory cytokines including IL-1β, IL-6, and TNF-α induce or worsen such symptoms as fatigue, anxiety, and depression, whereas IL-2 and IFN-α worsen depressive symptoms that are alleviated by antidepressants [62]. The most common sleep disorders in CFS patients are excessive daytime sleepiness and nighttime insomnia. These are exacerbated by IL-6 and / or TNF-α [63].

*Segment 4. Conclusion*

In summary, an increasing amount of evidence available shows that CFS is related to the CNS, but controversy remains because not only CFS but also several major symptoms of CFS are related to the CNS. The focus of CFS research should therefore be on the CNS and neurological mechanisms of CFS.

# Chapter 3. Brain Atrophy and Usefulness of Hochuekkito in a Mouse Model of Chronic Fatigue Syndrome

## Part 1. Introduction

CFS is a complex disorder characterized by combination of nonspecific symptoms and unexplained fatigue that interferes with activities of daily life. Most of the accompanying symptoms (including abnormal post-exertional malaise, insufficient sleep, notable memory/concentration impairment, headache, myalgia, joint pain, throat pain, and tender lymph nodes) are neurological/psychiatric symptoms [18, 64].

Nevertheless, the neurological basis of chronic fatigue is not fully understood. It was recently found that the absolute cortical blood flow was decreased in the right and left middle cerebral artery territories in patients with CFS [30]. In addition, clinical neuroimaging revealed that subjective feelings of fatigue were correlated with gray matter volume in some cortical regions [27] and with brain responses [31]. Therefore, investigation of the relationshp between the etiology of CFS and brain morphology/function is needed.

BDNF, a neurotrophic factor first isolated from porcine cerebrum by a German neuroscientist in 1982, [39] is widely found in the CNS including the hippocampus, cerebral cortex, basal forebrain nucleus, striatum, hypothalamus, brainstem, and cerebellum [65]. A previous study showed that exercise can increase hippocampal BDNF expression [66]. It has also been shown that BDNF can prevent programmed cell death of some neurons and promote cellular survival [67, 68].

In addition, exercise may increase the number of new hippocampal cells [69]. It was recently shown that the decreased BDNF expression (associated with major symptoms of CFS such as stress and major depressive disorder) might result in hippocampal atrophy and cell number decrease [42, 70]. It is evident that BDNF is related to major symptoms of CFS and neuronal survival and apoptosis, but no studies have investigated the relationship of CFS, BDNF, and neuron apoptosis directly.

Using a mouse model of CFS induced by two injections of BA antigen as described in Chapter 1, we previously showed TJ-41 increased the daily activity. Using another CFS model constructed by injecting BA antigen into BALB/c mice six times, we subsequently attempted to determine the relationships between running activity, BDNF, and brain atrophy and to investigate the mechanism of action of TJ-41 in CFS.

## Part 2. Experimental Materials and Methods

### *Section 1. Mice and Experimental Conditions*

See Part 2 of Chapter 1. Twenty-one mice were used.

### *Section 2 Induction of CFS by Brucella Abortus Antigen*

See Part 2 of Chapter 1. CFS was induced by six injections of undiluted BA antigen into the tail vein (one injection every 2 weeks, 0.2 mL/mouse) [71].

### *Section 3. Administration of Test Solution*

After acclimation of 21 BALB/c mice (including 6 mice in the normal control group) to the environment for 2 weeks, the mice began their regimen of injections. Five of 15 mice injected to induce CFS died during the 12-week model-construction period. After CFS was induced, TJ-41 dissolved in physiological saline was orally administered to 5 of the 10 surviving mice via a feeding needle inserted into the throat at a dose of 500 mg/kg (0.1 mL) once daily for 4 weeks [72]. Physiological saline was administered to the animals in the other two groups at a volume of 0.1 mL in the same manner every day.

### *Section 4. Running Activity, Body Weight, Food Consumption, Body Temperature, and Survival*

The level of voluntary running activity was determined based on the number of wheel turns. The daily running activity was recorded during the 12-week model-construction period and the following 4-week treatment period. For all mice, BW, food consumption, and body temperature were measured every week from the start to the completion of the experiment. The survival of all animals was monitored throughout the observation period.

### *Section 5. Morphology of the Brain and Hippocampus*

The mice in the three groups were killed by cervical dislocation 4 weeks after the start of treatment. At the time of sacrifice, the ratio of cerebrum weight to BW (CW/BW) was assessed in all groups. After the left half of the brain was fixed in 10% buffered formalin, sections were prepared and Nissl-stained for assessment.

### *Section 6. Real-time PCR*

The hippocampus was removed from the right half of the cerebrum and immediately frozen in liquid nitrogen or on a dry ice-cooled plate before being stored in a freezer at –80°C. RNA extraction from each frozen hippocampus was performed as described by the manufacturer (RNeasy Mini Kit, QIAGEN Inc., Tokyo, Japan). Reverse transcription with up to 4 μg of total RNA was carried out in a total volume of 20 μL containing 250 pmol of random primer, 100 U of SuperScript II RNase H-Reverse Transcriptase (Invitrogen Corporation), 50 mM Tris-HCl (pH 8.3), 40 mM KCl, 6 mM $MgCl_2$, 1 mM DTT, and 10 mM dNTPs. Initially, total RNA solution mixed with random primer was heated at 70°C for 10 min and immediately chilled on ice, then the other reagents were added. Single-strand cDNAs were obtained after 50 min at 42°C and 5 min at 98°C. Primers and TaqMan probes for target genes (BDNF and Bcl-2) and internal reference gene (GAPDH) were purchased from Applied Biosystems (TaqMan® Gene Expression Assays). Each TaqMan probe was labeled with a reporter dye 6-carboxyfluorescein (FAM) situated at the 5'end of the oligonucleotide and a quencher dye 6-carboxytetramethyl-rhodamine (TAMRA) situated at the 3'end. The TaqMan® Gene Expression Assay number was Mm00432069_m1 and Mm00432069_m1 for BDNF and Bcl-2 RT-PCR, respectively (Applied Biosystems Inc.). Quantification of target cDNAs (BDNF and Bcl-2) and internal reference gene (GAPDH) was performed in 96-well plates using an ABI PRISM7700 Sequence Detection System (ABI), and analyses were performed using the machine software. The PCR was carried out in a final volume of 25μL containing cDNA equivalent to 50 ng of total RNA, 12.5 μL of 1×TaqMan Universal PCR Master Mix, and 1.25 μL of 20×TaqMan Expression Assay reagent. Each sample was analyzed in triplicate. Thermal cycler conditions were 95°C for 10 min, followed by 40 cycles at 95°C for 15 sec and 60°C for 1 min. The comparative threshold cycle ($C_T$) method was used to analyze the data. The $C_T$ is the PCR cycle at which an increase in reporter fluorescence above the baseline level is first detected. The target gene $C_T$ and internal reference gene $C_T$ were calculated for each sample. $\Delta C_T$ is the difference in $C_T$ between target gene and reference gene. $\Delta\Delta C_T$ is the difference in $\Delta C_T$ between sample and calibrator sample. The expression level of target gene, normalized to an internal reference and relative to a calibrator, was given by $2^{-\Delta\Delta CT}$.

### *Section 7. Statistical Analysis*

The daily running activity, weekly food consumption, BW, and body temperature were analyzed using the Student's *t*-test. Comparisons were made between the groups before and after treatment using one-way analysis of variance (ANOVA). CW/BW and expression levels of Bcl-2 and BDNF mRNA were also assessed using one-way ANOVA. If a significant difference was found between the items of a specific factor, multiple comparison was made using the Bonferroni test in order to identify which items differed significantly from each other. A significance level of $P$ <0.05 was used.

## Part 3. Results

### *Section 1. Running Activity, Food Consumption, Body Temperature, Body Weight, and Number of Surviving Mice*

While the control mice were active, CFS model mice were sluggish with fluffy fur and became active after treatment with TJ-41 (Figure 4. A–C). The daily running activity at baseline and before and after treatment in the three groups is shown in Figure 5. The running activity was not significantly different between the groups at baseline and significantly decreased from the baseline level in mice after six injections of BA antigen, demonstrating that fatigue was induced. No difference was observed between the model and TJ-41 groups before treatment, but there were differences between the three groups after treatment ($P$=11.702, $P$=0.003). The daily running activity was significantly increased in the TJ-41 group and higher than that in the model group ($P$=0.011) but not significantly different from that in the normal control group.

At baseline and before and after treatment, no differences were observed between the three groups in the weekly food consumption or body temperature (Figs. 6 and 7). BW was significantly different between the three groups after treatment ($F$=7.200, $P$=0.009) but not at baseline or before treatment, and significantly lower in the normal control group than in the TJ-41 group after treatment ($P$=0.008, Figure 8).

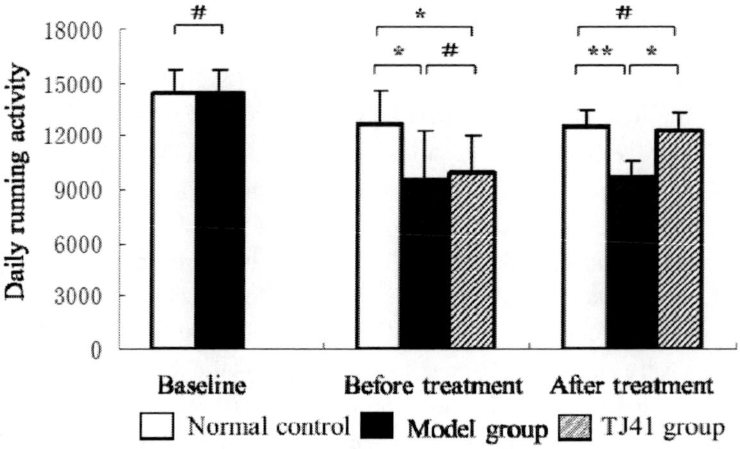


Figure 5. Daily running activity of the three groups at baseline, and before and after treatment.
At baseline, no significant difference was indicated between the daily running activity of each group. After six repeated injections of B. abortus antigen, a significant decrease was observed in the model mice, as compared with the baseline levels. No difference existed between the model and TJ-41 groups before treatment. After treatment, daily running activity in the model group was significantly lower than that in the normal control and TJ-41 groups, while no significant difference was shown between these two groups. Data are shown as mean ± SD. *P < 0.05, **P < 0.01 and #$P$ > 0.05.

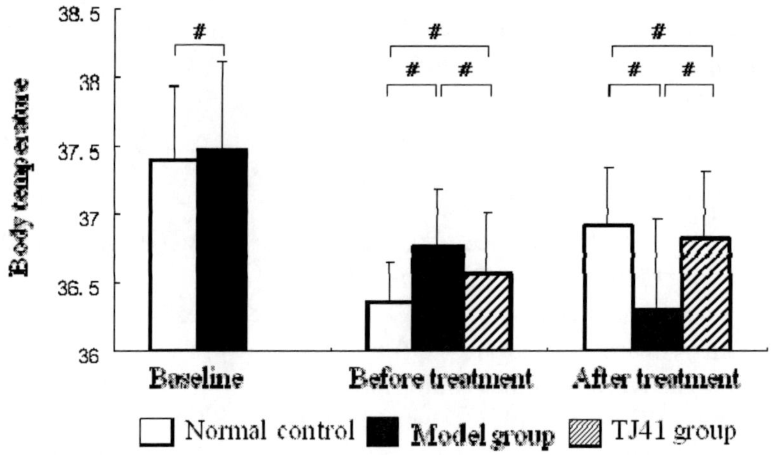


Figure 6. Body temperature of the three groups at baseline, and before and after treatment.
No significant difference was observed between the three groups at baseline, and before and after treatment. Data are shown as means ± SD. #$P$ > 0.05.

During the model-construction period, 5 mice died, all on the day after injection of BA antigen (1, 1, and 3 animals after the 3rd, 4th, and 6th injection, respectively). The number of animals before treatment was 6, 5, and 5 in the normal control, model, and TJ-41 groups, respectively. One animal died due to dehydration during the treatment period, but all animals in the other two groups survived.

### *Section 2. Body Weight-normalized CW*

Significant differences were observed in CW/BW ratio between the three groups ($F$=12.614, $P$=0.001). CW/BW was significantly lower in the model and TJ-41 groups than in the normal control group ($P$=0.001 and $P$=0.020), but similar in the model and TJ-41 groups (Figure 9).

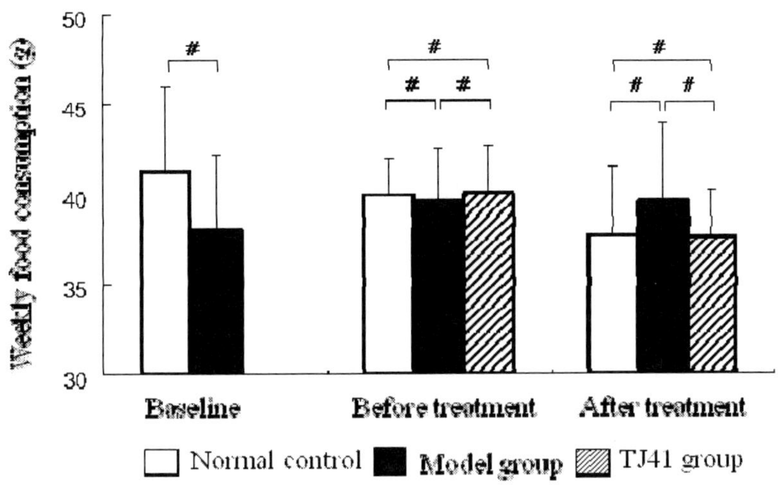


Figure 7. Weekly food consumption of the three groups at baseline, and before and after treatment.
No significant difference was observed between the groups at baseline, and before and after treatment. Data are shown as means ± SD. #$P$ > 0.05.

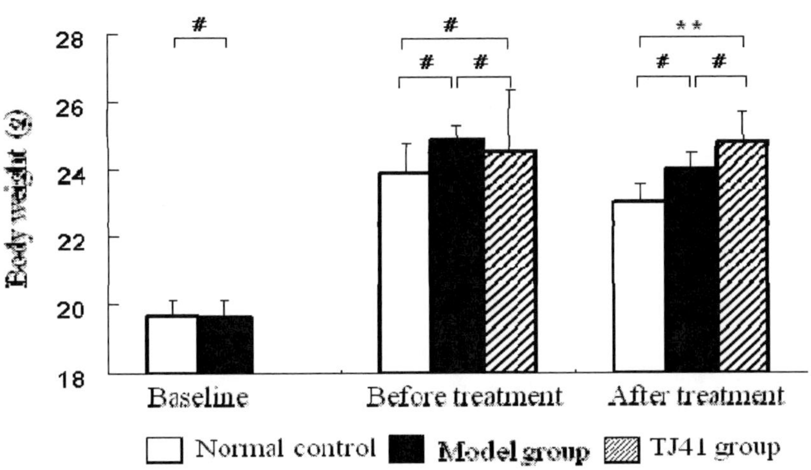


Figure 8. BW of the three groups at baseline, and before and after treatment.
No significant difference existed between the groups at baseline. On the other hand, before treatment, BW in the normal control group was significantly lower than that in the other two groups; and after treatment, the difference became more marked between the normal control and TJ-41 groups. Data are shown as means ± SD. **$P$ < 0.01 and #$P$ > 0.05.

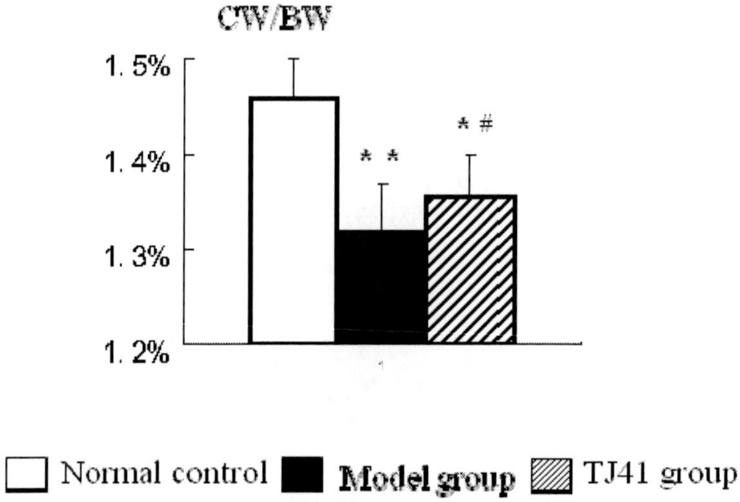


Figure 9. CW normalized by BW.
Data are shown as means ± SD. $*P < 0.05$, $**P < 0.01$ vs. normal control group, and $\#P > 0.05$ vs. model group.

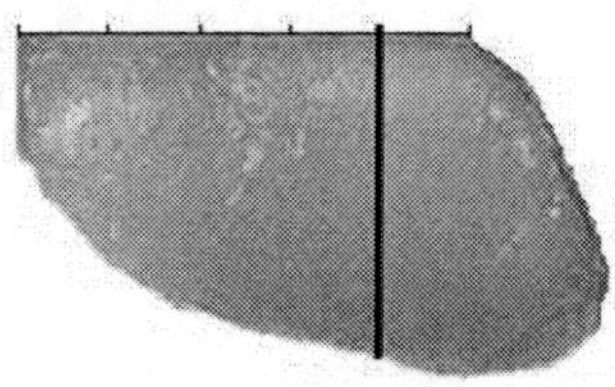

A

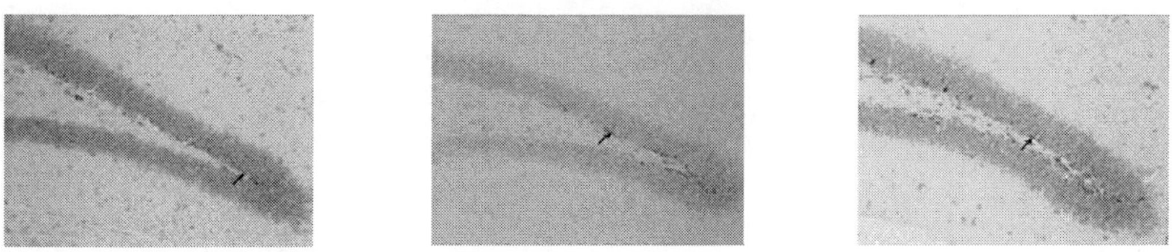

B C D

Figure 10A. Histological findings in the hippocampus of mice in each group.
A shows the slice-cutting line. The quintile point close to the cerebellum was chosen as the slice-cutting line. The thickness of the section was 4 μm along the direction from the cutting line to the olfactory bulb. B–D display the granule cells in the dentate gyrus of the hippocampus.

### *Section 3. Hippocampal Histological Findings*

There were more dead hippocampal granule and pyramidal cells in the model and TJ-41 groups than in the normal control group (Figure 10). Dead cells were primarily found in the dentate gyrus and dentate hilus. There were more dead cells in the CA region, especially in the CA3 region.

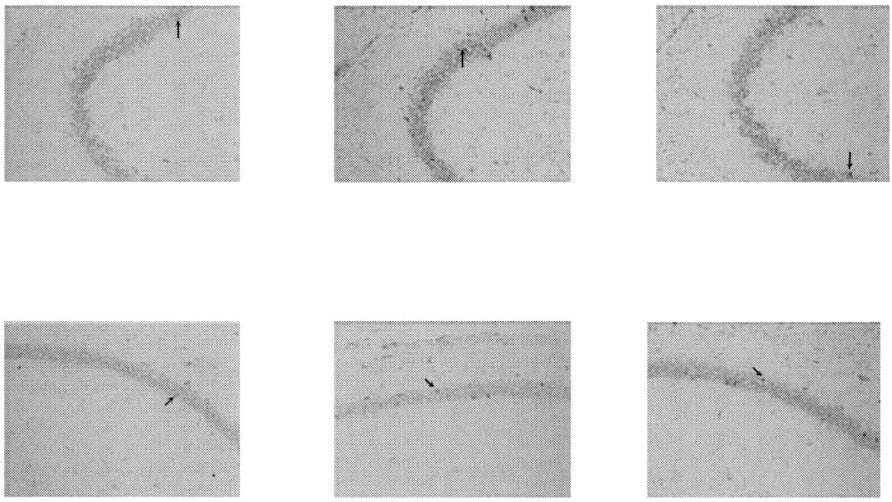

Figure 10B. Histological findings in the hippocampus of mice in each group. E–J show the pyramidal cells in the CA3–CA1 regions of the hippocampus. B, E, and H were from a normal control mouse; C, F, and I were from a model mouse; and D, G, and J were from a TJ-41-treated mouse. There were more dead granule cells and pyramidal cells in C, D, F, G, I, and J than in B, E, and H. Each black arrow points to a dead cell.

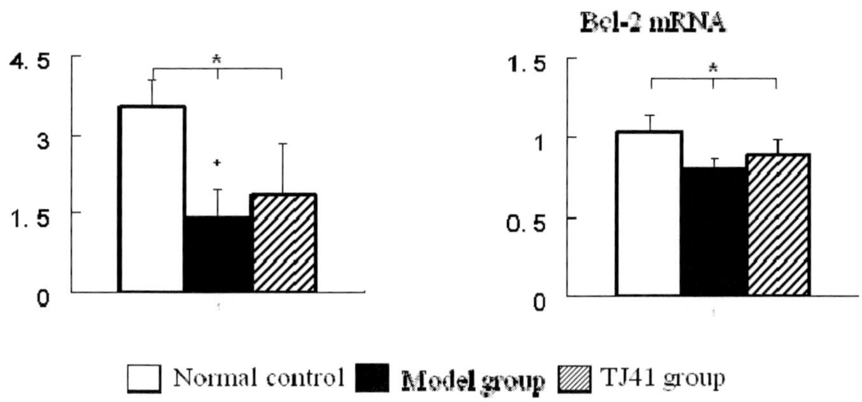


Figure 11. (A) Expression of BDNF mRNA in the hippocampus. Data are shown as means±SD. $+P > 0.05$ vs. normal control group and $*P < 0.05$ between the three groups. (B) Expression of Bcl-2 mRNA in the hippocampus. Data are shown as means±SD. $*P < 0.05$ between the three groups.

### *Section 4. Expression of BDNF and Bcl-2 mRNA in the Hippocampus*

Figure 11 compares the hippocampal expressions of BDNF and Bcl-2 mRNA between the groups and shows there were between-group differences (BDNF: $F$=7.701, $P$=0.022; Bcl-2: $F$=5.300, $P$=0.047). In multiple comparison, the BDNF mRNA level was significantly lower in the model group than in the normal control group ($P$=0.030), whereas the Bcl-2 mRNA level tended to be lower in the model group than in the normal control group ($P$=0.054). In the TJ-41 group, the expression level of neither BDNF nor Bcl-2 mRNA was significantly different from that in the other two groups.

## Part 4. Discussion

This study demonstrated that the daily running activity, CW/BW, and hippocampal expression of BDNF and Bcl-2 mRNA were decreased in BALB/c mice after six injections of *Brucella abortus* antigen. TJ-41 increased the daily running activity, but not CW/BW or hippocampal expression of BDNF or Bcl-2 mRNA. Many patients with CFS have a history of infections that act as a trigger, including colds, influenza-like illness, and infectious mononucleosis [57]. CFS-related pathogens include viruses [73], *Coxiella burnettii* [74], and other bacteria [75]. Therefore, post-viral fatigue syndrome is a useful model to investigate one of potential pathophysiological pathways of CFS [76]. In a previous study in 21 patients with chronic brucellosis, [77] 17 subjects had chronic disease, and no subject had a history of acute episode of brucellosis. The most common symptoms were fatigue, depressed state, joint pain, and muscle pain. Most subjects had already received psychiatric treatment, and laboratory test results were mostly negative. However, lymphadenoma was observed in 9 subjects. These clinical symptoms indicate that BA antigen-induced fatigue in the present study can serve as a model of CFS. In the mouse model of CFS in Chapter 1, CFS was induced using the method described by Ottenweller. However, the running activity was decreased for only 2 to 3 weeks after the first or second injection of BA antigen and recovered thereafter. The author successfully modified the model by administering six injections of BA antigen (one injection every 2 weeks). It was previously shown that the running activity decreased gradually over the period of mouse model construction, and the decrease was still notable 2 weeks after the sixth injection of antigen [71]. In addition, a gradual increase in spleen weight/BW, changes in Th1 and Th2 cytokine levels, and decreased NK cell activity were consistent with changes associated with CFS [71, 78]. Therefore, BALB/c mice injected six times with BA antigen resulting in decreased voluntary running activity may be regarded as a more stable animal model of CFS.

Five mice died on the day after injection of BA antigen, probably due to an acute immune response. As is the case with Q fever, the acute phase is associated with a fatality rate of 1% to 2%, and the chronic phase is associated with persistent sequelae of CFS [74]. In addition, the model group and control group had similar body temperature, which is inconsistent with the slight fever exhibited by patients with CFS. However, a previous study showed that subnormal body temperature and slight fever were frequently self-reported by patients with CFS, despite normal core body temperature [29].

The CNS plays an important role in the pathophysiology of CFS, as demonstrated by neuroimaging. The absolute cortical blood flow was found to be decreased in the right and left middle cerebral artery territories in patients with CFS as compared with healthy controls [30] and the global gray matter volume was found to be markedly decreased [79]. An association between subjective feelings of fatigue and brain responses was shown by functional magnetic resonance imaging [31]. Nonetheless, few studies have been conducted to establish the mechanism of the abovementioned brain changes in CFS. Since a significant decrease in CW in the mouse model of CFS constructed by the author was consistent with the abovementioned clinical data, a post hoc analysis was required to investigate the mechanism of brain atrophy for the first time.

In this mouse model, hippocampal Bcl-2 mRNA expression was decreased. Bcl-2 is an important regulator of programmed cell death in the development of the CNS and plays an important role in adult hippocampal neurogenesis [80]. Hippocampal Bcl-2 expression may be involved in emotional learning and memory [81] and has been used to measure the efficacy of tranquilizers such as lithium and valproic acid [82]. Decreased hippocampal Bcl-2 expression may result in neuron apoptosis [83], which, in turn, causes hippocampal nerve dysfunction. A previous study showed that hippocampal dysfunction was associated with major symptoms of CFS including neurasthenic fatigue [84], sleep disorder [85], and cognitive abnormality [86]. In the present study, the running activity and hippocampal Bcl-2 mRNA expression were decreased in the mouse CFS model, but sleep disorder and cognitive abnormality were not assessed.

The cause of decreased hippocampal Bcl-2 mRNA expression in CFS mice is another unresolved question. Peng et al. reported that small interfering RNA might significantly decrease the Bcl-2 protein level in hippocampus-derived neural stem cells by inhibiting BDNF expression [87]. The author showed that hippocampal BDNF mRNA expression in the mouse CFS model was significantly decreased, which is probably a cause of decreased Bcl-2 mRNA expression.

In previous studies, decreased BDNF levels were often connected with major symptoms of CFS. Exercise-induced neurogenesis is seen simultaneously with increased BDNF levels [43, 88-91], suggesting that BDNF may be involved in exercise and neurogenesis. Yasuhara et al. [43] recently showed that hindlimb suspension (a model of disuse) resulted in decreased hippocampal BDNF because of lack of exercise. In the present study, hippocampal BDNF expression was decreased in the mouse model of CFS, supporting the findings by Yasuhara. In addition, the author reviewed several reports about the relationship of BDNF with other features of CFS including depressed state, anxiety, cognitive disorder, pain, and sleep disorder, and found that depressed state and anxiety may result in decreased hippocampal BDNF mRNA expression [69]. In one study, rats with the lowest learning efficiency had the lowest hippocampal BDNF level, suggesting an effect of decreased cognitive function on BDNF level [92]. BDNF also locally plays an important role in the etiology of neurogenic pain secondary to peripheral nerve damage [93] and chronic pain in patients with fibromyalgia syndrome [45]. Hippocampal BDNF expression was decreased in sleep-deprived rats [94], indicating that major symptoms of CFS may result in decreased hippocampal BDNF mRNA expression.

As mentioned above, TJ-41 effectively reduced fatigue as reflected by the change in running activity in the mouse model of CFS, supporting the results in Chapter 1. However, TJ-41 did not change CW/BW or increase hippocampal expression of BDNF or Bcl-2 mRNA. Taken together with the results in Chapter 1, these findings suggest that the effect of TJ-41 on fatigue may be immunoregulatory. In addition, Astragalus root (*ogi*), Atractylodes lancea rhizome (*sojutsu*), and ginseng (*ninjin*), main components of TJ-41, effectively prevent nitric oxide-induced damage in the rat brain [95]. Shih et al. [96] showed that TJ-41 increased dopamine and noradrenaline in the cortical tissue and improved endurance, learning, and memory in mice at a dose of 500 mg/kg/day, indicating that TJ-41 can penetrate the blood-brain barrier. Therefore, the mechanism of action of TJ-41 in the treatment of CFS is not only related to increased hippocampal BDNF and Bcl-2, but also to its ability to penetrate the blood-brain barrier.

### Part 5. Conclusion

A new mouse model of chronic fatigue syndrome was established and used to investigate the relationship between brain dysfunction and CFS. Decreased daily activity was found to be related to decreased hippocampal BDNF mRNA expression, which may be a cause of hippocampal apoptosis and brain atrophy.

# Chapter 4. Evaluation of NK Cell Activity and Neuronal Protection after Combined Treatment with Hochuekkito and Interferon-Gamma

### Part 1. Introduction

CFS is defined as debilitating fatigue that persists for at least 6 months and is accompanied by various symptoms including neurocognitive symptoms, muscle pain, and joint pain [18]. The etiology of CFS was recently linked to infectious factors that impair immune function and CNS [97]. In particular, chronic activation of the immune response (predominantly the type 2 immune response) primarily reflects a decline in natural killer (NK) cell activity and abnormal regulation of cytokine production [98]. Neuroimaging findings suggest that the total hippocampal volume [29] and metabolism in hippocampal nerve cells/glial cells [99] are decreased in patients with CFS as compared with healthy controls.

As mentioned above, TJ-41 suppressed the marked decrease in the running activity but had no effect on hippocampal atrophy or decreased hippocampal expression of BDNF or Bcl-2 mRNA [71]. A recent study of cytokine gene polymorphism showed that the *IFNγ* gene was significantly decreased in patients with CFS [100], and another study reported that IFNγ protects hippocampal nerves [101], suggesting that combining TJ-41 with IFNγ may be more effective for CFS than TJ-41 alone. Therefore, an experiment was conducted using a modified mouse model of CFS to determine whether TJ-41 plus IFNγ could improve not only the daily running activity, but also immune system function and CNS function more effectively than TJ-41 alone.

### Part 2. Experimental Materials and Methods

#### *Mice and Experimental Conditions*

See Part 2 of Chapter 1.

#### *Induction of CFS by Brucella Abortus Antigen*

See Part 2 of Chapter 3.

#### *Drugs Used*

TJ-41 (24 g) was extracted with 600 mL of water at 100°C for 1 h. The decoction was filtered and then lyophilized. The yield of the resulting powdered extract was 8.84 g. Before administration, this product was dissolved in distilled water and diluted with water to the appropriate concentration. IFNγ (Shionogi & Co., Ltd., Osaka, Japan) was dissolved in physiological saline and diluted with saline to the appropriate concentration.

### *Administration of Test Solution*

The experimental design is shown in Figure 12. Twenty BALB/c mice were randomly assigned to three groups: the CFS model group ($n$=7), TJ-41 group ($n$=6), and TI group ($n$=7). During the 12-week model-construction period, 2, 1, and 2 mice in the model, TJ-41, and TI groups died, respectively. The animals in the TJ-41 and TI groups received TJ-41 at a dose of 500 mg/kg (0.1 mL) once daily for 4 weeks via a feeding needle inserted into the throat. At the same time, 0.1 mL of physiological saline was intraperitoneally administered to the animals in the TJ-41 group, and 0.1 mL of IFNγ (8.5 million U/kg) was intraperitoneally administered to those in the TI group. The animals in the model group received 0.1 mL of distilled water orally and 0.1 mL of physiological saline intraperitoneally.

### *Running Activity, Body Weight, Food Consumption, Body Temperature, and Number of Surviving Mice*

After the mice were acclimated to the environment for 2 weeks, measurement of their running activity was initiated. The daily running activity was recorded during the 12-week model-construction period and the following 4-week treatment period. For all mice, BW, food consumption, and body temperature were measured every week from the start to the completion of the experiment.

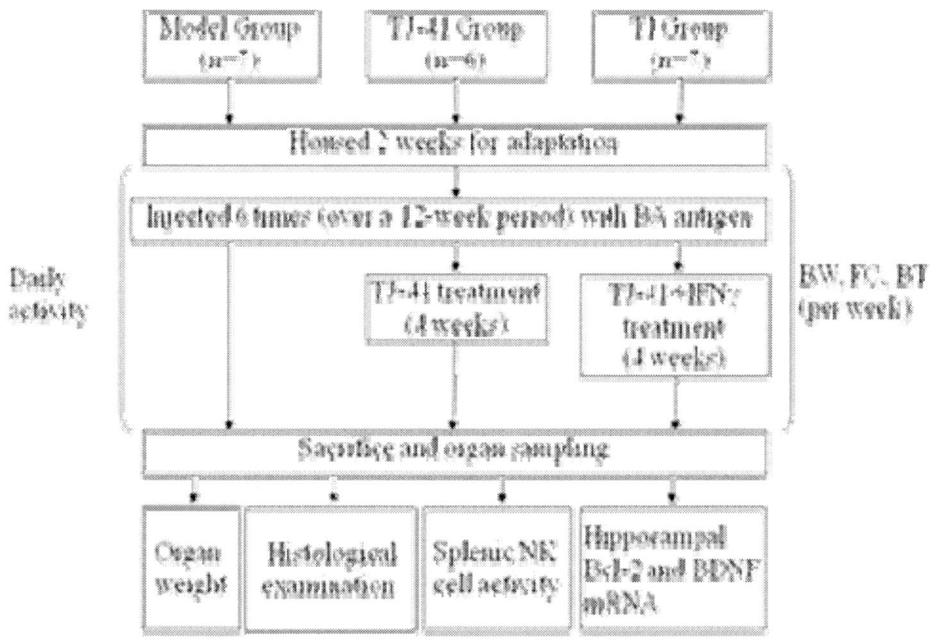


Figure 12. The sketch of the experimental design. TI, hochuekkito combined with interferon γ. Abbreviations: BW, body weight; FC, food consumption; BT, body temperature; BDNF, brain-derived neurotrophic factor; Bcl-2, B cell lymphoma-2.

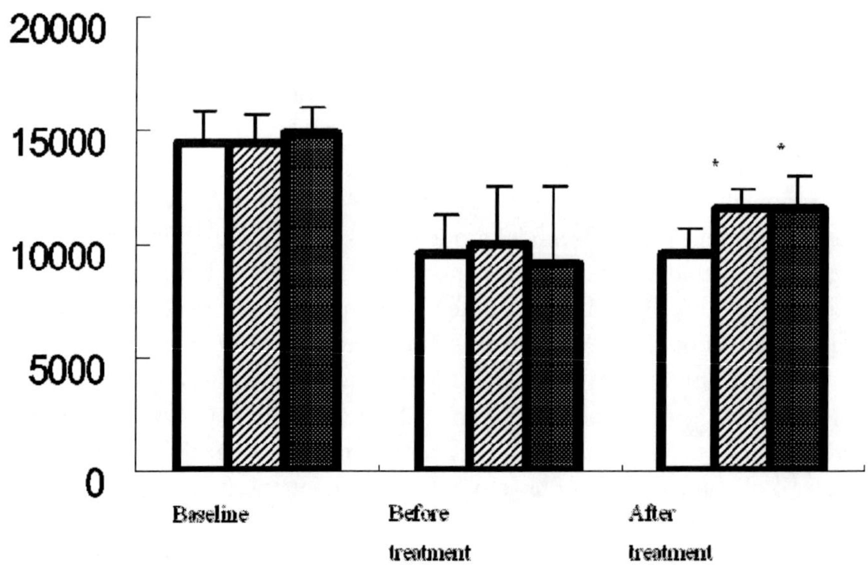


Figure 13. The daily running activity of the three groups at the baseline, before and after the treatment. Data are shown as Mean + SD. * $P < 0.05$ as compared with that of model group after the treatment.

### *Organ Weights and Pathological Examination of Brain, Spleen, and Thymus*

All mice were killed by cervical dislocation 4 weeks after the start of treatment. At the time of sacrifice, the ratio of cerebrum weight (CW) (mg) to BW (g) (CW/BW), ratio of spleen weight (SW) (mg) to BW (SW/BW), and ratio of thymus weight (TW) (mg) to BW (TW/BW) were assessed. For each group, half of the cerebrum and thymus from all animals and half of the spleen from 2 animals were fixed in 10% buffered formalin and processed for hematoxylin and eosin staining. The hippocampus was removed from the other half of the cerebrum and immediately frozen in liquid nitrogen or on a dry ice-cooled plate before being stored at –80°C for analysis of related gene expression. In addition, the splenic follicular area and thymic medullary area were measured and expressed as percentages of the total splenic or thymic area in the long-axis sections [9]. The splenic follicular area and thymic medullary area were also measured in 5 normal female BALB/c mice of the same age.

### *NK Cell Activity*

For each group, the spleen was removed from three animals, and the NK cell activity was measured using a $^{51}$Cr-release assay as reported by Morita [102].

### *Expression Levels of BDNF and Bcl-2 mRNA in the Hippocampus*

RNA extraction from each frozen hippocampus was performed as described by the manufacturer (RNeasy Mini Kit, QIAGEN Inc., Tokyo, Japan) and in Section 6 Real-time PCR (above).

### *Statistical Analysis*

The daily running activity before treatment was compared with that at baseline using Student's *t*-test. The daily running activity, food consumption, BW, and body temperature were compared between the groups before and after treatment using one-way analysis of variance (ANOVA). Between-group differences in CW/BW, SW/BW, TW/BW, splenic follicular area (%), thymic medullary area (%), and levels of BDNF and Bcl-2 mRNA were also assessed using one-way ANOVA. If a significant difference was found, post hoc multiple comparison analyses were performed using the Bonferroni test. A significance level of $P$ <0.05 was used.

## Part 3. Results

### *Section 1. Running Activity, Food Consumption, Body Temperature, Body Weight, and Number of Surviving Mice*

The daily running activity at baseline and before and after treatment in the three groups is shown in Figure 13. The running activity at baseline and before treatment was not significantly different between the groups and was significantly decreased from the baseline level after six injections of BA antigen. After treatment, the daily activity was significantly lower in the CFS model group than in the TJ-41 and TI groups but similar between the TJ-41 and TI groups. At baseline and before and after treatment, no differences were observed between the three groups in the weekly food consumption, body temperature, or body weight.

During the 12-week model-construction period, 5 mice died primarily from administration of BA. As a result, the number of animals per group before treatment was 5. After treatment, 1 animal in the model group died due to dehydration, but all animals in the other two groups survived until sacrifice.

**Table 3. Effect of hochuekkito combined with IFNγ on body weight and weight of organs including cerebrum, spleen, and thymus at the time of sacrifice**

| | BW (g) | TW (mg) | SW (mg) | CW (mg) |
|---|---|---|---|---|
| Model group** | 24.0±0.5 | 24.3±4.6 | 168.5±19.4 | 325.8±9.9 |
| | | (1.0±0.1) | (7.0±0.7) | (13.6±0.2) |
| TJ-41 group | 24.8±0.9 | 31.2±4.0* | 139.8±25.1* | 326.2±18.5 |
| | | (1.3±0.1*) | (5.6±0.8) * | (13.2±0.5) |
| TI group | 24.7±1.5 | 32.8±3.4* | 155.2±29.1 | 325.2±13.7 |
| | | (1.3±0.1*) | (6.3±1.4) | (13.2±0.6) |

Data are expressed as means ± SD.

Abbreviaitions: BW, body weight; TW, thymus weight; SW, spleen weight; CW, cerebrum weight. Parentheses show ratio of each organ weight to body weight (mg/g). *P < 0.05 compared with that in the model group. **One mouse died during the treatment.

### *Section 2. Organ Weights and Pathological Examination of Brain, Spleen, and Thymus*

CW/BW was lower in the TJ-41 and TI groups than in the model group, but not significantly lower. The mean thymus weight was markedly lower in the model group than in the TJ-41 or TI group ($P$ < 0.05) but similar in the TJ-41 and TI groups. The mean spleen weight was significantly lower in the TJ-41 group than in the model group ($P$ < 0.05), but no significant difference was observed between the TI and model groups (Table 3).

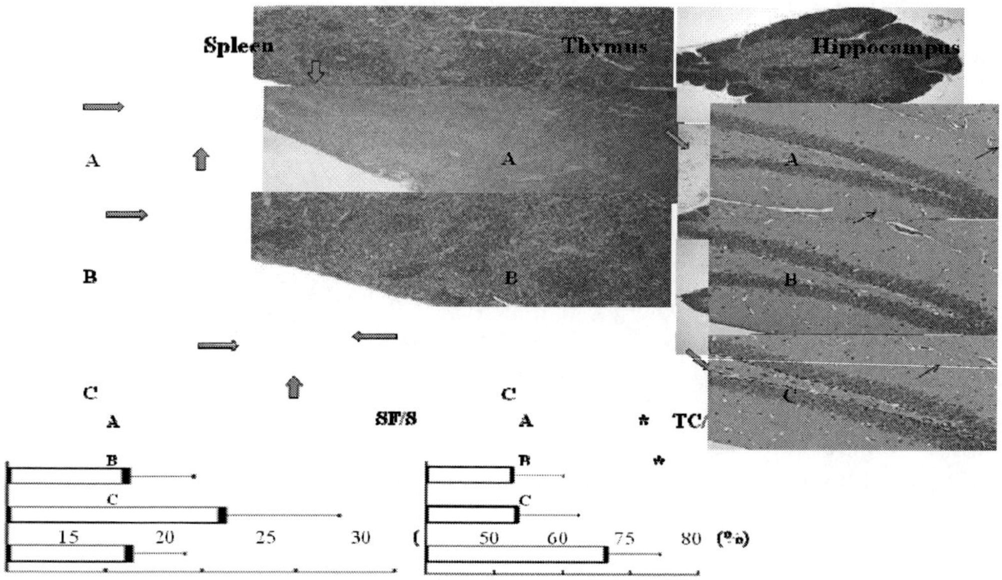


Figure 14. The pathological examination of the spleen, thymus, and dentate gyrus of the hippocampus and the percent of follicular area and cortex area in the spleen and thymus in the three groups. A, B, and C indicate the model, TJ-41 and TI group, respectively. SF/S and TC/T means the percent of follicular area and cortex area in the spleen and thymus, respectively. Data are shown as mean + SD. * $P < 0.05$ as compared with that of TI group. Hollow arrows show the follicular area in the spleen. Black arrows show the dead or granulovacuolar degenerated.

In normal female BALB/c mice of the same age, the percent splenic follicular area and percent thymic cortex area were 31.3 ± 6.7 and 82.9 ± 9.1, respectively. The percent splenic lymph follicular area was significantly lower in the TI (21.2 ± 3.2) and model (21.0 ± 3.6) groups than normal group ($P < 0.05$) but similar in the TJ-41 group (26.2 ± 6.0) and normal group (31.3 ± 6.7) ($P > 0.05$). As shown in Figure 13, the percent splenic follicular area was lower in the TI and model groups than in the TJ-41 group, but the difference between the three groups was not significant. The percent thymic cortex area was higher in the TI group (76.5.9 ± 7.8) than in the TJ-41 (63.3 ± 9.1) or model (62.6 ± 7.5) group (each $P < 0.05$).

As shown in Figure 14, more dead neurons or more granulovacuolar degeneration of neurons were found in the hippocampal dentate gyrus in the TI group than in the other two groups. However, no conclusion could be drawn on the difference from these images because they were not at the same slice level.

### *Section 3. NK Cell Activity*

The NK cell activity was significantly increased in the TI group than the model or TJ-41 group (5.6 ± 1.2 % vs. 1.4 ± 0.2 % or 2.6 ± 0.4 %, each $P < 0.05$) but not significantly different between the TJ-41 and model groups (Figure 15).

### *Section 4. Expression Levels of BDNF and Bcl-2 mRNA in the Hippocampus*

A between-groups comparison of Bcl-2 and BDNF mRNA levels in the hippocampus is shown in Figs. 16 A and C, respectively. No among-group differences in the mRNA levels of these two genes were significant (Bcl-2: 0.80 ± 0.06, 0.89 ± 0.10, 1.10 ± 0.35, respectively, *P* > 0.05; BDNF: 1.42 ± 0.52, 1.86 ± 0.97, 1.76 ± 0.81, respectively, *P* > 0.05).

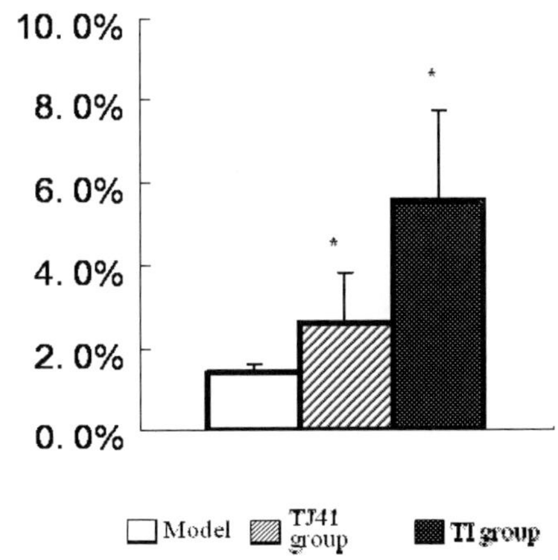


Figure 15. NK cell activity in the spleen in three groups.
Data are shown as mean + SD. * P < 0.05 as compared with that of TI group.

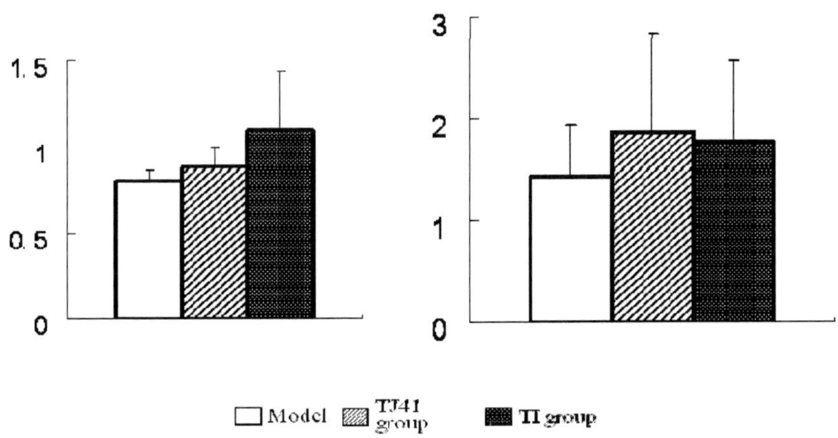


Figure 16. The expression level of Bcl-2 and BDNF mRNA in the hippocampus.
Data are shown as mean + SD.

## Part 4. Discussion

This study demonstrated that combined treatment with TJ-41 and IFNγ could moderately increase the daily activity in mice with CFS. Combined treatment compared with treatment with TJ-41 alone resulted in greater increase in splenic NK cell activity and thickness of thymic cortex. However, combined treatment and TJ-41 monotherapy had a similar effect on daily activity and no effect on CW or hippocampal expression of Bcl-2 or BDNF mRNA.

Imbalance of Thl/Th2-type cytokines has a very important role in the immunopathogenesis of CFS [103]. One of the main reasons for this imbalance is the reduction of NK cell activity [73]. NK cells play a key role in mediating Th1 polarization via secretion of high levels of IFNγ, and reduction in their activity results in a Th2 bias [74]. As mentioned above, combined treatment with TJ-41 and IFNγ resulted in increased splenic NK cell activity, which may be beneficial for restoring Th1/Th2- cytokines balance.

In addition, the thickness of thymic cortex was increased in the combined treatment group, but not in the TJ-41 monotherapy group. It has been reported that IFNγ itself has no effect *in vivo* or *in vitro* on thymocytes [75]. Hence, the thickening of the thymic cortex may be due to the combined effect of TJ-41 and IFNγ. On the other hand, there was no difference in the thickness of the splenic follicular area between the combined therapy group and monotherapy group, suggesting that measurement of the thickness of thymic cortex may be a useful indicator of improvement in immunostimulation during the treatment in this model.

The CNS plays a prominent role in the pathophysiology of CFS, as demonstrated by lines of evidence from neuroimaging and neuropathology. The results of functional magnetic resonance imaging show an association between subjective feelings of fatigue and brain responses in CFS patients [31]. BDNF is a member of the neurotrophin family and possesses the property of neuroprotection [108]. A recent study indicated that decreased BDNF expression associated with major symptoms of CFS (such as stress and depressed state) and might result in hippocampal atrophy and cell loss [42]. Bcl-2 is a crucial regulator for apoptosis and also plays an important role in adult hippocampal neurogenesis [80]. Decreased hippocampal expression of Bcl-2 is associated with neuron apoptosis and hippocampal dysfunction [83]. Hippocampal dysfunction is associated with major symptoms of CFS [86], and neuroprotection, especially hippocampal neuroprotection, is very important in the treatment of CFS.

In a study by Shih et al. [96], TJ-41 (500 mg/kg/day) increased the production of dopamine and noradrenaline in cortical tissues and improved endurance, learning, and memory in mice, suggesting that TJ-41 can penetrate the blood-brain barrier and may be beneficial for the treatment of CFS. The main components of TJ-41, Astragalus root (*ogi*), Atractylodes lancea rhizome (*sojutsu*), ginseng (*ninjin*), , are said to protect neurons by preventing oxidative injury. As described in Chapter 3, however, no significant changes were observed in CW/BW or hippocampal expression of Bcl-2 or BDNF mRNA in TJ-41-treated mice. IFNγ has also been reported to protect hippocampal neurons. *In vitro*, pretreatment of embryonic rat hippocampal cell cultures with IFNγ protected neurons from glutamate-induced death [101]. In IFNγ-knockout mice, moreover, a greater number of apoptotic cells in the brain was correlated with lower Bcl-2 expression [111]. In the present study, nevertheless, combined treatment had no beneficial effect on brain weight or hippocampal expression of Bcl-2 or BDNF mRNA, indicating that the mechanism of action of TJ-41 or IFNγ in treating CFS is not related to neuroprotection. Further studies are required to elucidate the interaction between the main components of TJ-41 and IFNγ.

## Part 5. Conclusion

Combined treatment with TJ-41 and IFNγ helped restore daily activity in the mouse model of CFS, but its efficacy in this respect was not superior to that of TJ-41 monotherapy. Nonetheless, the results indicate that combined treatment (more than monotherapy) increases the splenic NK cell activity and promotes some adaptive immune responses in the thymus. However, neither therapy could improve CFS pathogenesis in the CNS.

# Overall Conclusion

The experiments were designed to apply the technology of modern science (the foundation of modern Western medicine) to clarify the pharmacological effects of Kampo medicines known to be clinically efficacious. Chronic fatigue syndrome (CFS), a multifactorial disease of unknown etiology, was selected because it can be treated with Kampo medicine. Kampo medicines could potentially serve as complementary medicines to improve the efficacy and compensate for the weakness of modern medicines. CFS treatment is a challenge to modern medicine.

In this paper, the efficacy of hochuekkito (補中益気湯; TJ-41; ethical Kampo extract formulation manufactured by Tsumura & Co., Ltd.) for improving exercise capacity in a mouse model of CFS was evaluated as described in Chapter 1. CFS was induced by two BA antigen injections separated by an interval of 2 weeks. TJ-41 (500 mg/kg) was orally administered once daily for 4 weeks starting at 1 week before administration of BA. The daily running activity was significantly higher, body weight (BW), spleen weight (SW) and SW/BW were significantly lower, and splenic expression of IL-10 mRNA was suppressed in the TJ-41 group compared with the untreated group. These data suggest that hochuekkito may suppress the marked decrease in mouse running activity after injection of BA.

In Chapter 2, the effects of chronic fatigue syndrome on the central nervous system were discussed with a focus on the literature. Currently, many neuroimaging findings support the hypothesis that CFS stems from structural and/or functional abnormalities in the brain, and some neurotrophic factors, neurotransmitters, and cytokines have been assessed in order to explain abnormal neuropsychiatric findings in CFS. Therefore, the focus of CFS research should be on the CNS.

In Chapter 3, a study of the usefulness of hochuekkito as treatment for brain atrophy in a model of CFS (Balb/C mice injected six times with killed *Brucella abortus* antigen) was summarized. BDNF is related to major symptoms of CFS and neuron apoptosis, but no studies have directly investigated the relationship of CFS, BDNF, and neuron apoptosis. The daily running activity, BW, ratio of cerebrum weight to BW (CW/BW), and expression levels of BDNF and Bcl-2 mRNA in the hippocampus were assessed after treatment with TJ-41. The running activity and CW/BW were significantly decreased in the CFS model. Hippocampal expressions of BDNF and Bcl-2 mRNA were decreased in CFS model mice and TJ-41-treated mice with no significant difference between the two groups. The decreased daily running activity may have been related to decreased hippocampal expression of BDNF mRNA, hippocampal apoptosis, and brain atrophy. In the model, TJ-41 increased the daily running activity but had no effect on brain atrophy.

Finally in Chapter 4, the NK cell activity and neuroprotection as well as daily activity were evaluated after combined treatment with TJ-41 and IFNγ in the mouse model of CFS (constructed as described in Chapter 3). The running activity and thymus weight were increased in both the TJ-41 monotherapy group and TJ-41/IFNγ combined treatment group, whereas the thickness of thymic cortex and NK cell activity were increased only in the combined treatment group. Neither treatment affected hippocampal atrophy and decreased hippocampal expression of BDNF or Bcl-2 mRNA. These results suggest that combined treatment can restore activity via normalizing the host immune responses of CFS model mice but cannot protect neurons.

The relationship between BDNF and CFS pathology, which was studied by the author, has not been previously reported. Moreover, it was shown that the efficacy of the Kampo treatment for CFS, for which there is no established therapy, might be elucidated by analyzing changes in hippocampal expression of the BDNF precursor proBDNF and its promoter III as well as the BDNF receptor TrkB. A broader range of diseases involving BDNF decrease (depression, dementia) might be studied and new therapies for CFS consisting of Kampo medicines and immunotherapeutic agents (such as IFN) might be developed using this approach. In addition, it is suggested that such a therapy may be effective not only for CFS, but also for diseases with a similar brain pathology. Early social rehabilitation of patients with CFS, if achieved, can be expected to have positive economic effects and combined treatment can be expected to be cost-effective because herbal medicines are relatively inexpensive.

In the future, Kampo medicine and modern Western medicine will remain separate, but increasingly the former will function as a complement to Western medicine that compensates for its weaknesses. It is therefore important to apply modern science to the clarification of the pharmacological effects of Kampo medicine.

## References

[1] Eisenberg DM, Kessler RC, Foster C, Norlock FE, Calkins DR, Delbanco TL. Unconventional medicine in the United States. Prevalence, costs, and patterns of use. *N Engl J Med.* 1993;328:246–252.

[2] Motoo Y, Tsutani K. Is it Possible to Develop Global Clinical Practice Guidelines for Traditional Medicine?. Kampo Med. 2006;57:465–475.

[3] Kanda T, Yamakawa J, Moriya J, Saegusa S, Kawaura K, Yu F, et al. *J Kanazawa Med Univ.* 2005;30:297–301.

[4] Yu F, Takahashi T, Moriya J, Kawaura K, Yamakawa J, Kusaka K, et al. Traditional Chinese Medicine and Kampo: A Review from the Distant Past for the Future. *J Int Med Res.* 2006;34:231–239.

[5] Chen MK. The epidemiology of self-perceived fatigue among adults. *Prev Med.* 1986;15:74–81.

[6] Bates DW, Schmitt W, Buchwald D, Ware NC, Lee J, Thoyer E, et al. Prevalence of fatigue and chronic fatigue syndrome in a primary care practice. *Arch Intern Med.* 1993;153:2759–2765.

[7] Afari N, Buchwald D. Chronic fatigue syndrome: a review. *Am J Psychiatry.* 2003;160:221–236.

[8] Chao CC, DeLaHunt M, Hu S, Close K, Peterson PK. Immunologically mediated fatigue: a murine model. *Clin Immunol Immunopathol.* 1992;64:161–165.

[9] Ottenweller JE, Natelson BH, Gause WC, Carroll KK, Beldowicz D, Zhou XD, et al. Mouse running activity is lowered by Brucella abortus treatment: a potential model to study chronic fatigue. *Physiol Behav.* 1998;63:795–801.

[10] Svetić A, Jian YC, Lu P, Finkelman FD, Gause WC. Brucella abortus induces a novel cytokine gene expression pattern characterized by elevated IL-10 and IFN-gamma in CD4+ T cells. *Int Immunol.* 1993;5:877–883.

[11] Thomas KJ, Nicholl JP, Coleman P. Use and expenditure on complementary medicine in England: a population based survey. *Complement Ther Med.* 2001;9:2–11.

[12] Cho JM, Sato N, Kikuchi K. Prophylactic anti-tumor effect of Hochu-ekki-to (TJ41) by enhancing natural killer cell activity. *In vivo.* 1991;5:389–391.

[13] Kataoka T, Akagawa KS, Tokunaga T, Nagao S. Activation of macrophages with Hochu-ekkito. *Jpn J Cancer Chemother.* 1989;16:1490–1493.

[14] Mori K, Kido T, Daikuhara H, Sakakibara I, Sakata T, Shimizu K, et al. Effect of Hochu-ekki-to (TJ-41), a Japanese herbal medicine, on the survival of mice infected with influenza virus. *Antiviral Res.* 1999;44:103–111.

[15] Kido T, Mori K, Daikuhara H, Tsuchiya H, Ishige A, Sasaki H. The protective effect of hochu-ekki-to (TJ-41), a Japanese herbal medicine, against HSV-1 infection in mitomycin C-treated mice. *Anticancer Res.* 2000;20:4109–4114.

[16] Koshikawa N, Imai T, Takahashi I, Yamauchi M, Sawada S, Kansaku A. Effects of Hochu-ekki-to, Yoku-kan-san and Saiko-ka-ryukotsu-borei-to on behavioral despair and acetic acid-induced writhing in mice. *Methods Find Exp Clin Pharmacol.* 1998;20:47–51.

[17] Singh A, Naidu PS, Gupta S, Kulkarni SK. Effect of natural and synthetic antioxidants in a mouse model of chronic fatigue syndrome. *J Med Food.* 2002;5:211–220.

[18] Fukuda K, Straus SE, Hickie I, Sharpe MC, Dobbins JG, Komaroff A. The chronic fatigue syndrome: a comprehensive approach to its definition and study. International Chronic Fatigue Syndrome Study Group. *Ann Intern Med.* 1994;121:953–959.

[19] Lange G, Wang S, DeLuca J, Natelson BH. Neuroimaging in chronic fatigue syndrome. *Am J Med.* 1998;105:50S–53S.

[20] Yamamoto S, Ouchi Y, Onoe H, Yoshikawa E, Tsukada H, Takahashi H, et al. Reduction of serotonin transporters of patients with chronic fatigue syndrome. *Neuroreport.* 2004;15:2571–2574.

[21] Ichise M, Salit IE, Abbey SE, Chung DG, Gray B, Kirsh JC, et al. Assessment of regional cerebral perfusion by 99Tcm-HMPAO SPECT in chronic fatigue syndrome. *Nucl Med Commun.* 1992;13:767–772.

[22] Costa DC, Tannock C, Brostoff J. Brainstem perfusion is impaired in chronic fatigue syndrome. *QJM.* 1995;88:767–773.

[23] Tirelli U, Chierichetti F, Tavio M, Simonelli C, Bianchin G, Zanco P, et al. Brain positron emission tomography (PET) in chronic fatigue syndrome: preliminary data. *Am J Med.* 1998;105:54S–58S.

[24] Lange G, DeLuca J, Maldjian JA, Lee H, Tiersky LA, Natelson BH. Brain MRI abnormalities exist in a subset of patients with chronic fatigue syndrome. *J Neurol Sci.* 1999;171:3–7.

[25] Brooks JC, Roberts N, Whitehouse G, Majeed T. Proton magnetic resonance spectroscopy and morphometry of the hippocampus in chronic fatigue syndrome. *Br J Radiol.* 2000;73:1206–1208.

[26] Schmaling KB, Lewis DH, Fiedelak JI, Mahurin R, Buchwald DS. Single-photon emission computerized tomography and neurocognitive function in patients with chronic fatigue syndrome. *Psychosom Med.* 2003;65:129–136.

[27] Okada T, Tanaka M, Kuratsune H, Watanabe Y, Sadato N. Mechanisms underlying fatigue: a voxel-based morphometric study of chronic fatigue syndrome. *BMC Neurol.* 2004;4:14.

[28] Cleare AJ, Messa C, Rabiner EA, Grasby PM. Brain 5-HT1A receptor binding in chronic fatigue syndrome measured using positron emission tomography and [11C]WAY-100635. *Biol Psychiatry.* 2005;57:239–246.

[29] de Lange FP, Kalkman JS, Bleijenberg G, Hagoort P, van Der Meer JW, Toni I. Gray matter volume reduction in the chronic fatigue syndrome. *NeuroImage.* 2005;26:777–781.

[30] Yoshiuchi K, Farkas J, Natelson BH. Patients with chronic fatigue syndrome have reduced absolute cortical blood flow. *Clin Physiol Funct Imaging. 2006*;26:83–86.

[31] Cook DB, O'Connor PJ, Lange G, Steffener J. Functional neuroimaging correlates of mental fatigue induced by cognition among chronic fatigue syndrome patients and controls. *Neuroimage.* 2007;36:108–122.

[32] Schwartz RB, Garada BM, Komaroff AL, Tice HM, Gleit M, Jolesz FA, et al. Detection of intracranial abnormalities in patients with chronic fatigue syndrome: comparison of MR imaging and SPECT. *AJR Am J Roentgenol.* 1994;162:935–941.

[33] Lewis DH, Mayberg HS, Fischer ME, Goldberg J, Ashton S, Graham MM, et al. Monozygotic twins discordant for chronic fatigue syndrome: regional cerebral blood flow SPECT. *Radiology.* 2001;219:766–773.

[34] Natelson BH, Cohen JM, Brassloff I, Lee HJ. A controlled study of brain magnetic resonance imaging in patients with the chronic fatigue syndrome. *J Neurol Sci.* 1993;120:213–217.

[35] Poteliakhoff A. Adrenocortical activity and some clinical findings in acute and chronic fatigue. *J Psychosom Res.* 1981;25:91–95.

[36] Jerjes WK, Taylor NF, Wood PJ, Cleare AJ. Enhanced feedback sensitivity to prednisolone in chronic fatigue syndrome. *Psychoneuroendocrinology.* 2007;32:192–198.

[37] Jerjes WK, Taylor NF, Peters TJ, Wessely S, Cleare AJ. Urinary cortisol and cortisol metabolite excretion in chronic fatigue syndrome. *Psychosom Med.* 2006;68:578–582.

[38] Cleare AJ. The HPA axis and the genesis of chronic fatigue syndrome. *Trends Endocrinol Metab.* 2004;15:55–59.

[39] Barde YA, Edger D, Thoenen H. Purification of a new neurotrophic factor from mammalian brain. *EMBO J.* 1982;1:549–553.

[40] Tang SW, Chu E, Hui T, Helmeste D, Law C. Influence of exercise on serum brain-derived neurotrophic factor concentrations in healthy human subjects. *Neurosci Let.* 2008;431:62–65.

[41] Berchtold NC, Chinn G, Chou M, Kesslak JP, Cotman CW. Exercise primes a molecular memory for brain-derived neurotrophic factor protein induction in the rat hippocampus. *Neuroscience.* 2005;133:853–861.

[42] Martinowich K, Manji H, Lu B. New insights into BDNF function in depression and anxiety. *Nat Neurosci.* 2007;10:1089–1093.

[43] Wu A, Molteni R, Ying Z, Gomez-Pinilla F. A saturated-fat diet aggravates the outcome of traumatic brain injury on hippocampal plasticity and cognitive function by reducing brain-derived neurotrophic factor. *Neuroscience.* 2003;119:365–375.

[44] Pang PT, Teng HK, Zaitsev E, Woo NT, Sakata K, Zhen S, et al. Cleavage of proBDNF by tPA/plasmin is essential for long-term hippocampal plasticity. *Science.* 2004;306:487–491.
[45] Guzman-Marin R, Ying Z, Suntsova N, Methippara M, Bashir T,Szymusiak R, et al. Suppression of hippocampal plasticity-related gene expression by sleep deprivation in rats. *J Physiol.* 2006;575:807–819.
[46] Huang EJ, Reichardt LF. Trk receptors: roles in neuronal signal transduction. *Annu Rev Biochem.* 2000;72:609–642.
[47] Chen MJ, Nguyen TV, Pike CJ, Russo-Neustadt AA. Norepinephrine induces BDNF and activates the PI-3K and MAPK cascades in embryonic hippocampal neurons. *Cell Signal.* 2007;19:114–128.
[48] Kohara K, Kitamura A, Morishima M, Tsumoto T. Activity-dependent transfer of brain-derived neurotrophic factor to postsynaptic neurons. *Science.* 2001;291:2419–2423.
[49] Vaynman S, Ying Z, Gomez-Pinilla F. Interplay between brain-derived neurotrophic factor and signal transduction modulators in the regulation of the effects of exercise on synaptic-plasticity. *Neuroscience.* 2003;122:647–657.
[50] Chen MJ, Russo-Neustadt AA. Exercise activates the phosphatidylinositol 3-kinase pathway. *Brain Res Mol Brain Res.* 2005;135:181–193.
[51] Vasuta C, Caunt C, James R, Samadi S, Schibuk E, Kannangara T, et al. Effects of exercise on NMDA receptor subunit contributions to bidirectional synaptic plasticity in the mouse dentate gyrus. *Hippocampus.* 2007;17:1201–1208.
[52] Guan Z, Peng X, Fang J. Sleep deprivation impairs spatial memory and decreases extracellular signal-regulated kinase phosphorylation in the hippocampus. *Brain Res.* 2004;1018:38–47.
[53] Czarnecki A, Birtoli B, Ulrich D. Cellular mechanisms of burst firing-mediated long-term depression in rat neocortical pyramidal cells. *J Physiol.* 2007;578:471–479.
[54] Narita M, Nishigami N, Narita N, Yamaguti K, Okado N, Watanabe Y, et al. Association between serotonin transporter gene polymorphism and chronic fatigue syndrome. *Biochem Biophys Res Commun.* 2003;311:264–266.
[55] Katafuchi T, Kondo T, Take S, Yoshimura M. Brain cytokines and the 5-HT system during poly I:C-induced fatigue. *Ann N Y Acad Sci.* 2006;1088:230–237.
[56] Leonard BE. HPA and immune axes in stress: involvement of the serotonergic system. *Neuroimmunomodulation.* 2006;13:268–276.
[57] Prins JB, van der Meer JW, Bleijenberg G. Chronic fatigue syndrome. *Lancet.* 2006;367:346–355.
[58] Dantzer R, O'Connor JC, Freund GG, Johnson RW, Kelley KW. From inflammation to sickness and depression: when the immune system subjugates the brain. *Nat Rev Neurosci.* 2008;9:46–56.
[59] Rostène W, Kitabgi P, Parsadaniantz SM. Chemokines: a new class of neuromodulator? *Nat Rev Neurosci.* 2007;8:895–903.
[60] Natelson BH, Weaver SA, Tseng CL, Ottenweller JE. Spinal fluid abnormalities in patients with chronic fatigue syndrome. *Clin Diagn Lab Immunol.* 2005;12:52–55.
[61] Matsumura S, Shibakusa T, Fujikawa T, Yamada H, Inoue K, Fushiki T. Increase in transforming growth factor-beta in the brain during infection is related to fever, not depression of spontaneous motor activity. *Neuroscience.* 2007;144:1133–1140.

[62] Anisman H, Merali Z, Poulter MO, Hayley S. Cytokines as a precipitant of depressive illness: animal and human studies. *Curr Pharm Des.* 2005;11:963–972.

[63] Vgontzas AN, Chrousos GP. Sleep, the hypothalamic-pituitary-adrenal axis, and cytokines: multiple interactions and disturbances in sleep disorders. *Endocrinol Metab Clin North Am.* 2002;31:15–36.

[64] Reeves WC, Lloyd A, Vernon SD, Klimas N, Jason LA, Bleijenberg G, et al, Identification of ambiguities in the 1994 chronic fatigue syndrome research case definition and recommendations for resolution. *BMC Health Serv Res.* 2003;3:25–34.

[65] Kawamoto Y, Nakamura S, Nakano S, Oka N, Akiguchi I, Kimura J. Immunohistochemical localization of brain-derived neurotrophic factor in adult rat brain. *Neuroscience.* 1996;74:1209–1226.

[66] Neeper SA, Gomez-Pinilla F, Choi J , Cotman C. Exercise and brain neurotrophins. *Nature.* 1995;373:109.

[67] Lee R, Kermani P, Teng KK, Hempstead BL. Regulation of cell survival by secreted proneurotrophins. *Science.* 2001;294:1945–1948.

[68] Li HL, Li Z, Qin LY, Liu S, Lau LT, Han JS, et al. The novel neurotrophin-regulated neuronal development-associated protein, NDAP, mediates apoptosis. *FEBS Lett.* 2006;580:1723–1728.

[69] van Praag H, Kempermann G, Gage FH. Running increases cell proliferation and neurogenesis in the adult mouse dentate gyrus. *Nat Neurosci.* 1999;2:266–270.

[70] Schmidt HD, Duman RS. The role of neurotrophic factors in adult hippocampal neurogenesis, antidepressant treatments and animal models of depressive-like behavior. *Behav Pharmacol.* 2007;18:391–418.

[71] Moriya J. Establishment of Murine Model for Chronic Fatigue Syndrome and Efficacy of Kampo Medicine on Daily Activity. *J Kanazawa Med Univ.* 2006;31:263–268.

[72] Ottenweller JE, Natelson BH, Gause WC, Carroll KK, Beldowicz D, Zhou XD, et al. Mouse running activity is lowered by Brucella abortus treatment: a potential model to study chronic fatigue. *Physiol Behav.* 1998;63:795–801.

[73] Prins JB, van der Meer JW, Bleijenberg G. Chronic fatigue syndrome. *Lancet.* 2006;367:346–355.

[74] Parker NR, Barralet JH, Bell AM. Q fever. Lancet. 2006;367:679–688.

[75] Tarello W. Chronic fatigue syndrome (CFS) associated with Staphylococcus spp. bacteremia, responsive to potassium arsenite 0.5% in a veterinary surgeon and his coworking wife, handling with CFS animal cases. *Comp Immunol Microbiol Infect Dis.* 2001;24:233–246.

[76] Hickie I., Davenport T, Wakefield D, Vollmer-Conna U, Cameron B, Vernon SD, et al. Post-infective and chronic fatigue syndromes precipitated by viral and non-viral pathogens: prospective cohort study. *BMJ.* 2006;333:575–580.

[77] Sacks N, Van Rensburg AJ. Clinical aspects of chronic brucellosis. *S Afr Med J* 1976;50:725–728.

[78] Hamilos DL, Nutter D, Gershtenson J, Redmond DP, Clementi JD, Schmaling KB. et al. Core body temperature is normal in chronic fatigue syndrome. *Biol Psychiatry.* 1998;43:293–302.

[79] de Lange FP, Kalkman JS, Bleijenberg G, Hagoort P, van der Meer JW, Toni I. Gray matter volume reduction in the chronic fatigue syndrome. *Neuroimage.* 2005;26:777–781.

[80] Sasaki T, Kitagawa K, Yagita Y, Sugiura S, Omura-Matsuoka E, Tanaka S, et al. Bcl2 enhances survival of newborn neurons in the normal and ischemic hippocampus. *J Neurosci Res.* 2006;84:1187–1196.

[81] Fudge JL. Bcl-2 immunoreactive neurons are differentially distributed in subregions of the amygdala and hippocampus of the adult macaque. *Neuroscience.* 2004;127:539–556.

[82] Murray F, Hutson PH. Hippocampal Bcl-2 expression is selectively increased following chronic but not acute treatment with antidepressants, 5-HT(1A) or 5-HT(2C/2B) receptor antagonists. *Eur J Pharmacol.* 2007;569:41–47.

[83] Zhong LT, Sarafian T, Kane DJ, Charles AC, Mah SP, Edwards RH, et al. bcl-2 inhibits death of central neural cells induced by multiple agents. *Proc Natl Acad Sci USA.* 1993;90:4533–4537.

[84] Corrigan FM, MacDonald S, Brown A, Armstrong K, Armstrong EM. Neurasthenic fatigue, chemical sensitivity and GABAa receptor toxins. *Med Hypotheses.* 1994;43:195–200.

[85] Ponomarenko AA, Lin JS, Selbach O, Haas HL. Temporal pattern of hippocampal high-frequency oscillations during sleep after stimulant-evoked waking. *Neuroscience.* 2003;121:759–769.

[86] Vaynman S, Ying Z, Gomez–Pinilla F. The select action of hippocampal calcium calmodulin protein kinase II in mediating exercise-enhanced cognitive function. *Neuroscience.* 2007;144:825–833.

[87] Peng CH, Chiou SH, Chen SJ, Chou YC, Ku HH, Cheng CK, et al. Neuroprotection by Imipramine against lipopolysaccharide-induced apoptosis in hippocampus-derived neural stem cells mediated by activation of BDNF and the MAPK pathway. *Eur Neuropsychopharmacol.* 2008;18:128–140.

[88] Berchtold NC, Kesslak JP, Pike CJ, Adlard PA, Cotman CW. Estrogen and exercise interact to regulate brain-derived neurotrophic factor mRNA and protein expression in the hippocampus. *Eur J Neurosci.* 2001;14:1992–2002.

[89] Molteni R, Ying Z, Gómez-Pinilla F. Differential effects of acute and chronic exercise on plasticity-related genes in the rat hippocampus revealed by microarray. *Eur J Neurosci.* 2002;16:1107–1116.

[90] Kitamura T, Mishina M, Sugiyama H. Enhancement of neurogenesis by running wheel exercises is suppressed in mice lacking NMDA receptor epsilon 1 subunit. *Neurosci Res.* 2003;47:55–63.

[91] Farmer J, Zhao X, van Praag H, Wodtke K, Gage FH, Christie BR. Effects of voluntary exercise on synaptic plasticity and gene expression in the dentate gyrus of adult male Sprague-Dawley rats in vivo. *Neuroscience.* 2004;124:71–79.

[92] Wu A, Molteni R, Ying Z, Gomez-Pinilla F. A saturated-fat diet aggravates the outcome of traumatic brain injury on hippocampal plasticity and cognitive function by reducing brain-derived neurotrophic factor. *Neuroscience.* 2003;119:365–375.

[93] Marcol W, Kotulska K, Larysz-Brysz M, Kowalik JL. BDNF contributes to animal model neuropathic pain after peripheral nerve transection. *Neurosurg Rev.* 2007;30:235–243.

[94] Guzman-Marin R, Ying Z, Suntsova N, Methippara M, Bashir T, Szymusiak R, et al. Suppression of hippocampal plasticity-related gene expression by sleep deprivation in rats. *J Physiol.* 2006;575:807–819.

[95] Xuejiang W, Ichikawa H, Konishi T. Antioxidant potential of qizhu tang, a chinese herbal medicine, and the effect on cerebral oxidative damage after ischemia reperfusion in rats. *Biol Pharm Bull.* 2001;24:558–563.
[96] Shih HC, Chang KH, Chen FL, Chen CM, Chen SC, Lin YT, et al. Anti-aging effects of the traditional Chinese medicine bu-zhong-yi-qi-tang in mice. *Am J Chin Med.* 2000;28:77–86.
[97] Katafuchi T, Kondo T, Take S, Yoshimura M. Brain cytokines and the 5-HT system during poly I:C-induced fatigue. *Ann N Y Acad Sci.* 2006;1088:230–237.
[98] Rook GA, Zumla A. Gulf War syndrome: is it due to a systemic shift in cytokine balance towards a Th2 profile?. *Lancet.* 1997;349:1831–1833.
[99] Brooks JC, Roberts N, Whitehouse G, Majeed T. Proton magnetic resonance spectroscopy and morphometry of the hippocampus in chronic fatigue syndrome. *Br J Radiol.* 2000;73:1206–1208.
[100] Carlo–Stella N, Badulli C, De Silvestri A, Bazzichi L, Martinetti M, Lorusso L, et al. A first study of cytokine genomic polymorphisms in CFS: Positive association of TNF-857 and IFNgamma 874 rare alleles. *Clin Exp Rheumatol.* 2006;24:179–182.
[101] Lee J, Kim SJ, Son TG, Chan SL, Mattson MP. Interferon-gamma is up-regulated in the hippocampus in response to intermittent fasting and protects hippocampal neurons against excitotoxicity. *J Neurosci Res.* 2006;83:1552–1557.
[102] Kanda T, McManus JE, Nagai R, Imai S, Suzuki T, Yang D, et al. Modification of viral myocarditis in mice by interleukin-6. *Circ Res.* 1996;78:848–856.
[103] Becker PD, McGregor N, Meirleir KD. Possible triggers and mode of onset of chronic fatigue syndrome. *J Chronic Fatigue Syndr.* 2002;10:3–18.
[104] Natelson BH, LaManca JJ, Denny TN, Vladutiu A, Oleske J, Hill N, et al. Immunologic parameters in chronic fatigue syndrome, major depression, and multiple sclerosis. *Am J Med.* 1998;105:43S–49S.
[105] Chao CC, Janoff EN, Hu SX, Thomas K, Gallagher M, Tsang M, et al. Altered cytokine release in peripheral blood mononuclear cell cultures from patients with the chronic fatigue syndrome. *Cytokin*e. 1991;3:292–298.
[106] Tirelli U, Pinto A, Marotta G, Crovato M, Quaia M, De Paoli P, et al. Clinical and immunologic study of 205 patients with chronic fatigue syndrome: a case series from Italy. *Arch Intern Med.* 1993;153:116–117,120.
[107] Strowig T, Brilot F, Münz C. Noncytotoxic functions of NK cells: direct pathogen restriction and assistance to adaptive immunity. *J Immunol.* 2008;180:7785–7791.
[108] Kato Y, Morikawa A, Sugiyama T, Koide N, Jiang GZ, Lwin T, et al. Augmentation of lipopolysaccharide-induced thymocyte apoptosis by interferon-gamma. *Cell Immunol.* 1997;177:103–108.
[109] Beck T, Lindholm D, Castrén E, Wree A. Brain-derived neurotrophic factor protects against ischemic cell damage in rat hippocampus. *J Cereb Blood Flow Metab.* 1994;14:689–692.
[110] Geiger KD, Nash TC, Sawyer S, Krahl T, Patstone G, Reed JC, et al. Interferon-gamma protects against herpes simplex virus type 1-mediated neuronal death. *Virology.* 1997;238:189–197.

In: Traditional Medicine: New Research
Editor: Yoshiharu Motoo

ISBN: 978-1-62257-448-3


*Chapter 8*

# Study of Traditional Chinese Medicine Syndrome Classification in Hepatitis B and Liver Cirrhosis

***Shi-Bing Su***
Research Center for Traditional Chinese Medicine Complexity System,
Shanghai University of Traditional Chinese Medicine,
Shanghai, China

## Abstract

The traditional Chinese medicine (TCM) syndrome, also known as ZHENG or TCM pattern, is the basic unit and the key concept in TCM theory. TCM syndrome is the TCM theoretical abstraction of the symptom profiles of a disease as well as syndrome rather than a simple assemblage of disease symptoms. Because patients with this disease can be classifying into different TCM syndrome types, clinical diagnostic and therapeutic methods are based on the differentiation of TCM syndrome in TCM. The objective of this chapter is to clarify the experimental evidence for TCM syndrome classification of diseases, based on the research of single nucleotide polymorphisms (SNPs), transcriptomics and metabonomics in chronic liver diseases such as chronic hepatitis B (CHB) or liver cirrhosis (LC). The content includes that (1) TCM syndrome is a clinical special phenotype and there was the correlation between the some genotypes and different TCM syndrome types; (2) there were the differential gene expression profiles and the significantly differential expression genes in Excess and Deficiency syndromes; (3) there were the differential metabolite profiles and the significantly differential metabolites in TCM syndromes. In conclusion, we showed the evidence for TCM syndrome classification from some SNPs/genotypes, genes, metabolites and their phenotypes or profiles in CHB or LC. It was suggested that the systematic-omics technologies could be used to classify TCM syndromes, and the TCM syndrome could be a new classification of CHB or LC for clinical diagnosis and treatment.

**Keyword:** Traditional Chinese Medicine; TCM syndrome; Classification; Technology

The traditional Chinese medicine (TCM) ZHENG, also known as TCM syndrome or TCM pattern, is an integral and essential part of TCM theory. A TCM syndrome, or ZHENG, is, in essence, a characteristic profile of all clinical manifestations (or TCM theoretical abstraction of the symptom profiles) that can be identified by a TCM practitioner. Clinical treatments of a patient rely on the successful differentiation of a specific TCM syndrome. Recent advances in systems biology and medicine have allowed the application of new profiling technologies in the study of the TCM syndrome differentiation and its biological interpretation. Understanding the characteristic changes in biochemistry associated with a specific TCM syndrome will facilitate the development of TCM syndrome identification, a novel disease diagnostic and stratification approach that will potentially lead to personalized healthcare strategies for a range of diseases that lack therapeutic solutions.

Hepatitis B virus (HBV) infection is a major health problem in China. It is one of the important reasons for virus-related liver diseases, such as liver cirrhosis (LC) and hepatocellular carcinoma (HCC) [1, 2]. There are 350 million HBV-infected people worldwide who have a 15-25% risk of dying from the HBV-caused LC and HCC [3]. During the course of HBV infection, the human liver is gradually damaged by this hepatotropic DNA virus, presenting a wide variety of clinical manifestations ranging from an asymptomatic carrier state to chronic hepatitis B (CHB), and to CHB-caused cirrhosis [2, 4]. There is a five year survival rate of patients with severe CHB and it causes cirrhosis in about 50% of patients [5, 6]. Although several antiviral drugs have been approved for HBV infection, they cause significant side-effects and drug resistance [7]. In contrast, TCM treatment is one of the safe and effective methods for CHB and LC [8].

So far, an experiential diagnosis approach has been used to classify TCM syndromes in CHB or CHB-caused LC patients. TCM practitioners skilled in TCM diagnosis and treatment are often able to improve the symptoms of patients, which may be considered to be untreatable by conventional medicine [9]. It has been suggested that the effective rate increased when the treatment was appropriate to TCM syndrome in LC [8]. It was suggested that syndrome classification acts as a pivot in the therapeutic process and directly affects the therapeutic result of a specific disease. Instead of experiential diagnosis, therefore, it is necessary to standardize the diagnosis criteria of TCM syndrome in patients with CHB or CHB-caused LC by using a universally acceptable scientific approach.

The biological basis of TCM syndrome classification is the key scientific issue in the study of TCM diagnosis and treatment. In recent years, following the development of systematic-omics technologies and methods, it is used more frequently, such as new modalities for clinical characterization of TCM syndrome, molecular genetics and biologic diagnosis of TCM syndrome; new insights into TCM syndrome classification using genes, proteins, metabolites and their profiles; systems strategies in TCM syndrome classification and treatment evaluation. In this chapter, we clarified the experimental evidence for TCM syndrome classification of chronic liver diseases such as CHB or CHB-caused LC, based on the research of single nucleotide polymorphisms (SNPs), transcriptomics and metabonomics.

# 1. Study on the Correlation between CYP1A2 Genotypes and TCM Syndromes

As a ruler of hereditary susceptibility, SNPs account for approximately 90% of human DNA polymorphism [10]. The low mutation rate and essentially random nature of base-changing events make the SNP alleles very stable [11] and most (>80%) are common to all human populations, but allele frequencies are different in different persons and different diseases [29]. For the discovering and verifying of the correlations between SNPs and diseases as well as genotypes and phenotypes of diseases, it has been considered an approach for the personalized disease diagnostic and treatment.

In liver cirrhosis, the phenotypes have been presented as ZHENG type, a TCM syndrome as well as Child-Pugh classification, compensation or decompensation phase, hepatocellular function. However, whether TCM syndromes, Child-Pugh classification, compensation or decompensation phase in CHB-caused cirrhosis were affected by hereditary susceptibility of the patient, it remains poorly understood. In this study, we investigated the correlations between the CYP1A2 SNPs and CHB-caused cirrhosis, and the correlations between these polymorphisms and the phenotype of CHB-caused cirrhosis.

## 1.1. Characteristics of the Study Population

The CYP1A2 genes loci were assessed in 297 patients with CHB-caused cirrhosis in China. The Hardy-Weinberg equilibrium (HWE) test showed that distribution of these tested genotypes was not significantly different from the expected distribution ($P>0.05$). The ages of patients were from 18 to 65 years (mean ± SD, 49.15 ± 10.28). Furthermore, there were no significant differences of age and sex in gene polymorphisms in our study population ($P>0.05$). As Child-Pugh (Child-Pugh-Turcotte score) classification, there were 218 patients in A, 57 patients in B and 14 patients in C. As compensation or decompensation classification, there were 151 patients in compensation phase and 146 patients in decompensation phase.

## 1.2. Correlation between the Genotypes of CYP1A2 and Child-Pugh Classification and Compensation or Decompensation Phase in CHB-caused Cirrhosis

The correlation between CYP1A2-G2964A, -C733A and -T5347C and ZHENG types were analyzed by SNaPshot assay combined with the sequencing analysis in patients with CHB-caused cirrhosis. As shown in Table 1, there was no significant correlation between genotypes of CYP1A2 and Child-Pugh classification in CHB-caused cirrhosis. It showed that the P value were 0.181 and 0.198 between genotypes of CYP1A2-G2964A and CYP1A2-C733A and Child-Pugh classification (class A, class B+C), respectively. The P value was 0.605 between genotypes of CYP1A2-T5347C and Child-Pugh classification (class A, class B+C).

There was no significant correlation between genotypes of CYP1A2 and phase in CHB-caused cirrhosis. As shown in Table 1, the P values were 0.496 and 0.290 between genotypes of CYP1A2-G2964A and CYP1A2-C733A and phase (compensation, decompensation phase), respectively. The P value was 0.291 between genotypes of CYP1A2-T5347C and phase (compensation, decompensation phase).

**Table 1. Correlation between CYP1A2 and Child classification and phase in patients with CHB-caused cirrhosis**

| Gene/ genotype | Child classification | | | *P* | Phase | | *P* |
|---|---|---|---|---|---|---|---|
| | Class A (%) (n=218) | Class B (%) (n=57) | Class C (%) (n=14) | | Compensation (n=151) | Decompensation (n=146) | |
| *CYP1A2*-G2964A | | | | | | | |
| GG | 101(46.76) | 21(36.84) | 8(57.14) | 0.181 | 71(47.02) | 62(42.47) | 0.496 |
| AG | 93(43.06) | 31(54.39) | 3(21.43) | | 67(44.37) | 65(44.52) | |
| AA | 22(10.19) | 5(8.77) | 3(21.43) | | 13(8.61) | 17(11.64) | |
| *CYP1A2*-C733A | | | | | | | |
| CC | 19(8.76) | 6(10.53) | 4(28.57) | 0.198 | 11(7.28) | 18(12.33) | 0.290 |
| AC | 110(50.69) | 30(52.63) | 5(35.71) | | 76(50.33) | 73(50.00) | |
| AA | 88(40.55) | 21(36.84) | 5(35.71) | | 64(42.38) | 54(36.99) | |
| *CYP1A2*-T5347C | | | | | | | |
| TT | 4(1.83) | 2(3.51) | 0(0) | 0.605* | 5(3.31) | 1(0.68) | 0.291▲ |
| CT | 37(16.97) | 6(10.53) | 3(21.43) | | 26(17.22) | 23(15.75) | |
| CC | 177(81.19) | 49(85.96) | 11(78.57) | | 120(82.19) | 122(83.56) | |

* Fisher's exact test between class A and class B+C. ▲ Fisher's exact test.

## 1.3. Correlation between the Genotypes of CYP1A2 and TCM Syndromes in CHB-caused Cirrhosis

The correlation between CYP1A2-G2964A, CYP1A2-C733A, CYP1A2-T5347C and TCM syndromes were analyzed by SNaPshot assay combined with the sequencing analysis in patients with CHB-caused cirrhosis. As shown in Table 2, it was shown that AC heterozygous and AA homozygous genotypes at CYP1A2-C733A were significant differences compared to CC wild-type genotype ($P<0.05$) between the "damp abundance due to spleen asthenia syndrome" and other TCM syndromes. However, there was no significant correlation between the genotypes of CYP1A2-G2964A and CYP1A2-T5347C and the TCM syndromes.

The TCM syndrome type is a consequence of disease classification. According to TCM theory, the patients of same disease can be classifying into different syndrome types. A previous study reported that there is a relationship between gene polymorphisms of interleukin-10 and TCM syndromes in CHB-caused cirrhosis [12]. With the finding, there were significant correlations between AC plus AA genotype at CYP1A2-C733A mutation genotypes and the TCM syndrome "Spleen asthenia and damp abundance syndrome". In the study, these results provided an impersonal proof for TCM syndrome classification in CHB-caused cirrhosis and will be helpful to clinical diagnosis of TCM syndrome.

# 2. Analysis of Differential Gene Expression Profiles in CHB Patients with Excess and Deficiency Syndromes

"There is all inside, will show outside", the external development there will be the inherent law in disease. TCM syndromes are the clinical specific phenotype or expression patterns, which reflect the comprehensive changes of different levels including organs, systems, tissues, cells and molecules in the whole body. The changes of gene expression profiles reflect cell or tissue specific phenotype and expression patterns might be related to TCM syndromes, and appear in clinical signs and symptoms. In recent years, following the development of systematic-omics technologies and methods such as a high throughput technology, cDNA microarray, it is used more frequently as new modalities for the analysis of gene expression profiles of TCM syndrome and biologic diagnosis of TCM syndrome [13].

'Heat', 'Cold', 'Excess' and 'Deficiency' are the four basic syndromes of maladjustment nature in TCM [14]. Damp heat stasis syndrome and liver and kidney Yin deficiency syndrome, classified as Excess syndrome and Deficiency syndrome, respectively, are the common syndromes in CHB patients. A previous study suggested that Cold and Hot syndromes of rheumatoid arthritis have the distinct molecular signatures identified by microarray expression profiles [15]. However, it is still unclear in the gene profiles of TCM syndromes in CHB patients. Therefore, we investigated the differential gene expressions in CHB with the two typical TCM syndromes, Excess and Deficiency syndromes, and the relationship between various CHB with TCM syndromes and the gene expression.

**Table 2. Correlation between CYP1A2-G2964A, CYP1A2-C733A, CYP1A2-T5347C and TCM syndromes in patients with CHB-caused cirrhosis**

| TCM syndrome type | *CYP1A2*-G2964A | | *P* | *CYP1A2*-C733A | | *P* | *CYP1A2*-T5347C | | *P* |
|---|---|---|---|---|---|---|---|---|---|
| | GG | AG+AA | | CC | AC+AA | | TT | CT+CC | |
| Liver-*qi* stagnation syndrome | 29 | 32 | 0.759 | 5 | 61 | 0.566 | 2 | 59 | 0.630* |
| Damp abundance and spleen asthenia syndrome | 21 | 21 | 0.575 | 8 | 30 | **0.039** | 0 | 46 | |
| Damp-heat syndrome | 29 | 40 | 0.613 | 7 | 62 | 0.944 | 1 | 69 | 1.000* |
| Liver-kidney *yin* deficiency syndrome | 17 | 24 | 0.636 | 2 | 39 | 0.399* | 0 | 42 | |
| Blood stasis syndrome | 31 | 37 | 0.977 | 6 | 62 | 0.794 | 3 | 60 | 0.200* |
| *Yang* deficiency of spleen and kidney syndrome | 6 | 6 | 0.753 | 1 | 11 | 1.000* | 0 | 12 | |
| Totle | 133 | 160 | | 29 | 265 | | 6 | 288 | |

* Fisher's exact test.

## Analysis of Differential Gene Expression

Blood samples were collected from 10 CHB patients with Excess syndrome and Deficiency syndrome and 10 healthy volunteers. Total RNA was isolated from leukocyte. The gene expression profiles were detected by cDNA microarray (NimbleGen Homo sapiens 12×135K Array). Microarray analysis was carried out by a SAS Analysis System.

There were significant differences in gene expressions between CHB patients with Excess and Deficiency syndromes, as well as CHB patients and healthy volunteers. Patients with Excess and Deficiency syndromes could fully be distinguished by clustering of 403 differentially expressed genes ($P<0.05$). A total of 239 genes were significantly differentially expressed (foldchange≥2, $P<0.05$), among 142 were upregulated and 97 were downregulated. Moreover, there were 689 significantly differentially expressed (foldchange≥2, $P<0.05$) between Deficiency syndrome and healthy control, among which 396 were upregulated and 293 were downregulated. There were 1724 significantly differentially expressed (foldchange ≥2, $P<0.05$) between Excess syndrome and healthy control, among 854 were upregulated and 870 were downregulated. The regulated genes in Excess syndrome were more than that in Deficiency syndrome. The obvious differentially expressed genes between CHB patients with Excess and Deficiency syndromes were showed in Table 3. Furthermore, 10 genes in 40 CHB patients were tested and verified by real time RT-PCR. The changes of their mRNA expressions were accordance with that of microarray. Among these, there were significant differences in ABCC3 mRNA expressions between CHB patients with Excess and Deficiency syndromes ($P<0.05$), but it was no significant differences between CHB patients with syndromes and healthy controls ($P>0.05$).

**Table 3. Obvious differentially expressed genes between CHB patients with Excess and Deficiency syndromes**

| Probe ID | Gene symbol | Foldchange (Deficiency syndrome / Excess syndrome ) | Gene regulation |
|---|---|---|---|
| NM_030915 | LBH | 15.373 0 | up |
| BC051300 | PHYHD1 | 11.317 7 | up |
| NM_005098 | MSC | 9.840 3 | up |
| NM_003786 | ABCC3 | 8.759 2 | up |
| NM_018071 | FLJ10357 | 7.532 8 | up |
| NM_001001928 | PPARA | 3.921 1 | up |
| NM_176895 | PPAP2A | 3.3192 | down |
| AK055816 | PODXL | 0.161 1 | down |
| XM_933718 | LOC646576 | 0.148 1 | down |
| NM_016588 | NRN1 | 0.141 5 | down |
| NM_012338 | TSPAN12 | 0.139 3 | down |
| NM_002142 | HOXA9 | 0.119 3 | down |
| NM_016215 | EGFL7 | 0.115 5 | down |
| BC007600 | HOXA10 | 0.1106 | down |
| BC041772 | SPNS2 | 0.1046 | down |

### Gene Ontology (GO) and Pathway Analysis of Differential Genes

According to pathway analysis of differential genes between Excess or Deficiency syndromes compared to healthy controls, results showed that there are 254 same GO between Excess and Deficiency syndromes, including virus body combination, immune regulation, RNA polymerase Ⅲ transcription factors activity and neurotransmitter transporter activity, etc; 63 GO in Excess syndrome alone, including fat stored positive adjustment, protein lipid compounds and leukocyte-mediated cells toxicity, etc; 12 GO in Deficiency syndrome alone, including peroxides activity, nitric oxide syntheses adjustment factor activity and stem cell maintenance, etc.

According to pathway analysis of differential genes between Excess or Deficiency syndromes compared to healthy controsl, results showed that there are 296 same pathways between Excess and Deficiency syndromes, including MAPK pathways, metabolic pathways and endocytosis, etc; 101 pathways in Excess syndrome alone, including cytokines, immune and inflammatory responses, and amino acid, lipid and acetone metabolisms, etc; 22 pathways in Deficiency syndrome alone, including tryptophan metabolism, p27 phosphorylation regulation in cell cycle and mRNA adenosine acidification, etc.

In this study, differential gene expression was observed in CHB patients with Excess and Deficiency syndrome, indicating that there is a molecular foundation in the classification of TCM syndrome. The preliminary findings of this study suggested that TCM syndrome types are related to gene expression profiles. Moreover, genes specially regulated by Deficiency syndrome were mainly related to peroxidase activity and stem cell maintenance. Genes specially regulated by Excess syndrome are mainly related to cytokines, immune and inflammatory responses.

## 3. Study of Urine Metabolomics on TCM Syndrome Classification in Patients with CHB-Caused Cirrhosis

Metabonomics is an emerging subject together with genomics, transcriptomics and proteomics, jointly constitutes Systems Biology [16]. Metabonomics is concerned with the quantitative understandings of the metabolite component of integrated living systems and its dynamic responses to the changes of both endogenous and exogenous factors [17]. As a systemic approach, metabonomics adopts a “top-down” strategy to reflect the function of organisms from terminal symptoms of metabolic network and understand metabolic changes of a complete system caused by interventions in a holistic context [18].

In recent years, a wide range of metabonomic technologies are widely used in the modern research of TCM [19]. There are specific metabolism patterns in different physiological and pathological stages according to the metabonomics. The alteration of metabolism correlated closely with physiology and pathology of entrails, which is different from single index and could reflect the concept of TCM syndromes. At present, the most prevailing methods for TCM research are mainly nuclear magnetic resonance (NMR), gas chromatography-mass spectrometry (GC-MS), and liquid chromatography-mass spectrometry (LC-MS). With these techniques, metabonomics will help to understand TCM syndromes and treatment.

The metabolomic technology has been applied to classify TCM syndromes in hypertension [20], coronary heart disease [21] and rheumatoid arthritis [15, 22] that indicated that the characteristic metabolites identified by metabonomic analysis could study the essence of TCM syndrome. However, it has been not reported in the urinary metabolites profiles of TCM syndromes in patients with CHB-caused cirrhosis. Therefore, we analyzed the metabolic mode and differential urine metabolites on TCM syndromes in patients with CHB-caused cirrhosis.

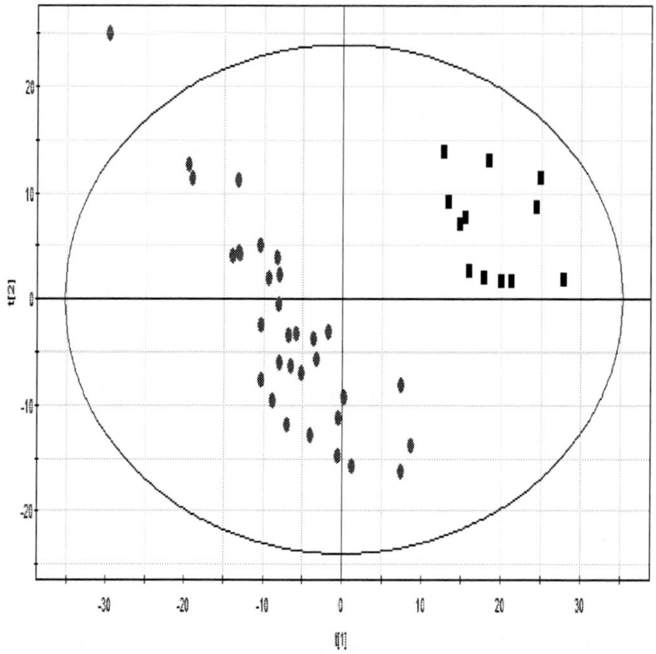


A

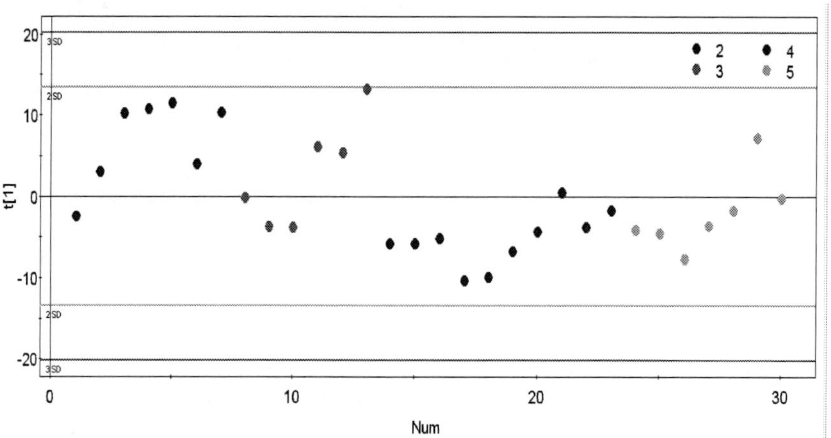


B

Figure 1. PLS-DA diagram of metabolic mode. A, comparison of patients with CHB-caused cirrhosis (red spot) and healthy control (black spot). B, comparison among TCM syndromes. 2, Damp abundance and spleen asthenia syndrome; 3, Damp heat stasis syndrome; 4, Liver and kidney Yin deficiency syndrome; 5, Blood stasis syndrome.

### 3.1. Comparison of Metabolic Mode among TCM Syndromes

In order to find the metabolic mode of urinary metabolites in different TCM syndromes, morning urine of 31 patients with CHB-caused cirrhosis and 12 healthy volunteers were collected. A combined GC–MS derived method was developed suitable for the urine sample treatment in aqueous phase with ethyl chloroformate (ECF) derivatization agents. And then the multivariate statistical analysis was carried out. Through the orthogonal noise filter combined with partial least squares discriminant analysis (PLS-DA), a complete differentiation was achieved between the patients with CHB-caused cirrhosis and healthy subjects (Figure 1A), as well as among patients with different TCM syndromes including Damp abundance and spleen asthenia syndrome, Damp heat stasis syndrome, Liver and kidney Yin deficiency syndrome and Blood stasis syndrome (Figure 1B).

### 3.2. Analysis of Differential Urinary Metabolites between Excess and Deficiency Syndromes

Excess syndrome such as Damp heat stasis syndrome and Deficiency syndrome such as liver and kidney Yin deficiency syndrome are also the common syndromes in patients with CHB-caused cirrhosis as well as in CHB patients [12]. In this study, to find the differential urinary metabolites of Excess and Deficiency syndromes, the PLS-DA analytic model was used through variables' importance of projection (VIP) for detecting differential urinary metabolites, which VIP>1.5 and $P<0.05$ (t' test) was set up as a significant difference. After the retrieval of NIST spectrum database, we found that the same part of differential urinary metabolites between TCM syndromes and healthy controls were amino acid metabolism related metabolites, such as, alanine, proline, etc, and energy metabolism related metabolites, such as citric acid, amber acid, etc (Table 4); The differential urinary metabolites between Excess and Deficiency syndromes compared to healthy controls were in the different content of branched chain amino acids (BCAA) such as leucine and valine (Table 4). In addition, there also were the different content in L-lysine and glycine between Excess and Deficiency syndromes (Table 4). In Table 4, ↑was indicated the increase of urinary metabolite content; ↓was indicated the decrease of urinary metabolite content.

In this study, TCM syndrome classification was investigated in patients with CHB-caused cirrhosis, through urinary metabolites detected by GC–MS combined with pattern recognition analysis and one- or multi-dimensional statistics methods. The results indicated that there are not only different metabolic mode and differential urine metabolites between healthy subjects and patients with CHB-caused cirrhosis, but also between Excess and Deficiency syndromes. Moreover, the differential urinary metabolites were mainly involved in amino acid and energy metabolism pathways, and the branched chain amino acids such as leucine and valine might be used to differentiate Excess and Deficiency syndromes. These differences of urinary metabolites and metabolic mode between Excess and Deficiency syndromes suggested that there are the biological characteristic of urinary metabolites in different TCM syndromes as well as above related genotype and differential genes.

**Table 4. Differential urine metabolites and content between Excess and Deficiency syndromes compared to healthy controls**

| No. | Metabolite name | Excess syndrome | Deficiency syndrome |
|---|---|---|---|
| 1 | Propanedioic acid | ↓ | ↓ |
| 2 | Phenol | ↑ | ↑ |
| 3 | D-Proline | ↑ | ↑ |
| 4 | 1H-Indole-7-carboxylic acid | ↑ | ↑ |
| 5 | l-Alanine | ↑ | ↑ |
| 6 | Benzeneacetic acid | ↑ | ↑ |
| 7 | Glycine | ↓ | ↑ |
| 8 | Succinic acid | ↑ | ↑ |
| 9 | Benzyl alcohol | ↑ | ↑ |
| 10 | 2-Furaldehyde diethyl acetal | ↑ | ↑ |
| 11 | Leucine | ↑ | — |
| 12 | Aspartic acid | ↑ | ↑ |
| 13 | Ethyl citrate | ↓ | ↓ |
| 14 | 4-Fluorobenzoic acid | ↑ | ↑ |
| 15 | Isobutyl 4-hydroxybenzoate | ↑ | ↑ |
| 16 | N-Benzoylglycine ethyl ester | ↓ | ↓ |
| 17 | L-Lysine | ↓ | — |
| 18 | l-Phenylalanine | ↑ | ↑ |
| 19 | Phthalic acid | ↑ | ↑ |
| 20 | Indolebutyric acid | ↑ | ↑ |
| 21 | Octanedioic acid | ↑ | ↓ |
| 22 | Pidolic Acid | ↑ | ↓ |
| 23 | dl-Isocitric acid lactone | ↑ | ↑ |
| 24 | Tyramine | ↑ | ↑ |
| 25 | histidine | ↑ | ↑ |
| 26 | Valine | ↑ | — |
| 27 | Cyclohexanol | ↑ | ↓ |
| 28 | Spermine | ↑ | ↑ |
| 29 | L-Tyrosine | ↑ | ↑ |
| 30 | Arginine | ↑ | ↑ |
| 31 | D-Tryptophan | ↑ | ↑ |
| 32 | Indole | ↑ | ↑ |

# Conclusion

In this chapter, we expounded the evidence for TCM syndrome classification from some SNPs/genotypes genes, metabolites and their phenotypes or profiles in CHB or LC. As a new research method of the post-genome era, systems biology including genomics, transcriptomics, and metabonomics, which is characterized with the global biological and functional status, is the best to fit the holistic concept of TCM syndromes. With systems biological technology, we can not only classify TCM syndromes and interpret its mechanism, but also elucidate the scientific connotation of "treatment based on syndrome differentiation". Our research results suggested TCM syndrome could be a new classification of CHB and LC for clinical diagnosis and treatment.

Further researches might implement quantitative and dynamical evaluation of TCM syndromes and treatment, with the further development of compositive analytical techniques, especially multi-analyzed techniques, which should combined genomics, transcriptomics, proteomics and metabonomics, will greatly promote TCM syndrome research and be beneficial to TCM diagnosis and treatment.

# References

[1] Zhang, X., Zhang, H., Ye, L. Effects of hepatitis B virus X protein on the development of liver cancer. *J Lab Clin Med.* 2006, 147:58–66.

[2] McMahon, B.J. Epidemiology and natural history of hepatitis B. *Seminars in Liver Disease* 2005, 1: 3–8.

[3] Margolis, H.S., Alter, M.J., Hadler, S.C. Hepatitis B: evolving epidemiology and implications for control. *Semin Liver Dis.* 1991, 11:84-92.

[4] Lee, W.M. Hepatitis B virus infection. *N Engl J Med.* 1997, 337:1733-1745

[5] Liaw, Y.F., Tai, D.I., Chu, C.M., Chen, T.J. The development of cirrhosis in patients with chronic type B hepatitis: a prospective study. *Hepatology.* 1988, 8:493-496.

[6] De Jongh, F.E., Janssen, H.L., de Man, R.A., Hop, W.C., Schalm, S.W., van Blankenstein, M. Survival and prognostic indicators in hepatitis B surface antigen-positive cirrhosis of the liver. *Gastroenterology.* 1992, 103:1630-1635.

[7] Cui, X., Wang, Y., Kokudo, N., Fang, D., Tang, W. Traditional Chinese medicine and related active compounds against hepatitis B virus infection. *Biosci Trends,* 2010, 4(2):39-47.

[8] Wang, Y., Ma, L., Liu, P. Feature selection and syndrome prediction for liver cirrhosis in traditional Chinese medicine. *Comput Methods Programs Biomed,* 2009, 95(3):249-257.

[9] Xu, W., Su, L.Q., Li, H.J. Research advances and clinical evaluation of drugs for hepatitis B. *Chin J Hosp Pharm.* 2008, 28(9):737-739.

[10] Collins, F.S., Brooks, L.D., Chakravarti, A. A DNA polymorphism discovery resource for research on human genetic variation. *Genome Res.* 1998, 8:1229-1231.

[11] Gra, I.C., Campbell, D.A., Spurr, N.K. Single nucleotide polymorphism as tools in human genetics. *Hum Mol Genet* 2000, 9:2402-2408.

[12] Jiang, Z.L., Zhang, W., Zhang, H., Liu, Y.B., Li, Q.Y., Su, S.B. Relationship between gene polymorphisms of interleukin-10 and syndrome types of traditional Chinese medicine in posthepatitis B cirrhosis. *J Chin Integr Med.* 2009, 7(11):1052-1056.

[13] Su, S.B., Hu, Y.Y., Zhao, L.P., Cao, Z.W., Ma, L.Z., Zhang, Y.Y,. Zhang, Q.H., Liu, P. Research approach for biological basis of Chinese medical syndromes of chronic viral hepatitis B. *Chin J Integr Trad West Med.* 2011, 31(2): 252-255.

[14] Jiang, W.Y. Therapeutic wisdom in traditional Chinese medicine: a perspective from modern science. *TRENDS in Pharm Sciences.* 2005, 26(11): 558-563.

[15] Cheng Lu, Cheng Xiao, Gao Chen, Miao Jiang, Qinglin Zha, Xiaoping Yan, Weiping Kong, Aiping Lu. Cold and heat pattern of rheumatoid arthritis in traditional Chinese medicine: distinct molecular signatures indentified by microarray expression profiles in CD4-positive T cell. *Rheumatol Int.* 2010, 32(1): 61-68.

[16] Nicholson, J.K., Wilson, I.D. Understanding "global" systems biology: metabonomics and the continuum of Metabolism. *Nature Reviews Drug Discovery.* 2003, 2(8):668–676.

[17] Tang, H.R., Wang, Y.L. Metabonomics: a revolution in progress. *Progress in Biochemistry and Biophysics.* 2006, 33(5): 401–417.

[18] Nicholson, J.K. Global systems biology, personalized medicine and molecular epidemiology. *Molecular Systems Biology,* 2006, 2, article 52.

[19] Zhu, C., Hu, P., Liang, Q.L., Wang, Y.M., Luo, G.A. Integration of metabonomics technology and its application in modernization of traditional Chinese medicine. *Acta Pharmaceutica Sinica.* 2008, 43, (7):683–689.

[20] Lu, Y.H., Hao, H.P., Wang, G.J., Chen, X.H., Zhu, X.X., Xiang, B.R. Metabolomics approach to the biochemical differentiation of Traditional Chinese Medicine syndrome types of hypertension. *Chin J Clin Pharmaco Ther.* 2007, 12(10):1144-1150

[21] Jian, W., Yuan, Z., Huang, X., Chen, Q., Zheng, J., Li, Y., Wang, L. Analysis on urine metabolomics of coronary heart disease patients with the heart blood stasis syndrome. *J Trad Chin Med.* 2010, 51(8):729-732.

[insert "22" in margin] Van Wietmarschen, H., Yuan, K., Lu, C., Gao, P., Wang, J., Xiao, C., Yan, X., Wang, M., Schroën, J., Lu, A., Xu, G., van der Greef, J. Systems biology guided by Chinese medicine reveals new markers for sub-typing rheumatoid arthritis patients. *J Clin Rheumatol.* 2009, 15: 330-337.

In: Traditional Medicine: New Research
Editor: Yoshiharu Motoo
ISBN: 978-1-62257-448-3


*Chapter 9*

# Mechanisms of Licorice-induced Pseudoaldosteronism, One of the Most Common Side Effects of Traditional Japanese Kampo Medicine and Traditional Chinese Medicine

***Toshiaki Makino**[*,1] **and Nobuhiro Ohtake**[2]*
[1]Department of Pharmacognosy, Graduate School of Pharmaceutical Sciences, Nagoya City University, Japan
[2]Tsumura Research Laboratories, Tumura Co. Ltd., Japan

## Abstract

One of the most common side effects of traditional Japanese kampo and traditional Chinese medicine is pseudoaldosteronism caused by licorice. In this review, we described pharmacological mechanisms of licorice-induced pseudoaldosteronism by the pharmacokinetics of chemical constituents and its metabolites containing licorice. Glycyrrhizin (GL), the main constituent of licorice, is absorbed as glycyrrhetinic acid (GA) that is a metabolite of GL by enterobacteria into circulation. Circulating GA is metabolized in liver to become 3-monoglucuronyl-glycyrrhetinic acid (3MGA), that is excreted into bile *via* multidrug resistance protein 2 (Mrp2). If Mrp2 function is damaged by some reasons, 3MGA is secreted from liver to the circulation, and excreted into urine *via* organic anion transporters expressed at the basolateral side of tubular epithelial cells. Circulating GA cannot be excreted into urine since GA highly binds to serum albumin not to pass through glomerular filtration and is not the substrate of transporters expressed on tubular epithelial cells. Licorice-induced pseudoaldosteronism is developed by the inhibition of type 2 11β-hydrosteroid dehydrogenase (11β-HSD2) to accumulate cortisol in tubular epithelial cells that activate mineral corticoid receptor to stimulate the

* Corresponding Author: Toshiaki Makino, Ph. D., Department of Pharmacognosy, Graduate School of Pharmaceutical Science, Nagoya City University, 3-1 Mizuho-ku, Nagoya 467-8603, Japan. E-mail: makino@phar.nagoya-cu.ac.jp. Tel. & Fax: +81 52 836 3416.

excretion of potassium and to cause hypokalemia. Since GA cannot pass through tubular epithelial cells and cannot inhibit the enzyme expressing in the cells but 3MGA can, the causative substance for licorice-induced pseudoaldosteronism would be 3MGA. In order to prevent the side effects when licorice is used, it may be important to monitor the concentration of 3MGA in plasma or urine.

# 1. Introduction

One of the most common side effects of traditional Japanese kampo medicine and traditional Chinese medicine (TCM) is pseudoaldosteronism caused by licorice. The onset of licorice-induced pseudoaldosteronism depends on a dose and the dosing period of licorice to some extent. However, it is inferred that there is some specific individual factors in the background of the patients suffering licorice-induced pseudoaldosteronism, since some patients do not develop it even if taking licorice for a long term while other patients develop it with minimum dosage in a short time. The authors are conducting experimental studies about the developing mechanisms of licorice-induced pseudoaldosteronism, and have obtained some new findings that we can apply to prevent the side effect of licorice.

# 2. What is Licorice-induced Pseudoaldosteronism?

Licorice is a crude drug prescribed in various herbal formulas in traditional Japanese and Chinese medicines. The origin of licorice is determined as root or stolon of *Glycyrrhiza uralensis* or *G. glabra* (Legminosae). In Japan, licorice is prescribed in 109 formulas among 148 items of ethical kampo extract formulation used as medical business. Therefore, licorice is a most frequently used crude drug in kampo medicine. Also, since taste of licorice is sweet, it is used as a natural sweetener for foods including salt such as soy sauce or pickle. Furthermore, glycyrrhizin (GL), one of the constituents in licorice provides detergency and is used in toothpastes or cosmetics. In Europe where they have used licorice as a food for a long time, it is reported that patients suffering from hypertension and edema are appeared by the intake of licorice frequently. In 1968, a syndrome with these symptoms is named for licorice-induced pseudoaldosteronism and is recognized not only as a simple side effect but as one disease [1]. Aldosterone, which is the origin of the name of pseudoaldosteronism, is a hormone playing regulative roles on the level of electrolytes in the body. Aldosterone binds to the intracytoplasmic mineral corticoid receptor in renal tubule cells, induces the expression of $Na^+/K^+$ pump, and then promotes reabsorption of urinary $Na^+$ and a secretion of $K^+$. When plasma aldosterone level rose up by some reason, primary aldosteronism occurs with symptoms such as hypertension, edema, hypokalemia, hypernatremia with the increase of the potassium secretional capacity in the renal tubule, metabolic alkalosis, low plasma renin, muscle ache or numbness by the myopathy. Since those symptoms can be occurred by the intake of licorice, it is named as licorice-induced pseudoaldosteronism as a side effect of licorice.

# 3. The Past Findings about the Developing Mechanisms of Licorice-induced Pseudoaldosteronism

Licorice contains glycyrrhizin (GL), which belongs to triterpenoidal saponin, as a major component. GL provides anti-inflammatory action and is used as not only the internal agent but also the injection to improve liver functions. GL is a glucoside having the structure that contains 2 molecules of glucuronic acid connected to a hydroxyl group of the third place of glycyrrhetinic acid (GA), which is an aglycone. When we took licorice orally, GL is hard to penetrate through gastrointestinal tract epithelium for its high hydrophilic sugar part, and is absorbed as GA after the sugar part is hydrolyzed by enterobacteria inhabiting in large intestine to convert from GL to GA. Therefore, it is considered that GA is the main body of the pharmacological activity of licorice (Figure 1).

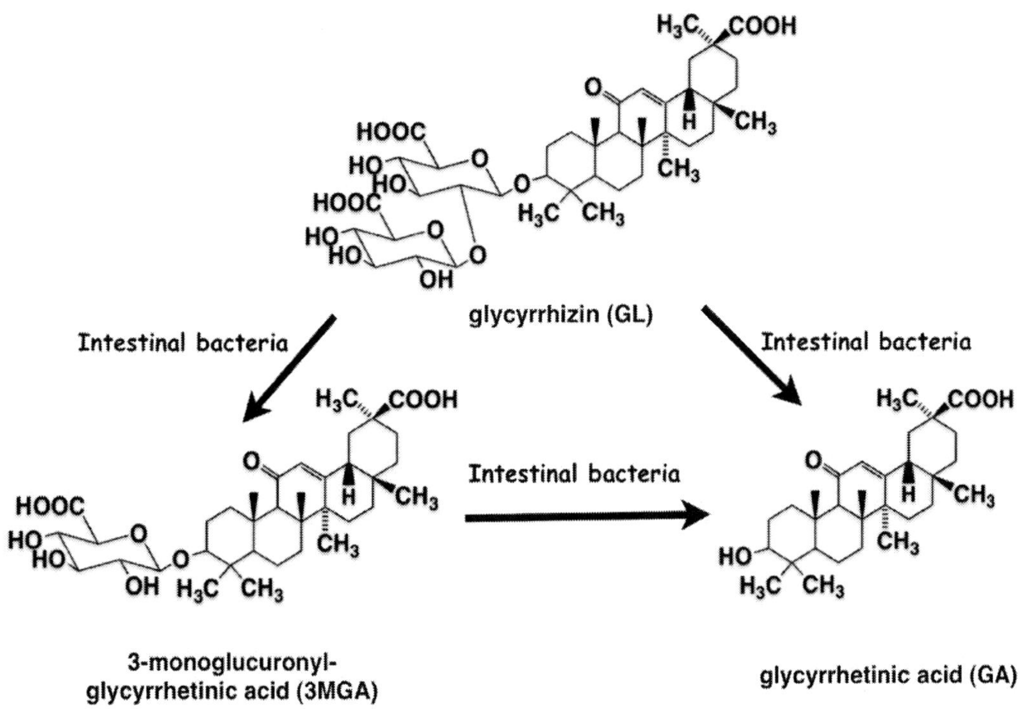


Figure 1. Chemical structures of glycyrrhizin and its metabolites by enterobacteria.

It has been well known that licorice has pharmacological activities similar to adrenal cortical hormones for a long time. In past, it had been thought that licorice-induced pseudoaldosteronism was occurred by the direct binding of GL or GA to mineral corticoid receptor. However, their affinity to the receptor is remarkably lower than aldosterone, which is an original substrate. Therefore, it is denied now that GL and GA directly bind to a receptor to cause cortical action at the level of real blood concentration. To a mineral corticoid receptor, cortisol, which is one of adrenal cortical hormones, also has the affinity with similar level of aldosterone. However, in the normal condition, cortisol is degraded into cortisone in the cytoplasm of renal tubular cells by type 2 11β-hydroxysteroid dehydrogenase (11β-HSD2). Since the affinity of cortisone to a mineral corticoid receptor is low, the activation of the receptor by cortisol is prohibited. GA and GL have the inhibitory effect on 11β-HSD2 [2]. It is reported that the inhibitory effect of GA on 11β-HSD1 was approximately 200 times than that of GL [3]. Furthermore, the compound which appears in blood when we ingest licorice is not GL but GA. Based upon the foregoing, it is thought that licorice-induced pseudoaldosteronism with hypokalemia and hypernatremia is caused as the results that GA inhibits 11β-HSD2 in renal tubular cells to accumulate cortisol that activates mineral corticoid receptor [4] (Figure 2).

However, from the above story, we cannot explain the individual differences of the onset of licorice-induced pseudoaldosteronism. In 1995, Kato *et al.* had reported the levels of licorice's metabolites in plasma of the patients using the kampo prescription containing licorice or using the preparation of GL, and they compared between those of the patients with or without licorice-included pseudoaldosteronism [5]. In their report, 3-monoglucronyl glychrrhetinic acid (3MGA), that contains 1 molecule of glucuronic acid connected to a hydroxyl group of the third place of GA (Figure 1), is detected in the plasma of the patients who developed licorice-induced pseudoaldosteronism, but is not detected in the plasma of the patients without pseudoaldosteronism. Therefore, it is supposed that the personal constitution to have 3MGA as a metabolite of GL might be associated with the onset of the pseudoaldosteronism. In contrast, in 2009, Harahap *et al.* had compared the gene sequencing of 11BHSD2 encoding 11β-HSD2 among the patients who had been treated with licorice and suffering from licorice-induced pseudoaldosteronism, and they found a point mutation of 11BHSD2 in genes collected from one of 15 patients [6].

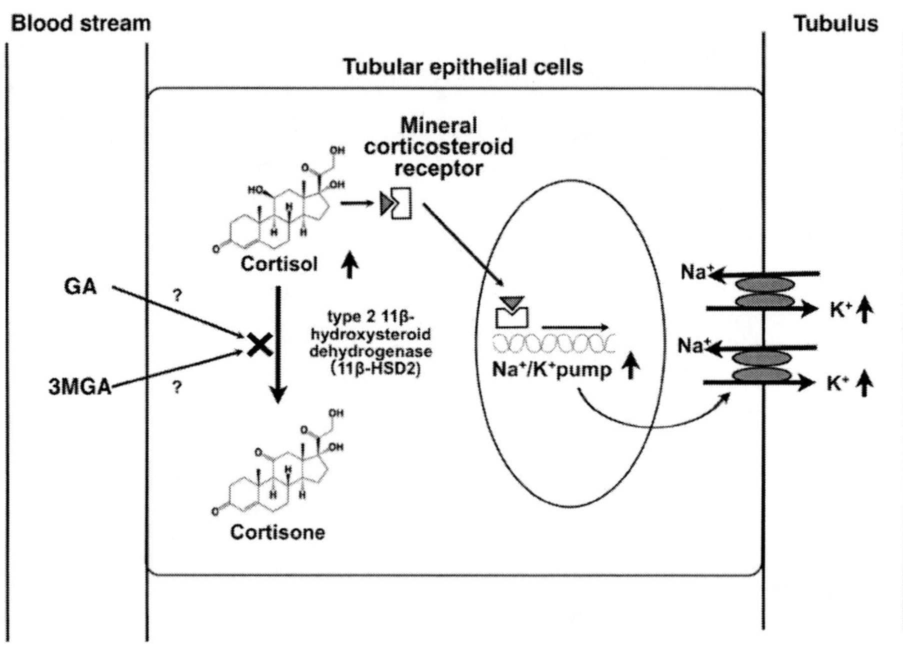


Figure 2. Estimated mechanisms of licorice-induced pseudoaldsteronism to cause hypokalemia.

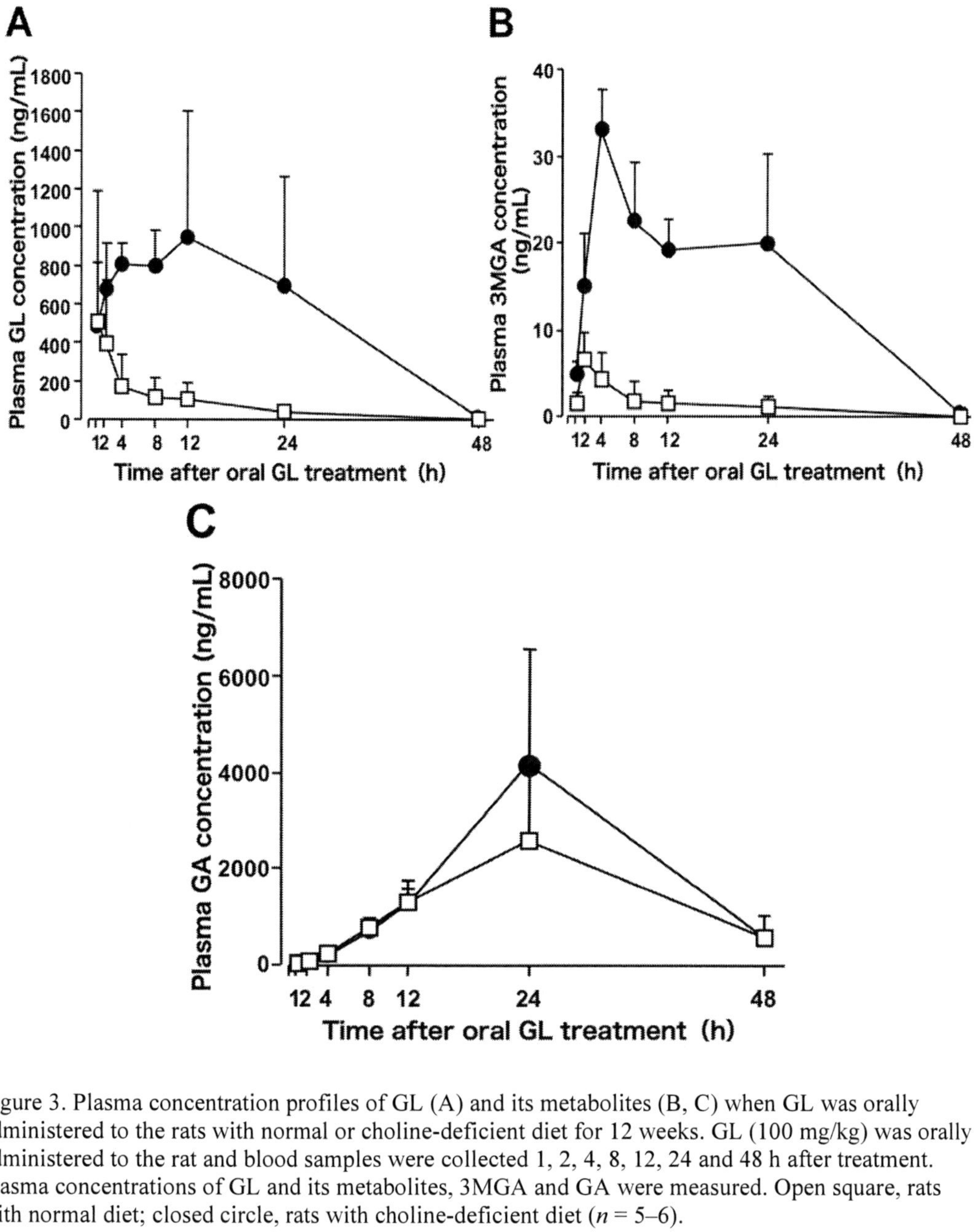


Figure 3. Plasma concentration profiles of GL (A) and its metabolites (B, C) when GL was orally administered to the rats with normal or choline-deficient diet for 12 weeks. GL (100 mg/kg) was orally administered to the rat and blood samples were collected 1, 2, 4, 8, 12, 24 and 48 h after treatment. Plasma concentrations of GL and its metabolites, 3MGA and GA were measured. Open square, rats with normal diet; closed circle, rats with choline-deficient diet ($n$ = 5–6).

# 4. Why Some Individuals Have 3mga in Blood as a Metabolite of Licorice, and Others Do not?

We paid our attention to the individual difference occurring in a blood level of 3MGA. We had bred rats in a choline-deficient diet for 12-13 weeks to make an animal model for hepatic fibrosis. Using this model, we examined the pharmacokinetics of licorice component and its metabolite [7]. We orally administered GL to the model rats of hepatic fibrosis or control rats, and we compared the profiles of plasma concentrations of each metabolite between these rats. As a result, higher levels of GL and 3MGA in the plasma of hepatic fibrosis model rats were found than those in control rats. However, there are no differences in plasma concentration profile of GA between these rats. Furthermore, in the hepatic fibrosis model rats, urinary excretion of GL and 3MGA showed higher values than those in control (Figure 3). Urinary excretion of GA in both hepatic fibrosis model rats and control was less than detection limit, and the difference was not found.

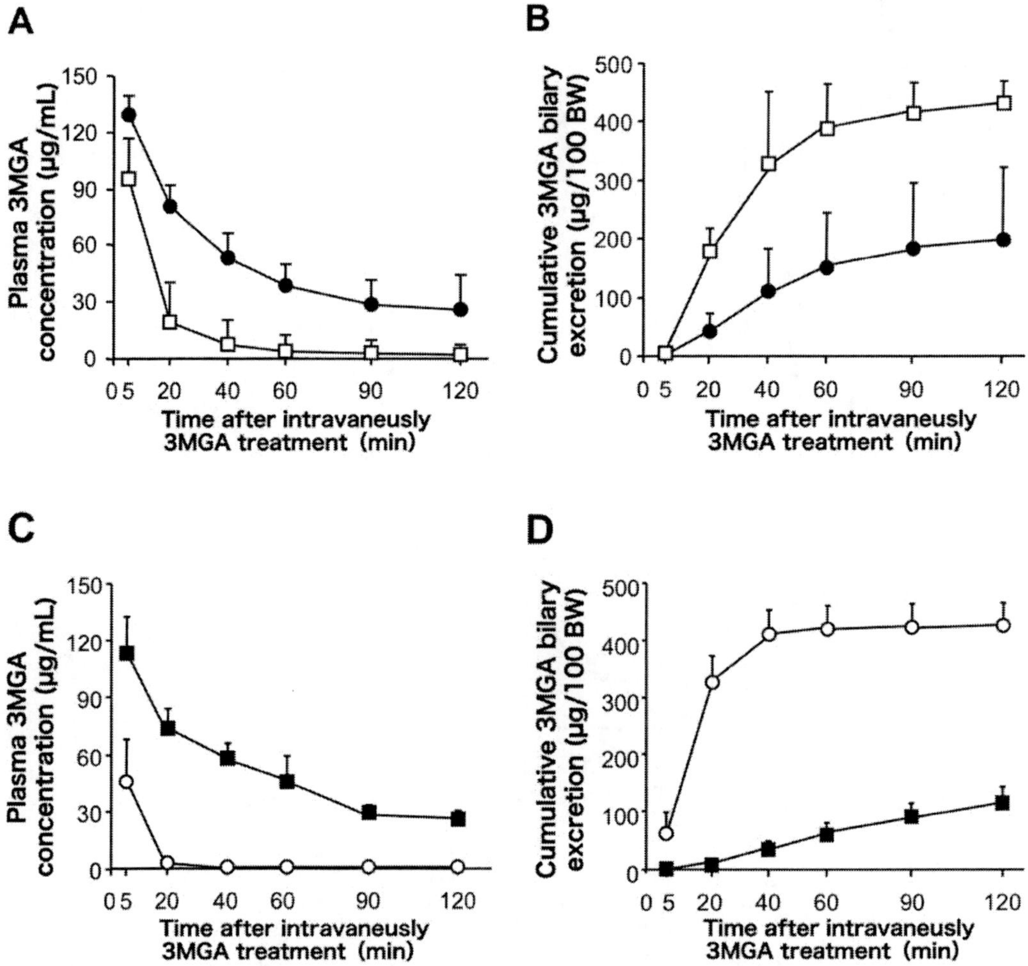


Figure 4. Plasma concentration profiles of 3MGA when 3MGA was intravenously infused to the rats with normal or choline-deficient diet for 13 weeks (A, B) and SD rats or EHBRs which have Mrp2 deficiency (C, D). 3MGA (5 mg/kg) was intravenously infused to the rats and blood samples were collected at 5, 20, 40, 60, 90, and 120 min (A, C), and bile samples were collected over a period of 120 min (B, D). Plasma and bile concentrations of 3MGA were measured as described in Materials and Methods. Open square, rats with normal diet; closed circle, rats with choline-deficient diet (A, B); open circle, SD rats; closed square, EHBRs (C, D); ($n = 6$).

3MGA has a chemical structure carrying glucuronic acid as a sugar moiety. That kind of the compounds may be excreted into bile from liver by some transporters such as the multidrug-resistant related protein (multidrug resistance protein 2, Mrp2). We found that the expression of Mrp2 in the bile duct pleural membrane of the liver was lower in hepatic fibrosis rat model than those in control. In another experiment, we intravaneously injected 3MGA into hepatic fibrosis rat model, and examined the profiles of its plasma and biliary levels. As a result, a decrease of plasma concentration and cumulative excretion of 3MGA in bile were found in hepatic fibrosis rat model compared with those in control. Furthermore, similar changes in plasma and biliary levels of 3MGA were found when we intravenously injected 3MGA into hyperbilirubinemia rats (EHBR), which have Mrp2 deficiency (Figure 4).

Based upon the foregoing, we can form following hypotheses about the pharmacokinetics of GL and its metabolites after the oral administration of licorice. When licorice was taken by oral, GL was hydrolyzed into GA by enterobacteria living in large intestine, and then GA is absorbed from gastrointestinal tract into the circulation. Therefore, the major component in blood is not GL but GA. GA is not excreted into urine. GA is metabolized by glucuronyltransferase expressed in liver into the conjugate, 3MGA. 3MGA is excreted into bile through at least Mrp2, which is a transporter taking biliary excretion from hepatocytes. Then a part of 3MGA is re-hydrolyzed into GA by enterobacteria, and is absorbed again to show enterohepatic circulation. And another part that was not absorbed is excreted into feces. Therefore, if liver function is in a normal state, 3MGA is not present in blood. However, when biliary excretion of 3MGA is prohibited by the decrease or the dysfunction of Mrp2 in liver, 3MGA would be returned from liver into blood by transporters such as Mrp3. In other words, in the background that 3MGA is present in blood, it is supposed that Mrp2 function or expression in liver would be interfered (Figure 5).

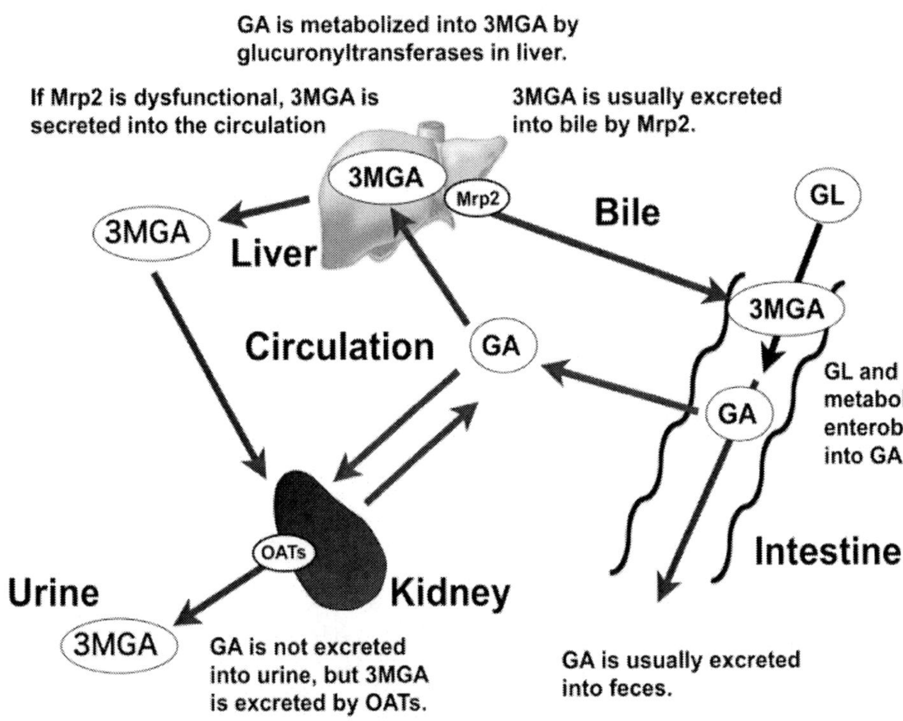


Figure 5. Estimated trip of glycyrrhizin (GL) in the body when it is orally administered.

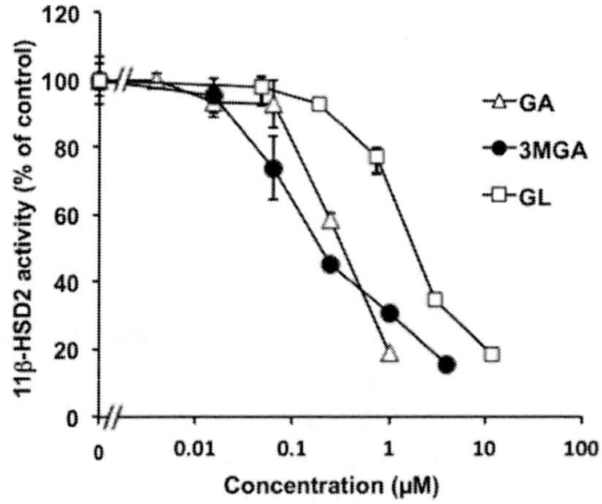


Figure 6. Inhibitory effect of glycyrrhizin (GL) and its metabolites on type 2 11β-hydroxysteroid dehydrogenase (11β-HSD2) in rat kidney microsome. Glycyrrhizin, 3MGA and glycyrrhetinic acid (GA) were added into the reaction mixture containing rat kidney microsome and cortisol, and the production of cortisone was measured. Open square, GL; closed circle, 3MGA; open triangle, GA. Data were expressed as mean of % of control ± S.E. ($n = 3$).

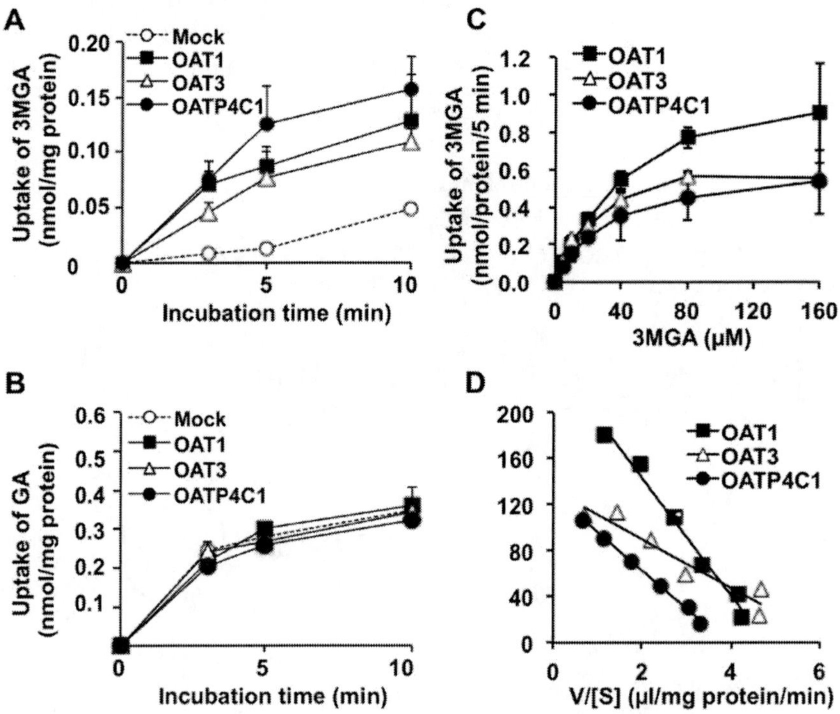


Figure 7. Uptake of 3MGA and glycyrrhetinic acid (GA) by HEK293 cells transfected with organic anion transporter (OAT) 1, OAT3 and organic anion transporting peptide (OATP) 4C1. HEK293 cells transfected with mock plasmid (open circle), OAT1 (closed square), OAT3 (open triangle) and OATP4C1 (closed circle) were incubated with 20 μM of 3MGA (A), 1 μM of GA (B) for 3–10 min and 5–160 μM of 3MGA for 5 min (C). The uptakes mediated with transporters were obtained by subtracting the uptake into mock cells from transporter-transfected cells (C). Data were expressed as mean ± S.E. ($n = 3$). The uptake kinetics was described as Eadie-Hofstee plots (D).

# 5. Relationships between Pseudoaldosteronism and 3MGA

Next, we conducted the experiments to reveal the relationships between pseudo-aldosteronism and 3MGA [8]. As described above, Kato *et al.*, who had reported that plasma 3MGA level had increased in the patients with pseudoaldosteronism, had compared the inhibitory effect of 3MGA on rat 11β-HSD2 activity with that of GA using rat kidney microsome fraction. At the concentration of 1 μM, the inhibitory titers of GA and 3MGA were similar (inhibition %, 96%), and at the concentration of 0.1 μM, that of GA was approximately 1.2 times stronger than that of 3MGA. From these results, it is suggested that 3MGA could inhibit 11β-HSD2 enough *in vitro* similar to GA to cause pseudoaldosteronism. We measured the dose-dependencies of the inhibition of GL, 3MGA and GA on 11β-HSD2 in rat kidney microsome fraction, and calculated their $IC_{50}$ values. As a result, we obtained 2.2 μM for GL, 0.26 μM for 3MGA and 0.32 μM for GA, respectively. Therefore, GA and 3MGA have approximately 10 times stronger than that of GL on 11β-HSD2 antagonism, and it was estimated that both GA and 3MGA could become the causative agent for pseudoaldosteronism (Figure 6).

We paid attention to the result that we could not detect GA in the urine collected from both liver fibrosis model rats and control rats. Because plasma and urinary levels of 3MGA in liver fibrosis model rats were higher than those in control, we examined the mechanism of the renal excretions of GA and 3MGA. At first, using bovine serum albumin and normal rat serum, we examined albumin-binding rates of 3MGA and GA by the ultrafiltration method. As a result, it was found that both 3MGA and GA were present as bounded form onto albumin in a ratio more than 99.9%. Therefore, it was suggested that both 3MGA and GA would hardly pass through the glomerular filtration to be excreted into urine. Since we could not detect GA but 3MGA in the urine of liver fibrosis model rats, it is supposed that GA could not be excreted through a tubular secretion but 3MGA could. We made rat renal slice segments and measured the uptakes of GA and 3MGA from the media into the specimen. Since 3MGA and GA adhered a lot to the renal tissue surface, kidney slices were incubated in the media containing GA and 3MGA at 4°C and 37°C environments and the part of active transport was calculated by the differences of uptakes between the temperature. As a result, the differences by the temperature were not found in the uptakes of GA from the media into kidney slices, but significantly higher uptakes of 3MGA at 37°C were observed compared with those at 4°C. It was supposed that the active transport of 3MGA was associated with the transition from the media into the renal tissue. 3MGA is an anionic organic compound. The transporters that express in the basolateral membrane of renal tubule epithelial cells and transport organic anions are OAT1, OAT3 and OATP4C1. Therefore, we conducted the uptake experiments using HEK293 cells that are transiently expressing those transporters. As a result, it is revealed that 3MGA is the substrates of those transporters, and the apparent Km values, 49.0 μM for OAT1, 30.1 μM for OAT3 and 41.8 μM for OATP4C1. However, the differences in the quantity of GA uptakes into between the mock cells and the cells transiently expressing these transporters were not observed (Figure 7). These results suggest that GA is hardly excreted into urine since GA has high albumin-binding property and is not the substrate for these transporters not to be excreted through glomerular filtration and tubular secretion.

The 11β-HSD2 antagonisms of GA and 3MGA using the kidney microsome fraction *in vitro* were almost similar levels. However, 11β-HSD2 is expressed in tubular cells in a real body, and it is estimated that only compounds that can be transferred into the cells can inhibit 11β-HSD2. Though most of both GA and 3MGA are present in blood as binding-form onto serum albumin, 3MGA can be transferred into the cells by active transporting systems through organic anion transporters, but GA would be hardly transferred into the tubular cells. Therefore, it is strongly suggested that 3MGA, not GA, exhibits the inhibitory effect on 11β-HSD2 in a real body; i.e., the causative agent of licorice-induced pseudoaldosteronism was supposed not to GA but more likely to 3MGA (Figure 8).

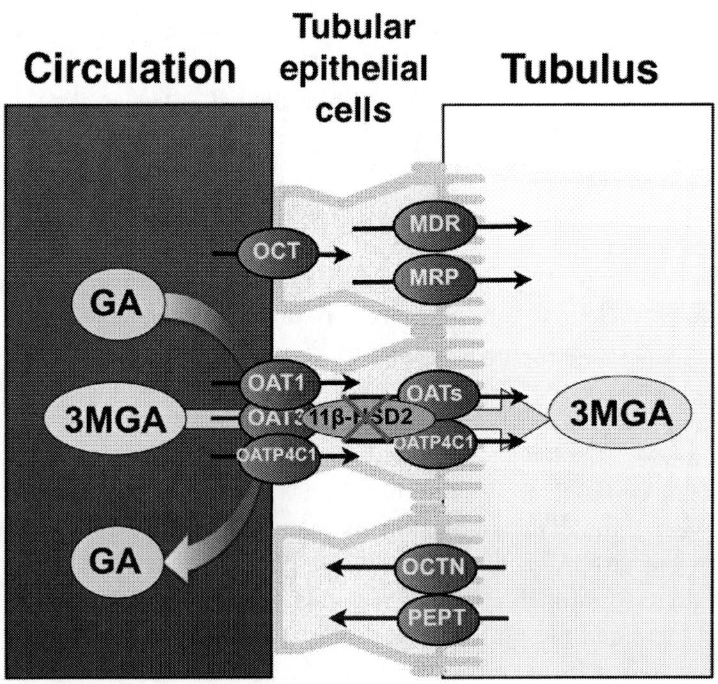


Figure 8. Estimated scheme to inhibit type 2 11β-hydroxysteroid dehydrogenase (11β-HSD2) in tubular epithelial cells by 3MGA or glycyrrhetinic acid (GA).

## Conclusion

As described in the first pragraph in this review, licorice-induced pseudoaldosteronism is the most common side effect of traditional Japanese kampo and Chinese medicines, and it is the most important subject in the medical care useing traditional medicine to prevent the onset beforehand. For pharmacists and physicians, the highly attention is required for the onset of the pseudoaldosteronism to use the prescription containing licorice more than 2.5 g per day. Physicians sometimes prescribe plural kampo formulas that containing licorice, and the dosage of licorice is excessive. In this case, pharmacists can check and solve the problems to prevent the side effects. However, since licorice is used as a food additive and the patients may ingest licorice unconsciously, it is very difficult to prevent pseudoaldosteronism only by the information about the dosage of licorice. In the present review, the authors find that

3MGA would play important roles to cause licorice-induced pseudoaldosteronism based on the clinical finding [5] of Kato *et al.* in 1995. Though our study is still limited by the experimental level, more large-scale clinical studies to reveal whether the onset of pseudoaldosteronism is related to the blood and urine level of 3MGA are demanded. In future, we are expecting that we can prevent the side effects of traditional Japanese kampo medicine and TCM containing licorice by measuring 3MGA levels in blood or urine.

# References

[1] Conn JW, Rovner DR, Cohen EL. Licorice-induced pseudoaldosteronism. Hypertension, hypokalemia, aldosteronopenia, and suppressed plasma renin activity. *JAMA* 1968:205:492–6.

[2] Edwards CR. Renal 11β-hydroxysteroid dehydrogenase: a mechanism ensuring mineralocorticoid specificity. *Horm Res* 1990:34:114–7.

[3] Monder C, Lakshmi V, Miroff Y. Kinetic studies on rat liver 11β-hydroxysteroid dehydrogenase. *Biochim Biophys Acta* 1991:1115: 23–9.

[4] Stewart PM, Wallace AM, Valentino R, Burt D, Shackleton CH, Edwards CR. Mineralocorticoid activity of liquorice: 11β-hydroxysteroid dehydrogenase deficiency comes of age. *Lancet* 1987:2:821–4.

[5] Kato H, Kanaoka M, Yano S, Kobayashi M. (1995) 3-Monoglucuronyl-glycyrrhetinic acid is a major metabolite that causes licorice-induced pseudoaldosteronism. *J Clin Endocrinol Metab* 1995:80:1929–33.

[6] Harahap IS, Sasaki, N., Gunadi, Yusoff S, Lee MJ, Morikawa S, Nishimura N, Sasaki T, Usuki S, Hirai M, Ohta M, Takaoka Y, Nishimoto T, Nishio H. Herbal medicine containing licorice may be contraindicated for a patient with an HSD11B2 mutation. *Evid Based Complement Alternat Med (in press).* doi: 10.1093/ecam/nep211.

[7] Makino T, Ohtake N, Watanabe A, Tsuchiya N, Imamura S, Iizuka S, Inoue M, Mizukami H. Down-regulation of a hepatic transporter multidrug resistance-associated protein 2 is involved in alteration of pharmacokinetics of glycyrrhizin and its metabolites in a rat model of chronic liver injury. *Drug Metab Dispos* 2008:36:1438–43.

[8] Makino T, Okajima K, Uebayashi R, Ohtake N, Inoue K, Mizukami H. 3-Monoglucuronyl-glycyrrhretinic acid is a substrate of organic anion transporters expressed in tubular epithelial cells and plays important roles in licorice-induced pseudoaldosteronism by inhibiting 11β-hydroxysteroid dehydrogenase 2. *J Pharmacol Exp Ther (in press).* doi; 10.1124/jpet.111.190009.

In: Traditional Medicine: New Research
Editor: Yoshiharu Motoo
ISBN: 978-1-62257-448-3


*Chapter 10*

# Gomisin N: A Herb-derived Compound that Enhances Death Receptor-mediated Apoptosis of Cancer Cells

***Pornthip Waiwut*** [1]**, *Hiroki Inoue*** [1]**, *Ikuo Saiki*** [1]
**and *Hiroaki Sakurai*** [1,2]
[1]Division of Pathogenic Biochemistry, Institute of Natural Medicine,
[2]Department of Cancer Cell Biology, Graduate School of Medicine
and Pharmaceutical Sciences, University of Toyama, Toyama, Japan

## Abstract

Tumor necrosis factor–α (TNF-α) is a pleiotropic cytokine that plays an important role in the control of cell proliferation, differentiation, and apoptosis. TNF-α-induced apoptosis is limited by TAK1-mediated activation of NF-κB (mainly p65-p50 heterodimer) signaling pathway. The kinase TAK1, a mitogen-activated protein kinase kinase kinase (MAP3K), has been widely accepted as a key kinase activating NF-κB and MAPKs in TNF-α signaling. We have recently reported that TAK1 regulates the transient phosphorylation and endocytosis of epidermal growth factor receptor (EGFR) in a tyrosine kinase activity-independent manner. Thr-669 and Ser-1046/7 were differently regulated via TAK1-ERK and TAK1-p38 pathways, respectively. In addition, p38, but not ERK, was involved in the endocytosis of EGFR. Surprisingly, modified EGFR was essential to prevent apoptotic cellular response: however, the EGFR was dependent of different signaling pathways, IκB kinase-NF-κB and MAPKs-EGFR, leading to the survival of cell exposed to the death signal from TNF-α receptor. We have recently screened gomisin N, a dibenzocyclooctadiene lignan isolated from the fruit of *Schisandra chinensis,* that influenced death receptor-mediated apoptotic response. Gomisin N strongly promoted TNF-α-induced cleavage of caspase-3 and PARP-1, which are key markers of apoptosis. We found that gomisin N inhibited the TNF-α-induced activation of NF-κB by suppressing the activation of IKKα. Gomisin N also inhibited p38-mediated phosphorylation of the EGFR at Ser-1046/7 and subsequent endocytosis of EGFR. Furthermore, gomisin N could protentiate TNF-related apoptosis-inducing ligand (TRAIL)-induced apoptosis through up-regulation of death receptore 4 (DR4) and DR5.

The findings suggested that gomisin N migh be useful to promote death receptor-mediated apoptosis in the treatment of malignant tumor.

# Introduction

In traditional Oriental medicine, the fruit of *Schisandra chinensis*, Schizandra berry, has been used to treat a variety of diseases. Pharmacological studies of lignans isolated from Schizandra berry have also revealed anti-cancer properties, anti-hepatocarcinogenesis, and antioxidant and anti-inflammatory activities [1-3]. Gomisin N, a dibenzocyclooctadiene lignan isolated from the fruit of *Schisandra chinensis*, has been reported as an anti-cancer drug candidate. A recent study demonstrated that gomisin N inhibits proliferation and induces apoptosis in human hepatic carcinomas through a mitochondrial (intrinsic) pathway by enhancing Bax protein expression and so inhibiting the anti-apoptotic activity of Bcl-2 [4]. Apoptosis, a programmed cell death, occurs during many important physiological conditions, such as embryonic development, tissue remodeling, the maintenance of homeostasis, and immune repertoires [5]. The deregulation of apoptosis results in diseases, including autoimmune diseases, cancer, and neurodegenerative disorders [6]. Apoptosis is also the basis for therapies designed to target cancerous cells and limit the cytotoxicity that results from drug treatment [7-8]. The efficacy of many chemotherapeutics is due to their ability to induce tumor cell death by apoptosis. Death receptor-mediated tumor cell death, either alone or in combination with other anticancer drugs, is considered a new strategy for anticancer therapy. Tumor necrosis factor (TNF)-α and TNF-related apoptosis-inducing ligand (TRAIL) are death ligands playing an important role in triggering apoptosis through death receptor pathways [9]. This article describes the effect of gomisin N on death receptor-mediated apoptosis in cancer cells by focusing on TNF-α- and TRAIL-mediated apoptosis.

# Gomisin N; Lignan Isolatated from *Schisandra chinensis*

Traditional Chinese medicines (TCMs) are essential components of alternative medicines. In China and Japan, the mainstream medical opinion is that supplementing chemotherapy with traditional herbal formulas can improve the survival rates and life expectancy of cancer patients. The fruit of *Schisandra chinensis* (Figure 1A) has been used in traditional Chinese medicine to treat a variety of diseases such as diabetes, asthma, respiratory infections and mental illnesses such as palpitation, insomnia, and forgetfulness. It is used to tone up and strengthen kidney function and to help the body to balance levels of fluid, making it helpful for treating excessive sweating. *Schisandra chinensis* has also been employed in the treatment and prevention of some chronic diseases such as inflammation, hepatitis, and cancer [10-11]. Pharmacological studies on animals have shown that Schizandra increases physical working capacity and affords a stress-protective effect against a broad spectrum of harmful factors including heat shock, skin burn, cooling, frostbite, immobilisation, swimming under load in an atmosphere with decreased air pressure, aseptic inflammation, irradiation, and heavy metal intoxication [12]. The major bioactive constituents of *Shisandra chinensis* are lignans, including gomisin A, B, C, E, F, G, K, N, and J, scisandrol B, and schisandrin C. [11]. Pharmacological studies revealed that lignans isolated from *Schisandra Chinesis* show anti-cancer, anti-hepatotoxic, anti-oxidative, and anti-inflammatory activities [13-15]. It has been reported that dibenzocyclooctadiene lignans inhibited cell proliferation in cancer cells. The most active and abundant dibenzo-cyclooctadiene derivative is schisandrin B (Sch B) [16]. This derivative has been used for the treatment of viral and chemical hepatitis. Schisandrin B has enantiomers [(+)Sch B and (-)Sch B], which exhibit different functions. (+)Sch B induces proliferation and apoptosis. This compound was found to significantly enhance doxorubicin-induced apoptosis in human hepatic carcinoma cells and breast cancer cells. In contrast, (-)Sch B is similar to gomisin N. Pretreatment with this compound significantly protected againt hypoxia/ reoxygeneration-induced apoptosis in H9c2 cells [17]. Gomisin N (Figure 1B) achieved the highest anticancer activity among the four compounds screened: gomisin N, schisandrin, schisandrin C, and gomisin A, suggesting that gomisin N is an anticancer drug candidate capable of inhibiting the proliferation and inducing the apoptosis of human hepatic carcinoma cells [18]. Moreover, gomisin N, the S-bihenyl configuration, the most abundant dibenzo-cyclooctadiene lignan correlated with increased antiproliferative activity, is shown to enhance doxorubicin-induced apoptosis in cancer cells but not normal cells [19]. We have recently demonstrated that gomisin N is able to sensitize cancer cells to TNF-α- and TRAIL- induced apoptosis [20].

## Death Receptor-mediated Apoptosis in Cancer Cells

Death receptors are cell-surface receptors belonging to the tumor necrosis factor (TNF) superfamily that includes CD95 (FAS/APO-1), TNF-R1 and TRAIL receptors (DR4 and DR5) (Figure 2). All death receptors carry a conserved cytoplasmic domain called the death domain (DD). The DD is a structurally conserved protein-interaction domain (consisting of six antiparallel α-helices) which is important for the initiation of apoptotic signals [21-22]. On ligand binding, death receptors trimerize and recruit adaptor molecules to form the death-inducing signaling complex (DISC); this initiates a cascade leading to caspase activation and finally to cell death. Although there are differences in the signaling pathways activated by the different death receptors, it is possible to outline a general apoptotic signaling pathway. Binding of the death-inducing ligand to its receptor leads to the generation of ceramide, typically produced by acid sphingomyelinase. Ceramide release is thought to promote lipid raft fusion which results in a large scale clustering of the death receptors. The receptor clustering is important because it helps amplification of the apoptotic signaling. Although some cells, such as lymphocytes, are still able to trigger apoptosis in the absence of receptor clustering, in most cases amplification of the signaling pathway is needed to activate the full apoptotic response [23-25]. Following ligand binding, a conformational change in the intracellular domains of the receptors allows the recruitment of various apoptotic proteins to the receptor. This protein complex is often called the DISC. The final step in this process is the recruitment of caspases-8 to the DISC via the adaptor protein Fas-associated death domain protein (FADD). This results in the activation of caspase 8, which triggers the initiation of apoptosis [26]. Many chemotherapeutic agents induce tumor cell death through death receptors. The death receptor ligands TNF-α, FasL and TRAIL are able to induce apoptosis by binding to their cell membrane receptors [27-28]. These ligands are capable of potentiating the effects of chemotherapeutic drugs *in vitro* and *in vivo* in the animal model. It is a major challenge to translate the current knowledge of these death receptor ligands into cancer therapeutics. For optimal effect, it is most likely that ligand therapy will be combined with chemotherapy, but even a combination of ligands for patient treatments can be envisioned. It is expected that compounds targeting these death receptors will be designed to lower toxicity and increase antitumor activity.

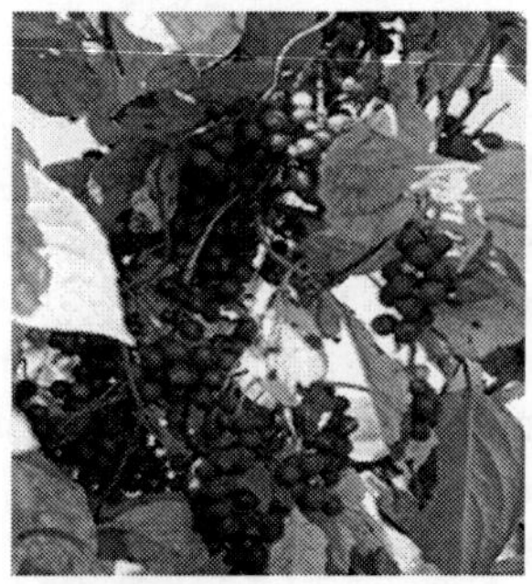

***Schisandra chinensis***

a

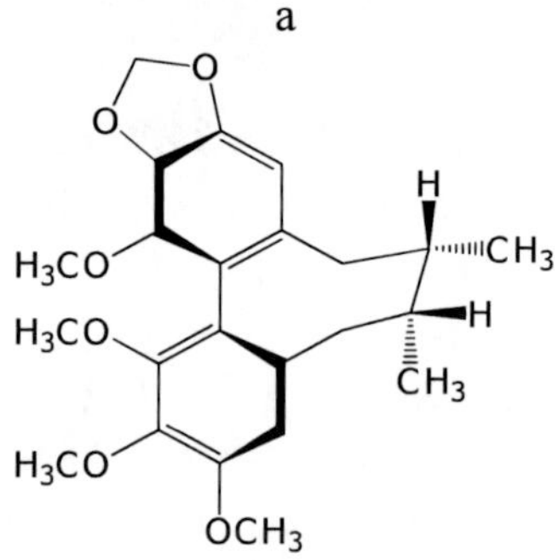


**Gomisin N**

b

Figure 1. Ilustration of Shisandra Chinensis (A) and chemical structure of gomisin N (B).

## TAK1 Regulates Two Independent Survival Pathways

TNF-α stimulates several intracellular signaling pathways, including nuclear factor-κB (NF-κB) and mitogen-activated protein kinases (MAPKs). TNF-α also triggers apoptosis via formation of the DISC [29], consisting of trimerized receptors, the death domain-containing adaptor protein FADD, and caspase-8. Activation of caspase-8 leads to the direct activation of downstream caspases, such as caspase-3, and subsequently the cleavage of a nuclear enzyme, poly (ADP-ribose) polymerase (PARP). Transforming growth factor-β-activated kinase (TAK1) is a common upstream regulator of NF-κB and MAPKs and prevents apoptotic responses. The IκB kinase (IKK) complex phosphorylates NF-κB at Ser-536 as well as IκBα at Ser-32/36 in cytokine-induced NF-κB activation [30-32]. NF-κB is involved in cell survival in a variety of cell types by up-regulating the expression of anti-apoptotic genes, including *c-FLIP* and *A20* [33]. We have recently demonstrated that TNF-α triggers a non-canonical epidermal growth factor receptor (EGFR) pathway in a TAK1-dependent fashion, in which EGFR Thr-669 and Ser-1046/7 are phosphorylated via extracellular signal-regulated kinase (ERK) and p38 MAPK, respectively. Moreover, p38-mediated Ser-1046/7 phosphorylation triggers transient endocytosis of the EGFR, which blocks the TNF-α-induced death signal [34-35]. Therefore, TAK1 regulates two independent survival pathways, the NF-κB and EGFR pathways, to prevent TNF-α-induced cell death.

## Gomisin N Enhances TNF-α-induced Apoptotic Responses

One of the key initiation elements of the apoptotic pathway is the activation of caspases followed by cleavage of the caspase substrates. The 113-kDa poly (ADP-ribose) polymerase 1 (PARP-1), which is normally involved in DNA repair, DNA stability, and other cellular events, is cleaved by members of the caspase family during early apoptosis [36]. TNF-α-induced apoptosis is associated with caspase activation and PARP degradation. Gomisin N has been shown to induce apoptotic responses in HeLa cells by activating pro-apoptotic cleavage of caspase-3 and PARP-1 [20].

## Gomisin N Enhances TNF-α-induced NF-κB Activation

In the death receptor-mediated apoptotic pathway, NF-κB is widely known for its ubiquitous roles as a cell survival transcription factor. NF-κB protects cells from apoptosis by transcriptional activation of survival genes encoding anti-apoptotic proteins [37]. It has been widely accepted that cells deficient in TAK1, IKKβ, or p65 are sensitive to TNF-α-induced apoptosis, indicating that the TAK1-NF-κB signaling pathway functions as a main survival signal [38-39]. In the TNF-α-induced NF-κB pathway, gomisin N inhibited the phosphorylation of IKKα and p65 but not TAK1, suggesting that gomisin N interferes with IKKα or multiple upstream kinases including MEKK3, PKC, and Akt [40].

## Effect of Gomisin N on TNF-α-induced Non-canonical EGFR Pathway

EGFR, a member of the receptor tyrosine kinase (RTK) family, has recently been a focus of molecular targeted cancer therapy, because overexpression, amplification, and mutations are involved in carcinogenesis and the progression of several types of cancer [41-42]. EGFR has been shown to be phosphorylated under cellular stress, including that caused by TNF-α, high osmotic stress, anisomycin, UV and cisplatin through p38[43]. We have identified two independent signaling pathways from the TNF-α receptor to EGFR via ERK and p38 MAPK pathways, which caused phosphorylation of EGFR at Thr-669 and Ser-1046/1047, respectively. Based on these findings, we describe this new EGFR function as a non-canonical pathway[34]. The independency of ligand binding and tyrosine kinase activation is the most important feature different from classical EGFR activation.

In the TNF-α-induced EGFR signaling pathway, treatment of HeLa cells with gomisin N resulted in inhibition of the phosphorylation of MKK3/6, p38, and MK2 as well as EGFR (pS1046/7). These results raise the possibility that gomisin N blocks the activation of MKK3/6 by interfering with some regulatory kinases including MEKK1-4, MLK, ASK1, and TAO, which have been shown to act as upstream kinases regulating MKK3/6 phosphorylation [20, 44]. Identification of the target molecules is essential and will contribute to our understanding of the molecular mechanisms of the anti-cancer activity of gomisin N. In addition, gomisin N is a powerful chemical probe with which to characterize the downstream signaling pathways of TAK1.

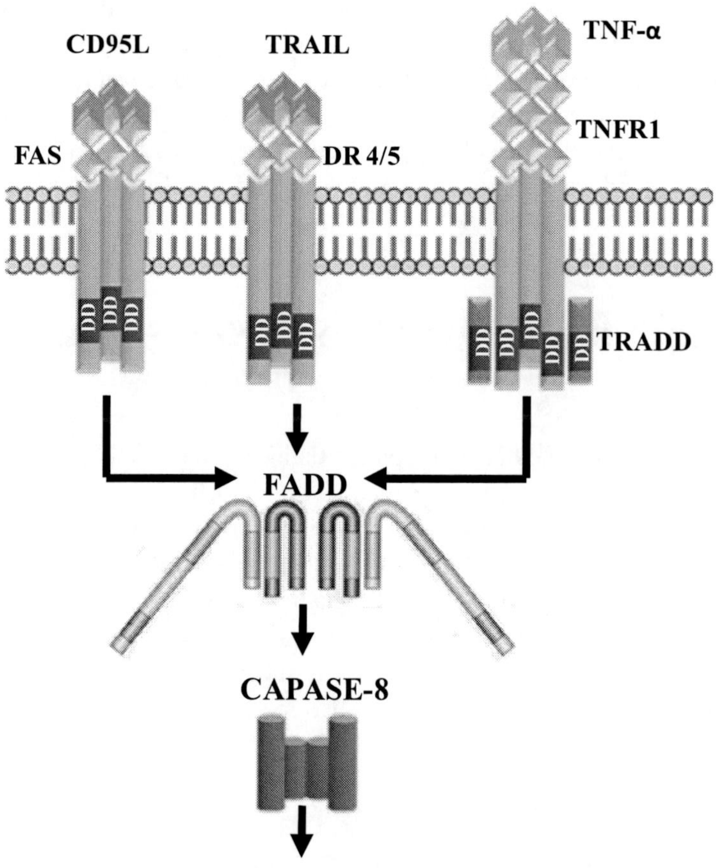


Figure 2. Death receptors and their ligands.

## Gomisin N Enhances TRAIL-induced Apoptosis

TRAIL is a cytokine inducing apoptosis in a variety of tumor cells through binding to its two distinct receptors, DR4 and DR5. These receptors interact with FADD, which leads to sequential activation of caspase-8 and caspase-3. Alternatively, TRAIL can also activate caspase-3 through mitochondrial bid cleavage, cytochrome *c* release, and caspase-9 activation [45]. Since TRAIL induces apoptosis in transformed or tumor cells but not in normal cells, it is considered to be a promising therapeutic agent for cancer. However, many types of cancer cells are resistant to TRAIL-induced apoptosis, therefore, it is important to overcome this resistance to expand the capabilities of TRAIL in cancer therapy [46]. We have recently demonstrated that gomisin N potentiated TRAIL-induced cell death via activation of caspase-8, caspase-3, and PARP-1. Moreover, gomisin N increased DR4 and DR5 expression. Generation of reactive oxygen species (ROS) has been proposed to be involved in the upregulation of TRAIL receptors by gomisin N, because an antioxidant agent, NAC, abolished the up-regulation [47].

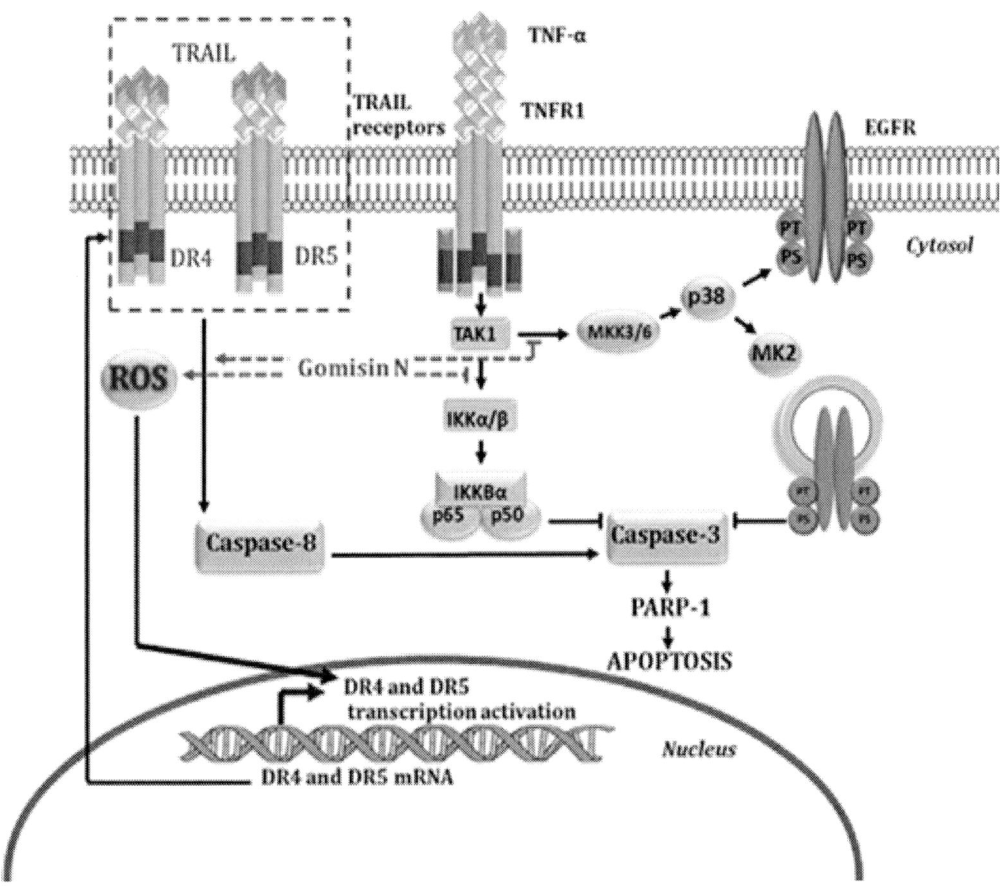


Figure 3. Schematic diagram of gomisin N-enhanced death receptor-induced apoptosis. Gomisin N enhances TNF-α-induced apoptosis via inhibition of the p65 and EGFR signaling pathways. Gomisin N sensitized cancer cells to TRAIL-induced apoptosis through ROS-mediated up-regulation of DR4 and DR5 expression.

# Conclusion

We have demonstrated that gomisin N sensitizes cancer cells to both TNF-α- and TRAIL-induced apoptosis (Figure 3). Gomisin N enhanced TNF-α-induced apoptosis by targeting TAK1-mediated anti-apoptotic pathways, including NF-κB and EGFR. Because TAK1 is normally activated by TNF-α even in the presence of gomisin N, gomisin N acted to suppress the activation of NF-κB through inhibition of IKKα phosphorylation and the p38-EGFR pathway through inhibition of MKK3/6. In addition, gomisin N sensitized cancer cells to TRAIL-induced apoptosis through ROS-mediated up-regulation of DR4 and DR5 expression. These findings provide a new molecular basis for the development of gomisin N as a potential anti-cancer drug.

# References

[1] Ikeya Y, Taguchi H, Yosioka I, Kobayashi H. The constituents of Schizandrachinensis Baill. I. Isolation and structure determination of five new lignans, gomisin A, B, C, F and G, and the absolute structure of schizandrin. *Chem Pharm Bull.* 1979; 27:1383–94.

[2] Lee YW, Voyksner RD, Pack TW, Cook CE, Fang QC, Ito Y. Application of countercurrent chromatography thermospray mass spectrometry for the identification of bioactive lignans from plant natural products. *Anal Chem.* 1990;62: 244–48.

[3] Opletal L, Sovov H, Brtlov M. Dibenzo[a,c]cyclooctadiene lignans of the genus Schisandra: importance, isolation and determination. *J Chromatogr B Analyt Technol Biomed Life Sci.* 2004;812: 357–71.

[4] Yim SY, Lee YJ, Lee YK, Jung SE, Kim JH, Kim HJ, et.al . Gomisin N isolated from Schisandra chinensis significantly induces anti-proliferative and pro-apoptotic effects in hepatic carcinoma. *Mol Med Rep.* 2009;2: 725-32.

[5] Evan GI, Vousden KH. Proliferation, cell cycle and apoptosis in cancer. *Nature.* 2001;411: 342–48.

[6] Okada H, Mak TW. Pathways of apoptotic and non-apoptotic death in tumour cells. *Nat Rev Cancer.* 2004;4: 592-603.

[7] Debatin KM, Krammer PH. Death receptors in chemotherapy and cancer. *Oncogene.* 2004;23: 2950–66.

[8] Irene GM, Thomas EW, Alex AA. Targeting Apoptosis Pathways in Cancer Therapy. *CA Cancer J Clin.* 2005;55:178-194.

[9] Smith CA, Farrah T, Goodwin RG. The TNF receptor superfamily of cellular and viral proteins: activation, costimulation, and death. *Cell.* 1994;76: 959-62.

[10] Štěrbová H, Ševčíková P, Kvasničková L, Glatz Z, Slanina J. Determination of lignans in Schisandra chinensis using micellar electrokinetic capillary chromatograph. *Electrophoresis.* 2002;23: 253-8.

[11] He X, Lian L, Lin L. Analysis of lignan constituents from Schisandra chinensis by liquid chromatography-electrospray mass spectrometry. *J Chromatogr A.* 1997;757: 81-7.

[12] Panossian A, Wikman G. Pharmacology of Schisandra chinensis Bail.: an overview of Russian research and uses in medicine. *J Ethnopharmacol.* 2008;23:183-212.

[13] Min HY, Park EJ, Hong JY, Kang YJ, Kim SJ, Chung HJ, et. al. Antiproliferative effects of dibenzocyclooctadiene lignans isolated from Schisandra chinensis in human cancer cells. *Bioorg Med Chem Lett.* 2008;18: 523-6.

[14] Choi MS, Kwon KJ, Jeon SJ, Go HS, Kim KC, Ryu JR, et. al. Schizandra chinensis Alkaloids Inhibit Lipopolysaccharide-Induced Inflammatory Responses in BV2 Microglial Cells. *Biomolecules & therapeutics.* 2009;17: 47-56.

[15] Oh SY, Kim YH, Bae DS, Um BH, Pan CH, Kim CY, et al. Anti-inflammatory effects of gomisin N, gomisin J, and schisandrin C isolated from the fruit of Schisandra chinensis. *Biosci Biotechnol Biochem.* 2010;74:285-91.

[16] Li XY. Bioactivity of neolignans from fructus Schizandrae. *Mem Inst Oswaldo Cruz.* 1991;2: 31-7.

[17] Chiu PY, Leung HY, Poon MK, Mak DH, Ko KM. (-)Schisandrin B is more potent than its enantiomer in enhancing cellular glutathione and heat shock protein production as well as protecting against oxidant injury in H9c2 cardiomyocytes. *Mol Cell Biochem.* 2006;289: 185-91.

[18] Yim SY, Lee YJ, Lee YK, Jung SE, Kim JH, Kim HJ, et al. Gomisin N isolated from Schisandra chinensis significantly induces anti-proliferative and pro-apoptotic effects in hepatic carcinoma. *Mol Med Report.* 2009;2: 725-32.

[19] Ling Li, Qinghua Lu, Yanwei Shen, Xun Hu. Schisandrin B enhances doxorubicin-induced apoptosis of cancer cells but not normal cells. *Biochemical Pharmacology.* 2006;71: 584-595.

[20] Waiwut P, Shin MS, Inujima A, Zhou Y, Koizumi K, Saiki I, et al. Gomisin N enhances TNF-α-induced apoptosis via inhibition of the NF-κB and EGFR survival pathways. *Mol Cell Biochem.* 2011;350: 169-75.

[21] Garofalo M, Condorelli GL, Croce CM, Condorelli G. MicroRNAs as regulators of death receptors signaling. *Cell Death Differ.* 2010;17: 200-8.

[22] Bodmer JL, Schneider P, Tschopp J. The molecular architecture of the TNF superfamily. *Trends Biochem Sci.* 2002;**27**: 19–26.

[23] Wehrli P, Viard I, Bullani R, Tschopp J, French LE. Death Receptors in Cutaneous Biology and Disease. *J Invest Der.* 2000;115: 141–48.

[24] Fulda S, Debatin KM. Extrinsic versus intrinsic apoptosis pathways in anticancer chemotherapy. *Oncogene.* 2006;7:4798-811.

[25] Ashkenazi A. Targeting death and decoy receptors of the tumour-necrosis factor superfamily. *Nature Reviews Cancer***.** 2002;**2**: 420-30 .

[26] Thorburn A. Death receptor-induced cell killing. *Cellular Signalling.* 2004;16: 139–44.

[27] Fulda S, Debatin KM. Resveratrol modulation of signal transduction in apoptosis and cell survival: a mini-review. *Cancer Detect Prev.* 2006;30: 217-23.

[28] Jacquemin G, Shirley S, Micheau O. Combining naturally occurring polyphenols with TNF-related apoptosis-inducing ligand: a promising approach to kill resistant cancer cells. *Cell Mol Life Sci.* 2010;67:3115-30.

[29] Wajant H, Pfizenmaier K, Scheurich P. Tumor necrosis factor signaling. *Cell Death Differ.* 2003;10: 45-65.

[30] Sakurai H, Suzuki S, Kawasaki N, Nakano H, Okazaki T, Chino A, et al. Tumor necrosis factor-alpha-induced IKK phosphorylation of NF-κB p65 on serine 536 is mediated through the TRAF2, TRAF5, and TAK1 signaling pathway. *J Biol Chem.* 2003;278: 36916-23.

[31] Perkins ND. Integrating cell-signalling pathways with NF-κB and IKK function. *Nat Rev Mol Cell Biol.* 2007;8: 49-62.
[32] Takaesu G, Surabhi RM, Park KJ, Tsuji JN, Matsumoto K, Gaynor RB. TAK1 is Critical for IκB Kinase-mediated Activation of the NF-κB Pathway. *J Mol Biol.* 2003;326: 105-115.
[33] Chariot A. The NF-κB-independent functions of IKK subunits in immunity and cancer. *Trends Cell Biol.* 2009;19:404-413.
[34] Nishimura M, Shin MS, Singhirunnusorn P, Suzuki S, Kawanishi M, Koizumi K, et al. TAK1-mediated serine/threonine phosphorylation of epidermal growth factor receptor via p38/extracellular signal-regulated kinase: NF-κB-independent survival pathways in tumor necrosis factor alpha signaling. *Mol Cell Biol.* 2009;29: 5529-39.
[35] Shin MS, Shinghirunnusorn P, Sugishima Y, Nishimura M, Suzuki S, Koizumi K, et al. Cross interference with TNF-α-induced TAK1 activation via EGFR-mediated p38 phosphorylation of TAK1-binding protein 1. *Biochim Biophys Acta.* 2009;793: 1156-64.
[36] Lazebnik YA, Kaufmann SH, Desnoyers S, Poirier GG, Earnshaw WC. Cleavage of poly(ADP-ribose) polymerase by a proteinase with properties like ICE. *Nature.* 1994;371: 346-7.
[37] Jo Luo J, Kamata H, Karin M. IKK/NF-κB signaling: balancing life and death-a new approach to cancer therapy. *J Clin Invest.* 2005;115: 2625–32.
[38] Beg AA, Baltimore D. An essential role for NF-κB in preventing TNF-α-induced cell death. *Science.* 1996;274: 782-4.
[39] Omori E, Matsumoto K, Sanjo H, Sato S, Akira S, Smart RC, et al. TAK1 is a master regulator of epidermal homeostasis involving skin inflammation and apoptosis. *J Biol Chem.* 2006;281: 19610-7.
[40] Hayden MS, Ghosh S. Signaling to NF-κB. *Genes Dev.* 2004;18: 2195-224.
[41] Schneider MR, Wolf E. The epidermal growth factor receptor ligands at aglance. *J Cell Physiol.* 2009;218: 460-6.
[42] Sebastian S, Settleman J, Reshki SJ, Azzariti A, Bellizzi A, Paradiso A. The complexity of targeting EGFR signalling in cancer: from expression to turnover. *Biochim Biophys Acta.*2006;1766: 120-39.
[43] Singhirunnusorn P, Ueno Y, Matsuo M, Suzuki S, Saiki I, Sakurai H. Transient suppression of ligand-mediated activation of epidermal growth factor receptor by tumor necrosis factor-α through the TAK1-p38 signaling pathway. *J Biol Chem.* 2007;282: 12698-706.
[44] Coulthard LR, White DE, Jones DL, McDermott MF, Burchill SA. p38 (MAPK): stress responses from molecular mechanisms to therapeutics. *Trends Mol Med.* 2009;15: 369-79.
[45] Kim K, Fisher MJ, Xu SQ, el-Deiry WS. Molecular determinants of response to TRAIL in killing of normal and cancer cells. *Clin Cancer Res.* 2000;6: 335-46.
[46] Zhang L, Fang B. Mechanisms of resistance to TRAIL-induced apoptosis in cancer. *Cancer Gene Ther.* 2005;12: 228-37.

[47] Zhang L, Fang B. Mechanisms of resistance to TRAIL-induced apoptosis in cancer. *Cancer Gene Ther.* 2005;12: 228-37.

[48] Inoue H, Waiwut P, Saiki I, Shimada Y, Sakurai H. Gomisin N enhances TRAIL-induced apoptosis via reactive oxygen species-mediated up-regulation of death receptors 4 and 5. *Int J Oncol.* 2012:1048-65.

In: Traditional Medicine: New Research
Editor: Yoshiharu Motoo
ISBN: 978-1-62257-448-3


*Chapter 11*

# Clinical Risk Management of Interactions between Kampo Medicines and Western Medicines

***Peter A. G. M. De Smet*** *
Departments of IQ Healthcare and Clinical Pharmacy, Radboud University Nijmegen Medical Centre, Nijmegen, The Netherlands

## Abstract

Clinical risk management offers a systematic approach to minimize healthcare-related risks by paying attention to: (1) risk identification and assessment; (2) development and execution of risk reduction strategies; (3) evaluation of risk reduction strategies. This paper reviews these key areas for the risk of interactions between Kampo medicines and Western drugs (KMWDIs) to explore how the impact of these interactions on public health can be minimized. It argues that specific components of clinical risk management need to be evaluated, before adoption, and then actively implemented if proven valuable.

## Introduction

The concept of clinical risk management aims at the reduction of healthcare-related risks by shifting care-providing processes from organisational vulnerability towards organisational integrity. It offers a systematic approach by combining a focus on the following basic issues: (1) risk identification and assessment; (2) development and execution of risk reduction strategies; (3) evaluation of risk reduction strategies. In drug therapy, clinical risk management is often directed at the immediate post-licensing phase of newly licensed medicines. However, its principles are also relevant for reducing adverse drug reactions, drug-drug interactions and herb-drug interactions of older medicines.

* pdesmet@knmp.nl.

To demonstrate this important point, this chapter reviews key areas in the clinical risk management of interactions between Kampo medicines and Western drugs (KMWDIs). It summarizes two general reviews of the clinical risk management of herb-drug interactions. For a detailed background and underlying references, the interested reader is referred to these earlier reviews [1;2]. In addition, this chapter overviews prospective clinical studies of KMWDIs, in so far as they have been published in the English language.

## Risk Identification and Assessment

This first basic step in clinical risk management requires that hazards are identified and stratified in terms of evidence, probability and significance.

### Spontaneous Reporting

Spontaneous reporting systems are not only a relatively inexpensive cornerstone of the early detection of adverse drug reactions (ADRs) but they can also provide valuable insights into the contribution of drug-drug and herb-drug interactions to the development of ADRs.

It goes without saying that the higher the quality of spontaneous case reports, the more useful they can be. It is therefore important to educate healthcare professionals on the guidelines of the International Society for Pharmacoepidemiology and the International Society of Pharmacovigilance for the submission of adverse event reports to biomedical journals. These guidelines specify which information should be considered when describing the patient, the drug therapy, the adverse event, and the evaluation [3;4]. For reports attributing ADRs to herbal medicines, the guidelines recommend that their exact composition, details of processing, legal status and manufacturer are carefully specified. This is particularly important in those parts of the world, where it is possible to prescribe or buy herbal preparations that are not sufficiently regulated and therefore have a product quality that cannot be guaranteed. This does not appear to be a serious problem in Japan, however, because the market of Kampo medicines is dominated by 148 formulas which are officially licensed as medicines [5;6].

A major limitation of spontaneous reporting systems is the risk of considerable underreporting. The number of case reports on KMWDIs will depend directly on the perceptivity and willingness to come forward of every professional who comes into contact with such adverse events. Since Kampo medicines are prescribed by approximately 85% of the physicians trained in Western biomedicine, it is important to convey the message to these professionals that Kampo medicines are not free from adverse effects by definition and that it is important to report suspected adverse events to this type of medicines.

The volume of case reporting on Kampo medicines could also be increased by encouraging patients and their lay caregivers to submit cases directly. In recent years, favourable experiences have been gained with direct patient reporting of ADRs of Western drugs. This strategy appears to have more potential benefits than drawbacks, and may lead to the identification of adverse effects that have not previously been reported by healthcare professionals.

## Clinical Studies

The advantages and limitations of different types of experimental studies (*in vitro*, animal and human studies) have been recently reviewed [7]. Only the latter type of studies provides a definitive answer but it is generally much more costly than the other two types [8;9]. A number of clinical studies of KMWDIs have already appeared in the English-language literature (Table 1).

Among the factors to be taken into consideration when assessing the potential relevance of studies of individual herbs and compounds for the use of finished Kampo formulas are potential differences in the levels of exposure. For instance, the usual oral dose of the Kampo formula Orengedokuto is 7.5 g of granules per day corresponding to 1.5 g of a dried extract from a mixture of crude drugs consisting for 23.5% (i.e. 353 mg per day) of Coptis rhizome [37]. If Coptis rhizome is assumed to contain 3.5-9% of berberine [38], this corresponds to 12-32 mg of berberine per day, which is much lower than the 300-900 mg/day tested in the clinical studies listed in Table 1.

Prospective clinical studies are generally rated as more valuable than case reports but one should remain aware of the risk that they may lead to non-generalizable conclusions, when relevant risk modifiers (e.g., infrequent genotypes, frailness, renal or hepatic insufficiency, comorbidities, additional natural products or conventional drugs) have been underrepresented in the test population. Well-documented case reports (especially those with a positive re-challenge) do not necessarily constitute a lower level of evidence than a negative controlled interaction study [1].

Although there are several clinical studies which do not reveal significant interactions between Kampo medicines and Western drugs, some other clinical studies indicate that such interactions are possible and can be clinically relevant (Table 1). Various *in vitro* and animal experiments raise the possibility that these positive studies may represent the tip of an iceberg [39-51]. *In vitro* and animal data do not obviate the need of well-designed clinical investigations, but they do indicate the necessity of such investigations and may serve as guidance as to which KMWDIs deserve priority when planning human studies.

## Pharmacoepidemiological Studies

Pharmacoepidemiological studies help to overcome the limitations of spontaneous case reports and clinical studies. Generally speaking, however, epidemiological evaluations of the nature, volume and risk modifiers of herb-drug interactions have been scarce. One of the likely underlying reasons is that in many parts of the world herbal preparations are available without a prescription and are not registered systematically by professional healthcare providers. Japan might offer an advantage in this respect, since the prescribing of Kampo medicines by physicians and their coverage by national health insurance [5;6] could provide a stimulus to include these products routinely in healthcare records.

As suggested before, an alternative way forward would be to collect data within the context of a specific pharmacoepidemiological study in high risk patients (e.g., on the contribution of herbal preparations to the haemorrhagic and thrombotic complications of patients on oral anticoagulants) [1;2].

**Table. Prospective clinical studies of the effects of Kampo medicines on Western drugs (a)**

| Name | Western Drug(s) (b) | Effect on Western Drug(s) (c) | Reference |
|---|---|---|---|
| Finished Formulae | | | |
| Hochuekkito<br>(1x 2.5g of granules po) | Levofloxacin<br>(1x 200 mg po) | $AUC_{0\text{-}24\,h}$: –5% (NS) | (10) |
| Kakkonto<br>(tested as two different single doses) | Paracetamol<br>(1x 5 g po) | $AUC_{0\text{-}7\,h}$: –1% (NS) | (11;12) |
| Juzentaihoto<br>(1x 2.5g of granules po) | Levofloxacin<br>(1x 200 mg po) | $AUC_{0\text{-}24h}$ : +7% (NS) | (10) |
| Rikkunshito<br>(1x 2.5g of granules po) | Levofloxacin<br>(1x 200 mg po) | $AUC_{0\text{-}24h}$: +2% (NS) | (10) |
| (1x 2.5g of granules po) | Ofloxacin<br>(1x 200 mg po) | $AUC_{0\text{-}\infty}$ : +6% (NS) | (13) |
| Saibokuto<br>(3x 2.5g of granules po per day for 3 days) | Prednisolone<br>(10 mg po on day 3) | $AUC_{0\text{-}10h}$ +15% (S) | (14) |
| Saireito<br>(3x 3.0 g of granules po per day for 3 days) | Prednisolone<br>(10 mg po on day 3) | $AUC_{0\text{-}10h}$ – 4% (NS) | (14) |
| (1x 3.0g of granules po) | Ofloxacin<br>(1x 200 mg po) | $AUC_{0\text{-}\infty}$ : +4% (NS) | (13) |
| Shosaikoto<br>(3x 2.5g of granules po per day for 3 days) | Prednisolone<br>(10 mg po on day 3) | $AUC_{0\text{-}10h}$ –17% (S) | (14) |
| (2x 2.5 g for five days) | Caffeine<br>(150 mg po on day 1 and on day 5) | CYP1A2 activity –16%<br>xanthine oxidase activity –20-25% | (15) |
| (1x 3.0 g of granules po) | Ofloxacin<br>(1x 200 mg po) | $AUC_{0\text{-}\infty}$ : +7% (NS) | (13) |
| Shoseiryuto (TJ-19)<br>(9.0 g po equivalent to 5.0 g of dried aqueous extract per day for 7 days) | Caffeine (1x 150 mg po) | Ln [(AAMU+1U+1X)/17U] (e): +11% (NS)<br>Ln [AAMU/(AAMU+1X+1U)] (e): +7% (NS)<br>Ln [1U/(1U+1X)] (e): –1% | (16) |

| Name | Western Drug(s) (b) | Effect on Western Drug(s) (c) | Reference |
|---|---|---|---|
| (idem) | Dextromethorphan (1x 30 mg po) | Ln (DM/DX) (e): +30% (NS) in EMs and +13% (NS) in IMs (f)<br>Ln (DM/MM) (e): +14% (NS) in EMs and +22% (NS) in IMs (f) | (16) |
| Individual Herbs and Herbal Compounds | | | |
| *Angelica dahurica* root (Byakushi)<br>(4 g of aqueous extract 3x per day on days 3 to 13) | Six different drug probes (either on day 1 and day 13 or on day 2 and day 14)<br>Midazolam (7.5 mg po)<br>Omeprazole (40 mg po)<br>Dextromethorphan (30 mg po)<br>Losartan (50 mg po)<br>Caffeine (100 mg po)<br>Chlorzoxazone (400 mg po) | Midazolam (CYP3A4 probe): plasma level after 4 hrs: +2% (NS)<br>Omeprazole (CYP2C19 probe): 5-hydroxyomeprazole/ omeprazole plasma ratio after 4 hrs: +2% (NS)<br>Dextromethorphan (CYP2D6 probe): 0–12 hrs urinary dextrorphan/ dextromethorphan ratio: +14% (NS)<br>Losartan (CYP2C9 probe): 0–12 hrs urinary E-3174/losartan ratio:<br>–5% (NS)<br>Caffeine (CYP1A2 probe): paraxanthine/caffeine plasma ratio after 6 hrs: –90% (S)<br>Chlorzoxazone (CYP2E1 probe): 6-hydoxychlorzoxazone/chlorzoxazone plasma ratio after 2 hrs: +8% (NS) | (17) |
| Baicalin (*Scutellaria* root)<br>(3x 50 mg po for 14 days) | Rosuvastatin<br>(20 mg po) | Effect on $AUC_{0\text{-}72h}$ in different haplotypes of OATP1B1 (organic anion-transporting polypeptide 1B1):<br>–9% in subjects with OATP1B1*15/*15<br>–21% in subjects with OATP1B1*1b/*15<br>–47% in subjects with OATP1B1*1b/*1b | (18) |
| Berberine ( *Coptis* rhizome)<br>(3x 200 mg for 12 days) | Ciclosporin<br>(2x 3 mg/kg po per day in renal transplant recipients) | $AUC_{0\text{-}12h}$ : +34% | (19) |
| A: (1x 300 mg po)<br>B: (2x 300 mg po for 10 days) | Ciclosporin<br>A: (1x 3 mg/kg po)<br>B: (6 mg/kg po on day 10) | A: $AUC_{0\text{-}12h}$ +19%<br>B: $AUC_{0\text{-}12h}$ NS | (20) |

**Table. (Continued)**

| Name | Western Drug(s) (b) | Effect on Western Drug(s) (c) | Reference |
|---|---|---|---|
| (3x 300 mg po for 2 weeks) | Single dose of cocktail after 2 weeks:<br>Midazolam (2 mg po)<br>Omeprazole (20 mg po)<br>Dextromethorphan (30 mg po)<br>Losartan (30 mg po)<br>Caffeine (93 mg po) | Midazolam (CYP3A4 probe): $AUC_{0-\infty}$ +40%<br>Omeprazole (CYP2C19 probe): $AUC_{0-\infty}$ −2% (NS)<br>Dextromethorphan (CYP2D6 probe): 0–8 h urinary dextromethorphan/dextrorphan ratio: +879%<br>Losartan (CYP2C9 probe): 0–8 h urinary losartan/E-3174 ratio: +102%<br>Caffeine (CYP1A2 probe): $AUC_{0-\infty}$ −15% (NS) | (21) |
| *Citrus aurantium* unripened fruit (Kijitsu)<br>(350 mg standardized to 4% synephrine 2x per day on days 1 to 28) | Four different drug probes (either on day −1 and day 27 or on day 0 and day 28)<br>Midazolam (8 mg po)<br>Caffeine (100 mg po)<br>Chlorzoxazone (250 mg po)<br>Debrisoquin (5 mg po) | Midazolam (CYP3A4 probe): 1-hydroxymidazolam/midazolam serum ratio after 1 hr: NS<br>Caffeine (CYP1A2 probe): paraxanthine/caffeine serum ratio after 6 hrs: NS<br>Chlorzoxazone (CYP2E1 probe) 6-hydroxychlorzoxazone/chlorzoxazone serum ratio after 2 hrs: NS<br>Debrisoquin (CYP2D6 probe): 0-8 hrs urinary 4-hydroxydebrisoquin/ (debrisoquin plus 4-hydroxydebrisoquin) ratio: NS | (22) |
| Curcumin (*Curcuma* rhizome)<br>(300 mg po per day for 6 days) | Talinolol<br>(1x 50 mg po) | $AUC_{0-\infty}$ −33% (S) | (23) |
| (1000 mg po per day for 14 days) | Caffeine (1x 100 mg po) | CYP1A2 activity: UCMR of (AFMU+1X+1U)/17U: −29% (S) (g)<br>CYP2A6 activity: UCMR of 17U/(17U+17X+1U+1X+AFMU): +44% (S) (g)<br>N-acetyltransferase 2 activity: UCMR of AFMU/(AFMU+1U+1X): NS (g)<br>Xanthine oxidase activity: UCMR of 1U/(1X+1U): NS (g) | (24) |

| Name | Western Drug(s) (b) | Effect on Western Drug(s) (c) | Reference |
|---|---|---|---|
| Ephedrine (*Ephedra* herb)<br>(1x 25 mg po) | Caffeine (1x 200 mg po) | $AUC_{0-\infty}$ – 2.5% (NS)<br>Ephedrine plus caffeine (EC) significantly increased systolic blood pressure 30 min after dosing, whereas ephedrine alone (E) did not.<br>EC gave a similar peak in heart rate 120 min after dosing as E alone | (25) |
| Glycyrrhizin (*Liquiritia* root)<br>A: (1x 200 mg po)<br>B: (4x 50 mg po) | Prednisolone<br>(0.075 mg/kg iv) | A: Insignificant increase in $AUC_{0\text{-}24h}$ of total plasma prednisolone<br>Significant increase in $AUC_{0\text{-}24h}$ of free plasma prednisolone<br>B. Significant increases in $AUC_{0\text{-}24h}$ of total and free plasma prednisolone | (26;27) |
| (150 mg of monopotassium glycyr-rhizinate po 2x per day for 14 days) | Midazolam po (CYP3A probe) | $AUC_{0-\infty}$ : –23% (S) | (28) |
| *Panax ginseng* root (Ninjin)<br>(extract equivalent to 1.0 g ginseng root and 18 mg ginsenosides 3x per day for 7 days) | *Rac*-warfarin (25 mg po) | $AUC_{0-\infty}$ of S-warfarin: –12% (NS)<br>$AUC_{0-\infty}$ of R-warfarin: –11% (NS) | (29) |
| (extract equivalent to 0.5 g ginseng root and 25 mg ginsenosides 3x per day on days 1 to 28) | Four different drug probes (either on day –1 and day 27 or on day 0 and day 28)<br>Midazolam (8 mg po)<br>Caffeine (100 mg po)<br>Chlorzoxazone<br>(500 mg po)<br>Debrisoquin (5 mg po) | Midazolam (CYP3A4 probe): 1-hydroxymidazolam/midazolam serum ratio after 1 hr: NS<br>Caffeine (CYP1A2 probe): paraxanthine/caffeine serum ratio after 6 hrs: NS<br>Chlorzoxazone (CYP2E1 probe) 6-hydroxychlorzoxazone/ chlorzoxazone serum ratio after 2 hrs: NS<br>Debrisoquin (CYP2D6 probe): 0-8 hrs urinary 4-hydroxydebrisoquin/ (debrisoquin plus 4-hydroxydebrisoquin) ratio: NS | (30) |
| (extract equivalent to 0.5 g ginseng root and 25 mg ginsenosides 3x per day on days 1 to 28) (d) | Four different drug probes (either on day –1 and day 27 or on day 0 and day 28)<br>Midazolam (8 mg po)<br>Caffeine (100 mg po)<br>Chlorzoxazone (500 mg po)<br>Debrisoquin (5 mg po) | Midazolam (CYP3A4 probe): 1-hydroxymidazolam/midazolam serum ratio after 1 hr: NS<br>Caffeine (CYP1A2 probe): paraxanthine/caffeine serum ratio after 6 hrs: NS<br>Chlorzoxazone (CYP2E1 probe) 6-hydroxychlorzoxazone/ chlorzoxazone serum ratio after 2 hrs: NS<br>Debrisoquin (CYP2D6 probe): 0-8 hrs urinary 4- | (31) |

**Table. (Continued)**

| Name | Western Drug(s) (b) | Effect on Western Drug(s) (c) | Reference |
|---|---|---|---|
| | | hydroxydebrisoquin/ (debrisoquin plus 4-hydroxydebrisoquin) ratio: –7% (S) | |
| *Paeonia* root (Shakuyaku)<br>(1.2 g of powdered extract 1x per day for 7 days) | Valproic acid (200 mg po) | $AUC_{0-\infty}$ of valproic acid: +4% (NS) | (32) |
| *Scutellaria* root (Ōgon)<br>(4 g of aqueous extract 3x per day on days 3 to 13) | Six different drug probes (either on day 1 and day 13 or on day 2 and day 14)<br>Midazolam (7.5 mg po)<br>Omeprazole (40 mg po)<br>Dextromethorphan (30 mg po)<br>Losartan (50 mg po)<br>Caffeine (100 mg po)<br>Chlorzoxazone (400 mg po) | Midazolam (CYP3A4 probe): plasma level after 4 hrs: +5% (NS)<br>Omeprazole (CYP2C19 probe): 5-hydroxyomeprazole/omeprazole plasma ratio after 4 hrs: –11% (NS)<br>Dextromethorphan (CYP2D6 probe): 0–12 hrs urinary dextrorphan/ dextromethorphan ratio: +11% (NS)<br>Losartan (CYP2C9 probe): 0–12 hrs E-3174/losartan ratio: –29% (S)<br>Caffeine (CYP1A2 probe): paraxanthine/caffeine plasma ratio after 6 hrs: –32% (NS)<br>Chlorzoxazone (CYP2E1 probe): 6-hydoxychlorzoxazone/ chlorzoxazone plasma ratio after 2 hrs: +42% (S) | (17) |
| *Zingiber* rhizome (Shokyō)<br>(extract equivalent to 1.2 g of gingerrhizome powder 3x per day for 7 days) | *Rac*-warfarin (25 mg po) | $AUC_{0-168\ hrs}$ of S-warfarin: NS<br>$AUC_{0-168\ hrs}$ of R-warfarin: NS<br>Platelet aggregation: NS<br>INR: NS | (33) |

(a) Based on various searches in Pubmed [http://www.ncbi.nlm.nih.gov/pubmed/] and several recent reviews (12;34-36)
(b) Tested in healthy volunteers (unless stated otherwise)
(c) AUC = area under the plasma/blood concentration-time curve
NS = no(t) significant
(d) In elderly healthy subjects aged 60-76 years
(e) AAMU = 5-acetylamino-6-amino-3-methyluracil; 17U, 1U and 1X are caffeine metabolites
The formulas are logarithmic transformed urinary molar concentration ratios as probes for CYP1A2, xanthine oxidase and N-acetyltransferase 2, respectively.
(f) DM = Dextromethorphan; DX = dextrorphan; MM = 3-methoxymorphinan
The formulas are logarithmic transformed urinary molar concentration ratios as probes for CYP2D6 and CYP3A, respectively.
(g) UCMR = Urinary Caffeine Metabolite Ratio 1U = 1-methylurate; 1X = 1-methylxanthine; 17U = 1,7-dimethylurate; 17X = 1,7-dimethylxanthine; AFMU = 5-acetylamino-6-formylamino-3-methyluracil

An example of such a specific study has been reported from a Canadian research hospital, where 171 adult warfarin users were asked to complete a 16-week diary by recording prospectively bleeding events and exposure to factors previously reported to increase the risk of bleeding and supratherapeutic INRs, including the use of herbal medicines. Multivariate analysis showed that the Kampo herb ginger was independently associated with an increased risk of self-reported bleeding [OR = 3.2; 95% CI 2.4-4.2] [52]. This finding should be interpreted with caution, as the study was not without limitations. For instance, there may have been uncontrollable variation in patients' interpretations of what warranted recording, and the significant association between ginger use and bleeding was based on only 7 self-reported events in 25 users (whereas 6 events in 23 users of willow bark produced no significant association). Notwithstanding such reservations, this study demonstrated that is feasible to perform specific epidemiological evaluations of KMWDIs. Such studies could be performed either among users of drugs that are known for an increased risk on drug interactions (e.g. antithrombotics, HIV medications) or among patient groups known to have a high use of Kampo medicines.

## Risk Assessment

The first step in the clinical risk assessment of KMWDIs is a systematic collection of the available data on their nature, incidence and consequences. Comprehensive search strategies which are not restricted to general terms but also include names of specific Kampo herbs and their major constituents are needed for this purpose. Also, Pubmed is certainly not the only database that should be used, as it does not adequately cover all sources that provide potentially useful information about KMWDIs.

After the collection of all available data, it is important to consider the following principles in their evaluation:

(1) The quality of the evidence is often variable and must therefore be carefully assessed. For instance, how well-designed, well-performed and generalizable is a clinical study and to which extent does a case report comply with current guidelines for submitting adverse event reports to biomedical journals? Consistency of data from different sources may further add to the validity of the evidence.
(2) The clinical impact of an adverse KMWDI at the population level will depend both on its seriousness and on the probability that it actually occurs.
(3) Are there any data on potential risk modification by factors such as certain genotypes, frailness, comorbidities, renal or hepatic insufficiency, additional natural products or conventional drugs? Such data can help to identify the drug users who are at the highest risk. For instance, in a recent study of the pharmacokinetics of rosuvastatin in healthy volunteers, the addition of baicalin (a flavone glucuronide in the Kampo medicine Scutellariae Radix) depended on the haplotype of OATP1B1 (organic anion-transporting polypeptide 1B1, the expression of which is considered the main uptake mechanism for rosuvastatin into the liver) reduced the $AUC_{0-\infty}$ of rosuvastatin by 42%, 24% and 2%, respectively, in OATP1B1*1b/*1b, OATP1 B1*1b/*15, and OATP1B1 *15/*15 subjects [18].

(4) The risk of an adverse KMWDI may extend beyond the natural Kampo-drug pair for which there is actual clinical evidence. For instance, if a certain herb is a well-established potent inducer of CYP 3A4, it would be wise to be careful with combining this herb with any CYP 3A4 substrate, even in the absence of concrete clinical data to underpin such interactions.

(5) Evaluations of KMWDIs have a shelf life of their own: any systematic assessment of NPDIs must comprise an adequate method for collecting and assessing new emerging evidence without unnecessary delay.

## Development and Execution of Risk Reduction Strategies

This phase of clinical risk management aims at the definition of operational strategies needed to reduce health risks, at the identification of resources, and at the execution of selected strategies. Regulatory authorities, manufacturers, prescribers, dispensers and users of Kampo medicines and Western drugs should all contribute to this goal without shifting their responsibility to other parties involved.

### Product Information

Commercially available Kampo medicines should carry appropriate warnings concerning KMWDIs in their product information. If specific data are not available, a general cautionary note should be included that conclusive data are mostly absent and that the safety of combining the Kampo medicine with Western drugs has therefore not been adequately established. Mutatis mutandis, similar warnings should be included in the product information of Western drugs.

### Professional Contributions

Physicians and pharmacists should make their customers aware of the possibility that an adverse drug event or herb-drug interaction might occur, which is not yet described in the product information. They should register Kampo medicines in the same healthcare records, in which Western medicines are registered.

### Computerised Screening

The registration of Kampo medicines in healthcare records opens the door to computerised screening for adverse KMWDIs, which is a more efficient and reliable strategy than depending on the ready knowledge and perceptivity of an individual healthcare professional. To benefit optimally from such screening, the healthcare professional must know exactly what the computerised system can and cannot do. For instance, a computerised system can more readily produce an alert when a CYP 3A4 inducer is being added to a CYP 3A4 substrate than detect another equally important risk moment, viz. when the inducer is being withdrawn again.

Ideally, computerised systems should identify clinically relevant KMWDIs with high specificity (i.e., low rate of false positive alerts) as well as high sensitivity (i.e. low rate of the false negative absence of alerts). Unfortunately, each of these parameters decreases when the other increases, so a kind of trade-off between the two will be needed. Some researchers argue that reducing current numbers of false positive DDI alerts should be given priority. However, other researchers point out that physicians' reasons for overriding alerts are not always convincing and that turning off certain alerts systematically (nation-wide or even hospital-wide) could be problematic because of differences in physicians' drug knowledge, routine drug monitoring practices, and so on.

### Patient-oriented Communication

Further research in this domain is warranted to guide product information and professional counseling about Kampo medicines. A particular point of attention should be that patients may find it difficult to deal with uncertainties that arise from the lack of good quality information. For instance, how are patients supposed to deal with a general warning that the safety of combining their Kampo medicine with Western drugs has not been adequately established?

In daily practice, physicians and pharmacists should aim for a middle ground between paternalism and consumerism by making room not only for their professional views but also for the values of the individual patient.

### Evaluation of Risk Reduction Strategies

The third phase in clinical risk management is the evaluation of the impact of risk minimization strategies, i.e. do these strategies actually work effectively and efficiently. This final phase is crucial in the clinical risk management of Western drug-drug interactions and should not be overlooked either in the risk management of KMWDIs.

### Product Information

As the package inserts of Kampo medicines and Western drugs are a main tool for informing consumers about KMWDI risks, it should be monitored whether the KMWDI information in such inserts is accurate, complete and useful for consumers. The least that should be done to make consumers more aware is the inclusion of a general advice in the product information about Kampo medicines to contact a physician or pharmacist in case of an unexpected adverse event. Judging from some product information examples of Kampo medicines retrieved from the internet, such a general statement is not yet always included. The same applies to published human data on KMWDI risks (e.g. the differential effects of Saiboku-to and Sho-saiko-to on the pharmacokinetics of prednisolone) [53;54].

### Professional Resources

The development and maintenance of KMWDI information in professional reference books and computerised databases should be organized in such a way that the quality, consistency and usefulness of the information is adequately assured. Among the important points of attention are: (1) how timely and consistently are KMWDIs included; (2) has the KMWDI information been evaluated by a well-structured method before inclusion; (3) what is the scientific quality of the descriptions and of the recommendations on how to deal with each KMWDI; (4) how unambiguous and practicable are the recommendations in the eyes of busy end users?

With respect to computerised systems for KMWDI screening, it is important to know how these systems perform in theory (to which degree do they allow end users to adjust default settings, how regularly is the software updated, etc.) and how they perform in daily practice (to which degree have end users actually adjusted default settings, how correctly has the software been actually updated, etc.). Among the methods used to research such issues is testing systems by means of mock patient profiles containing potentially hazardous drug-drug and herb-drug pairs.

### Professional Performance

It should be monitored whether healthcare professionals have adequate knowledge about KMWDIs and to which extent they apply this knowledge correctly. If actual performance of healthcare providers turns out to be poor, potential reasons for this finding should be explored. Experts of quality improvement recommend that, after underlying barriers have been identified, educational and organizational interventions tailored to the most relevant barriers should be performed, even though the evidence does not conclusively suggest that tailored interventions are consistently effective.

If computerised screening for KMWDIs is used, it should be monitored how often alerts are overridden or another action than the recommended one is taken.

### Consumer Performance

Questions in this domain that can be addressed by active monitoring include: are consumers aware of the existing KMWDI risks; what are their sources of information on these issues and how intensively do they consult them; how well informed does this make them; and how does this affect their actual behaviour?

## Conclusion

Clinical pharmacologists, health services researchers and governmental scientists can further the risk management of KMWDIs by contributing to the above-mentioned domains: the collection and interpretation of spontaneous reports; the design and interpretation of prospective clinical studies; the development of pharmacoepidemiological investigations; the synthesis and weighing of the available evidence; the expert counseling of regulatory authorities and manufacturers on relevant issues; and the evaluation of existing and emerging risk reduction strategies.

## References


[1] De Smet PAGM. Clinical risk management of herb-drug interactions. *Br.J Clin Pharmacol.* 2007;63:258-67.

[2] De Smet PAGM, Floor-Schreudering A, Bouvy ML, Wensing M. Clinical risk management of interactions between natural products and drugs. *Curr.Drug Metab* 2008;9:1055-62.

[3] Kelly WN, Arellano FM, Barnes J, Bergman U, Edwards RI, Fernandez AM, et al. Guidelines for submitting adverse event reports for publication. *Drug Saf* 2007;30:367-73.

[4] Kelly WN, Arellano FM, Barnes J, Bergman U, Edwards RI, Fernandez AM, et al. Guidelines for submitting adverse event reports for publication. Pharmacoepidemiol. *Drug Saf* 2007;16:581-7.

[5] Motoo Y, Seki T, Tsutani K. Traditional Japanese medicine, Kampo: its history and current status. *Chin J Integr.Med* 2011;17:85-7.

[6] Watanabe K, Matsuura K, Gao P, Hottenbacher L, Tokunaga H, Nishimura K, et al. Traditional Japanese Kampo Medicine: Clinical Research between Modernity and Traditional Medicine-The State of Research and Methodological Suggestions for the Future. Evid.Based. *Complement Alternat.Med* 2011;2011:513842

[7] Venkataramanan R, Komoroski B, Strom S. In vitro and in vivo assessment of herb drug interactions. *Life Sci* 2006;78:2105-15.

[8] Farkas D, Greenblatt DJ. Influence of fruit juices on drug disposition: discrepancies between in vitro and clinical studies. *Expert.Opin.Drug Metab Toxicol.* 2008;4:381-93.

[9] Markowitz JS, von Moltke LL, Donovan JL. Predicting interactions between conventional medications and botanical products on the basis of in vitro investigations. *Mol.Nutr.Food Res.* 2008;52:747-54.

[10] Hasegawa T, Yamaki K, Muraoka I, Nadai M, Takagi K, Nabeshima T. Effects of traditional Chinese medicines on pharmacokinetics of levofloxacin. *Antimicrob.Agents Chemother.* 1995;39:2135-7.

[11] Qi J, Toyoshima A, Honda Y, Mineshita S. Pharmacokinetic study on acetaminophen: interaction with a Chinese medicine. J Med Dent.Sci. 1997;44:31-5.

[12] Mills E, Wu P, Johnston BC, Gallicano K, Clarke M, Guyatt G. Natural health product-drug interactions: a systematic review of clinical trials. *Ther Drug Monit.* 2005;27:549-57.

[13] Hasegawa T, Yamaki K, Nadai M, Muraoka I, Wang L, Takagi K, et al. Lack of effect of Chinese medicines on bioavailability of ofloxacin in healthy volunteers. *Int J Clin Pharmacol.Ther* 1994;32:57-61.

[14] Homma M, Oka K, Ikeshima K, Takahashi N, Niitsuma T, Fukuda T, et al. Different effects of traditional Chinese medicines containing similar herbal constituents on prednisolone pharmacokinetics. *J Pharm Pharmacol.* 1995;47:687-92.

[15] Saruwatari J, Nakagawa K, Shindo J, Nachi S, Echizen H, Ishizaki T. The in-vivo effects of sho-saiko-to, a traditional Chinese herbal medicine, on two cytochrome P450 enzymes (1A2 and 3A) and xanthine oxidase in man. *J Pharm Pharmacol.* 2003;55:1553-9.
[16] Nakao M, Muramoto Y, Hisadome M, Yamano N, Shoji M, Fukushima Y, et al. The effect of Shoseiryuto, a traditional Japanese medicine, on cytochrome P450s, N-acetyltransferase 2 and xanthine oxidase, in extensive or intermediate metabolizers of CYP2D6. *Eur.J Clin Pharmacol.* 2007;63:345-53.
[17] Yi S, Cho JY, Lim KS, Kim KP, Kim J, Kim BH, et al. Effects of Angelicae tenuissima radix, Angelicae dahuricae radix and Scutellariae radix Extracts on Cytochrome P450 Activities in Healthy Volunteers. *Basic Clin Pharmacol.Toxicol.* 2009; May 5. [Epub ahead of print]
[18] Fan L, Zhang W, Guo D, Tan ZR, Xu P, Li Q, et al. The effect of herbal medicine baicalin on pharmacokinetics of rosuvastatin, substrate of organic anion-transporting polypeptide 1B1. *Clin Pharmacol.Ther* 2008;83:471-6.
[19] Wu X, Li Q, Xin H, Yu A, Zhong M. Effects of berberine on the blood concentration of cyclosporin A in renal transplanted recipients: clinical and pharmacokinetic study. *Eur.J Clin Pharmacol.* 2005;61:567-72.
[20] Xin HW, Wu XC, Li Q, Yu AR, Zhong MY, Liu YY. The effects of berberine on the pharmacokinetics of cyclosporin A in healthy volunteers. *Methods Find.Exp.Clin Pharmacol.* 2006;28:25-9.
[21] Guo Y, Chen Y, Tan ZR, Klaassen CD, Zhou HH. Repeated administration of berberine inhibits cytochromes P450 in humans. *Eur.J Clin Pharmacol.* 2012;68:213-7.
[22] Gurley BJ, Gardner SF, Hubbard MA, Williams DK, Gentry WB, Carrier J, et al. In vivo assessment of botanical supplementation on human cytochrome P450 phenotypes: Citrus aurantium, Echinacea purpurea, milk thistle, and saw palmetto. *Clin Pharmacol.Ther* 2004;76:428-40.
[23] Juan H, Terhaag B, Cong Z, Bi-Kui Z, Rong-Hua Z, Feng W, et al. Unexpected effect of concomitantly administered curcumin on the pharmacokinetics of talinolol in healthy Chinese volunteers. *Eur.J Clin Pharmacol.* 2007;63:663-8.
[24] Chen Y, Liu WH, Chen BL, Fan L, Han Y, Wang G, et al. Plant polyphenol curcumin significantly affects CYP1A2 and CYP2A6 activity in healthy, male Chinese volunteers. *Ann Pharmacother.* 2010;44:1038-45.
[25] Haller CA, Jacob P, III, Benowitz NL. Enhanced stimulant and metabolic effects of combined ephedrine and caffeine. *Clin Pharmacol.Ther* 2004;75:259-73.
[26] Chen MF, Shimada F, Kato H, Yano S, Kanaoka M. Effect of glycyrrhizin on the pharmacokinetics of prednisolone following low dosage of prednisolone hemisuccinate. *Endocrinol.Jpn.* 1990;37:331-41.
[27] Chen MF, Shimada F, Kato H, Yano S, Kanaoka M. Effect of oral administration of glycyrrhizin on the pharmacokinetics of prednisolone. *Endocrinol.Jpn.* 1991;38:167-74.
[28] Tu JH, He YJ, Chen Y, Fan L, Zhang W, Tan ZR, et al. Effect of glycyrrhizin on the activity of CYP3A enzyme in humans. *Eur.J Clin Pharmacol.* 2010;66:805-10.
[29] Jiang X, Williams KM, Liauw WS, Ammit AJ, Roufogalis BD, Duke CC, et al. Effect of St John's wort and ginseng on the pharmacokinetics and pharmacodynamics of warfarin in healthy subjects. *Br.J Clin Pharmacol.* 2004;57:592-9.

[30] Gurley BJ, Gardner SF, Hubbard MA, Williams DK, Gentry WB, Cui Y, et al. Cytochrome P450 phenotypic ratios for predicting herb-drug interactions in humans. *Clin Pharmacol.Ther* 2002;72:276-87.

[31] Gurley BJ, Gardner SF, Hubbard MA, Williams DK, Gentry WB, Cui Y, et al. Clinical assessment of effects of botanical supplementation on cytochrome P450 phenotypes in the elderly: St John's wort, garlic oil, Panax ginseng and Ginkgo biloba. *Drugs Aging* 2005;22:525-39.

[32] Chen LC, Chou MH, Lin MF, Yang LL. Lack of pharmacokinetic interaction between valproic acid and a traditional Chinese medicine, Paeoniae Radix, in healthy volunteers. *J Clin Pharm Ther* 2000;25:453-9.

[33] Jiang X, Williams KM, Liauw WS, Ammit AJ, Roufogalis BD, Duke CC, et al. Effect of ginkgo and ginger on the pharmacokinetics and pharmacodynamics of warfarin in healthy subjects. *Br.J Clin Pharmacol.* 2005;59:425-32.

[34] Hu Z, Yang X, Ho PC, Chan SY, Heng PW, Chan E, et al. Herb-drug interactions: a literature review. *Drugs* 2005;65:1239-82.

[35] Kennedy DA, Seely D. Clinically based evidence of drug-herb interactions: a systematic review. *Expert.Opin.Drug Saf* 2010;9:79-124.

[36] Tarirai C, Viljoen AM, Hamman JH. Herb-drug pharmacokinetic interactions reviewed. *Expert.Opin.Drug Metab Toxicol.* 2010;6:1515-38.

[37] Anonymous. Tsumura Orengedokuto extract granules for ethical use 5th version (May 2007). Available at: http://www.tsumura.co.jp/english/products/pi/JPR_T015.pdf [accessed Oct 23 2011] . 2007.

[38] Hoppe HA. Drogenkunde. *Band 1 Angiospermen.* 8. Auflage. Berlin: Walter de Gruyter. 1975:338

[39] Imai T, Sakai M, Ohtake H, Azuma H, Otagiri M. In vitro and in vivo evaluation of the enhancing activity of glycyrrhizin on the intestinal absorption of drugs. *Pharm Res.* 1999;16:80-6.

[40] Ishihara K, Kushida H, Yuzurihara M, Wakui Y, Yanagisawa T, Kamei H, et al. Interaction of drugs and Chinese herbs: pharmacokinetic changes of tolbutamide and diazepam caused by extract of Angelica dahurica. *J Pharm Pharmacol.* 2000;52:1023-9.

[41] Makino T, Wakushima H, Okamoto T, Okukubo Y, Deguchi Y, Kano Y, Pharmacokinetic interactions between warfarin and kangen-karyu, a Chinese traditional herbal medicine, and their synergistic action. *J Ethnopharmacol.* 2002;82:35-40.

[42] Makino T, Wakushima H, Okamoto T, Okukubo Y, Deguchi Y, Kano Y, Pharmacokinetic and pharmacological interactions between ticlopidine hydrochloride and Kangen-Karyu - Chinese traditional herbal medicine. *Phytother.Res.* 2003;17:1021-4.

[43] Nose M, Tamura M, Ryu N, Mizukami H, Ogihara Y. Sho-saiko-to and Saiko-keisi-to, the traditional Chinese and Japanese herbal medicines, altered hepatic drug-metabolizing enzymes in mice and rats when administered orally for a long time. *J Pharm Pharmacol.* 2003;55:1419-26.

[44] Guo LQ, Yamazoe Y. Inhibition of cytochrome P450 by furanocoumarins in grapefruit juice and herbal medicines. *Acta Pharmacol.Sin.* 2004;25:129-36.

[45] Nishimura N Effects of Chinese herbal medicines on intestinal drug absorption [in Japanese]. *Yakugaku Zasshi* 2005;125:363-9.

[46] Ikegami F, Sumino M, Fujii Y, Akiba T, Satoh T. Pharmacology and toxicology of Bupleurum root-containing Kampo medicines in clinical use. *Hum.Exp.Toxicol.* 2006;25:481-94.

[47] Kinoshita N, Yamaguchi Y, Hou XL, Takahashi K, Takahashi K. Experimental Adjustment on Drug Interactions through Intestinal CYP3A Activity in Rat: Impacts of Kampo Medicines Repeat Administered. *Evid.Based.Complement Alternat.Med* 2009; Nov 1. [Epub ahead of print]

[48] Nakagawa N, Katoh M, Yoshioka Y, Nakajima M, Yokoi T. Inhibitory effects of Kampo medicine on human UGT2B7 activity. *Drug Metab Pharmacokinet.* 2009;24:490-9.

[49] Satoh T, Watanabe Y, Ikarashi N, Ito K, Sugiyama K. Effects of Kampo medicines on P-glycoprotein. *Biol.Pharm Bull.* 2009;32:2018-21.

[50] Iwanaga K, Hayashi M, Hamahata Y, Miyazaki M, Shibano M, Taniguchi M, et al. Furanocoumarin derivatives in Kampo extract medicines inhibit cytochrome P450 3A4 and P-glycoprotein. *Drug Metab Dispos.* 2010;38:1286-94.

[51] Yokooji T, Kida M, Mori M, Akashi H, Mori N, Yoshihara S, et al. Interaction of Rhei Rhizoma extract with cytochrome P450 3A and efflux transporters in rats. *Pharmazie* 2010;65:367-74.

[52] Shalansky S, Lynd L, Richardson K, Ingaszewski A, Kerr C. Risk of warfarin-related bleeding events and supratherapeutic international normalized ratios associated with complementary and alternative medicine: a longitudinal analysis. *Pharmacotherapy* 2007;27:1237-47.

[53] Anonymous. Tsumura Saibokuto extract granules for ethical use 6th version (May 2007). Available at: http://www.tsumura.co.jp/english/ products/pi/ JPR_T096.pdf [accessed Oct 23 2011] . 2007.

[54] Anonymous. Tsumura Shosaikoto extract granules for ethical use 7th version (May 2007). Available at: http://www.tsumura.co.jp/english/ products/pi/JPR_T009.pdf [accessed Oct 23 2011] . 2007.

In: Traditional Medicine: New Research
Editor: Yoshiharu Motoo

ISBN: 978-1-62257-448-3


*Chapter 12*

# How Do Drug-Herb Interaction Studies Lead to Safer Traditional Medicine?

***Renke Dai[1,*], Feng Wu[2,†] and Chi-Wai Wong[2,‡]***
[1]PharmaSS Corporation, Bio-Building, National Health Technology Park, Zhongshan City, Guangdong, China
[2]NeuMed Pharmaceuticals Limited, Shatin, New Territories, Hong Kong

## Abstract

Alternative medicines including those derived from traditional remedies are gaining popularity; particularly, when used as supplements with prescription drugs to enhance efficacious or reduce side effects. Many traditional remedies were developed and refined through practical experience over long periods of time. They are well tolerated in patients; thus, presumed to have superior safety profiles. This assumption should be more vigorously challenged as herbs used in traditional remedies may induce undesirable drug-herb interaction to alter the pharmacokinetic profile of the prescription drug in use, resulting in unnecessary risk. A rational guideline acceptable by both traditional remedy developers and regulatory agencies needs to be developed to fully examine the risk involved so that patients are better served.

In recent years, alternative medicines including those derived from traditional remedies are gaining popularity among the general public and raising intrigues among the medical community; particularly, when used as supplements. Across the world, many cultures develop and refine traditional remedies through practical experience over long periods of time. Herbal based traditional remedies are noticeably common among Asian countries with the Chinese, Indian, Japanese, Korean and Tibetan being documented in written texts and passed on through oral tradition. In fact, the theories and uses of these herbal remedies are extensively

* renke.dai@pharmass.com.cn.
† wuf@neumedpharma.com.hk.
‡ wongcw@neumedpharma.com.hk.

trained in medical colleges and practiced at local hospitals. In China alone, the market of Traditional Chinese Medicine is estimated to be around 1 billion USD annually.

Primarily composed of a mixture of herbs, many traditional remedies are well tolerated in patients, as herbs that induce strong side effects are screened out through practical experience. Additionally, most people perceive these herbal remedies as more natural compared to prescription drugs that are composed of synthetic chemicals. These factors contribute to the presumption that herbal remedies are safe. This assumption perhaps remains valid within a certain context; namely, when these herbal remedies are used as stand alones and in moderate doses. However, modern day usages of these herbal remedies often extend beyond their historic contexts. More often than not, herbal remedies are taken together with synthetic chemical based prescription drugs. The rationale is that herbal remedies, serving as complements, can either enhance the efficacious or reduce the side effects associated with prescription drugs. However, this hypothesis has rarely been investigated by well designed and controlled clinical trials. In fact, it should be more vigorously challenged as herbs may induce undesirable drug-herb interactions.

Drug-herb interactions are herein defined as alterations of the pharmacokinetic profiles of prescription drugs when herbal remedies are used in conjunctions. Over the course of drug development, the pharmacokinetic profiles of a drug are to be established in both preclinical and early clinical phases. These types of data constitute integral parts for designing drug dosage regiments for later phase clinical trials and eventually submitting information for regulatory approval. Alterations in pharmacokinetic profile may result in over- or under-dosage; neither is desirable for matching the appropriate amount of drug exposure originally established, instead potentially reducing the efficacy or enhancing the side effects putting patients at unnecessary risk.

Mechanistically, drug-herb interactions are typically manifested from changes in the absorption, distribution, metabolism, and excretion (ADME) of those drugs in use. The expression and activity levels of drug transporters and metabolizing enzymes in the intestine, liver, and kidney play major roles in determining the ADME profile. Ingredients or phyto-chemicals within herbal remedies may induce the expression and activity levels of these transporters and metabolizing enzymes. In addition, these phyto-chemicals may themselves serve as substrates or inhibitors of drug transporters and metabolizing enzymes. Combinations of these effects are likely contributing to changes in the ADME profiles of drugs used in conjunction. For example, the plant species *Hypericum perforatum*, commonly known as Saint John's wort used as an herbal treatment for depression, causes drug-herb interactions through the inductions of drug efflux transporter such as P-glycoprotein (P-gp) and cytochrome P450 drug metabolizing enzymes such as CYP3A4 and CYP2C9 [1].

Recent progress in understanding the mechanism responsible for this type of induction points to xenobiotic sensor pregnane X receptor (PXR) as a key factor [2]. PXR belongs to the nuclear hormone receptor superfamily of transcription factors which bind to response elements located on the promoters or enhancers of their target genes. PXR contains a ligand binding domain with broad specificity, recognizing a great variety of drugs and phyto-chemicals. Binding of these substances to PXR leads to its activation; namely, PXR turns on the expression of detoxifying enzymes at the transcriptional level. These detoxifying enzymes include phase I cytochrome P450 oxidases such as CYP3A4, phase II conjugating enzymes such as glutathione S-transferase and UDP-glucuronosyltransferases, and phase III transport uptake and efflux proteins such as P-gp that are collectively responsible for the metabolism and excretion of many drugs. Besides PXR, another nuclear hormone receptor constitutive androstane receptor (CAR) also plays a role in guiding the expression levels of detoxifying enzymes. The activity of CAR is subjected to modulation by binding to xenobiotics including phyto-chemicals. Therefore, whether an herbal remedy contains phyto-chemicals that modulate the activities of PXR and CAR is likely a major determinant of the extent of drug-herb interaction potentially elicit by that herbal remedy.

Besides inducing their expressions, phyto-chemicals within herbal remedies may act directly as substrates or sometimes even as inhibitors of detoxifying enzymes. Saint John's wort serves once again as an example of herb containing phyto-chemicals that inhibits detoxifying enzymes including CYP1A1, CYP1B1, CYP2D6, and CYP3A4 [3]. By inhibiting their activities, Saint John's wort effectively increases the doses of drugs that are normally metabolized by these enzymes, leading to over-dosing.

While the sale of herbal remedies brings considerable profits to herbal remedy developers/manufacturers, particularly in Asian countries, a rational guideline acceptable by both developers/manufacturers and regulatory agencies to inform the general public how to avoid unnecessary risk due to inappropriate combinatorial use of herbal remedies with prescription drugs does not exist. In part, this is due to the lack of a database listing the drug-herb interaction potentials of herbal remedies. Developing and agreeing upon a set of standard assays that readily and reliably detect the PXR, CAR, and detoxifying enzyme modulating activities of herbal remedies/phyto-chemicals is perhaps one way towards constructing such a database [4]. This database can in turn help herbal remedy developers/manufacturers improve the safety profiles of their products by either avoiding the inclusion of herbs that have strong drug-herb interaction potentials or putting labels on their products stating the types of prescription drug to avoid being used with. This database can also serve as references for the regulatory agencies to start monitoring the safety of selective herbal remedies. Ultimately, the general public is better served having safer herbal remedies as health supplements or alternative medicines.

## References

[1] Mannel, M. Drug interactions with St John's wort : mechanisms and clinical implications. Drug Saf 2004; 27(11): 773-97.

[2] Miller, RT, Willson, TM. Regulation of xenobiotic metabolism by orphan nuclear receptors. Toxicol Pathol 2001; 29(1): 3-5.

[3] Obach, RS. Inhibition of human cytochrome P450 enzymes by constituents of St. John's Wort, an herbal preparation used in the treatment of depression. J Pharmacol Exp Ther 2000; 294(1): 88-95.

[4] Strandell, J, Neil, A, Carlin, G. An approach to the in vitro evaluation of potential for cytochrome P450 enzyme inhibition from herbals and other natural remedies. *Phytomedicine* 2004; 11(2-3): 98-104.

In: Traditional Medicine: New Research
Editor: Yoshiharu Motoo
ISBN: 978-1-62257-448-3


*Chapter 13*

# Pharmacoeconomic Evaluations on Kampo Medicine and Development of Structured Abstracts

***Wentao Tang and Kiichiro Tsutani***
The University of Tokyo, Japan

## Abstract

The current state of increasing demands for health services and scarce health resources poses a big challenge for medical practice in Japan. To improve the overall quality of health services while inhibiting the rapid increase of health expenditures, the optimal allocation of health resources is required. Guided by the principle of evidence-based medicine (EBM), decision-making in health practices and the allocation of health resources should be based on the best, available economic evidence reflecting the cost-effectiveness of health services.

Kampo medicine (Japanese traditional herbal medicine) [1], which plays a certain role in the current health practices in Japan, has a potential to be more cost-effective than other alternatives due to its features including unique therapeutic approach, certain effectiveness in specific therapeutic areas, and comparatively low cost. Although Kampo medicine may be one of key roles in the optimum allocation of health resources, lack of clinical and economic evidence for Kampo medicine impedes its further use in health practices. Conducting pharmacoeconomic evaluations on Kampo medicine and establishing economic evidence for it is significant in facing the challenges imposed on health practices in Japan.

In this chapter, we introduce the review of the pharmacoeconomic evaluations on Kampo medicine in Japan currently under way. Two examples of pharmacoeconomic evaluations on Kampo medicine summarized in structured abstracts (SA) are included as well. This review and the use of SA are believed to contribute to the future establishment of the evidence from pharmacoeconomic evaluations on Kampo medicine, and a database assisting in the management and utilization of the evidence.

# 1. Introduction

According to the statistical report from Ministry of Health, Labour and Welfare (MHLW), the national health expenditures of Japan in 2009 have reached 36 trillion Japanese Yen (US$450 billion, US$1=80 Yen) and this number has increased by approximately 17.3% compared with that ten years ago [2]. Considering the aging society and the continual introduction of new but expensive health technologies into Japan, the increasing trend of National health expenditures is expected to continue in future. On the other hand, affected by the economic downturn in recent years and the aging trend of the society, the GDP and National Income of Japan have turned to decrease since 2008 [2]. It is shown that the contradiction between people's increasing demand for health services and scarce health resources is becoming a more and more serious problem in the health system of Japan. In this context, we have to consider how to maximize the health benefits produced from health services available with limited health resources and will always be confronted with the following questions:

1) What are the costs of alternative treatments for specific patients and what are the expected benefits of those alternatives?
2) Are the benefits generated by Treatment A worth the cost, or is the incremental effectiveness of Treatment A compared with Treatment B worth the incremental cost needed to pay for A if A is more expensive than B?
3) Among all the feasible alternative treatments, which should be chosen to maximize the benefit for patients and the whole society?

When faced with such questions, careful consideration and wise decision-making are always needed to make the optimum allocation of health resources. However, given the large amount of health technologies and drugs existing now, comparing the alternative treatments and making the best choice is often confusing and by no means an easy work.

# 2. EBM and Economic Evaluation

Evidence-based Medicine (EBM) has been developing very quickly since the middle of the 1990s. EBM means the integration of best research evidence with clinical expertise and patient values [3]. The development of EBM provides us with a strong guide to make our decisions on the allocation of health resources and health practices with the best, available evidence.

Generally, there are two types of evidence: "clinical evidence" and "economic evidence" [4]. The "clinical evidence" refers to the "efficacy" (Can it work?), "effectiveness" (Does it work?) and "safety" (Is it safe?) of drugs and other interventions which can be produced from clinical evaluation. However, the resources consumed by health practices are not evaluated and cannot be reflected in clinical evidence. On the other hand, "economic evidence" pays more attention to "efficiency" (Is it worth?), which is also called "cost-effectiveness". Cost-effectiveness focuses on the balance between costs and consequences (effectiveness) of health services [5]. Economic evidence is produced from economic evaluation which is defined as the comparative analysis of alternative courses of action in terms of both their costs and consequences [6]. Economic evaluation focused on drugs is specified as 'pharmaco-economics'. There are also economic evaluations focused on health technologies other than drugs, such as devices and surgeries.

Although both clinical evaluation and economic evaluation belong to health technology assessment, they are very different in their aims and nature. Clinical evaluation is aimed to generate clinical evidence informing the relative efficacy by explanatory trials, or the relative effectiveness by pragmatic trials. The explanatory trials are aimed to test causal research hypotheses (i.e., that a given intervention causes a particular benefit) and primarily designed to determine the effects of an interventions under ideal circumstances, while the pragmatic trials are aimed to help users choose between options for care and designed to determine the effects of an intervention under the usual conditions in which it will be applied [7].

However, costs of interventions are neither considered in pragmatic trials, nor in explanatory trials. Given the condition of scarce health resources, not only effectiveness but also costs will play an important role in the choices among interventions in health practices. Under this situation, results of clinical evaluation only are not enough reference for wise decision-making. We must also conduct economic evaluations. The economic evaluation, which analyzes both costs and consequences, is aimed to generate the economic evidence on cost-effectiveness of health services. Thus the economic evaluation can provide reference for decision-making in health practices and the allocation of health resources from the perspective of relative cost-effectiveness of comparing interventions, which cannot be reflected from clinical evaluation. Of course, there are also many factors other than effectiveness and costs which have influence on the decision-making in health practices and need to be considered, such as patient preferences, clinical expertise, feasibility of specific health interventions and so on. What we want to mention additionally is that, the clinical evaluation is the basis for economic evaluation and the generation of economic evidence. Because without reliable clinical evidence informing the certain effectiveness of health services in question, analysis of cost-effectiveness in economic evaluation will be meaningless. You have to first make sure whether a treatment really does more good than harm, and then consider whether its benefit worth the money paid for it. This should not be forgotten when conducting or evaluating an economic evaluation.

# 3. Main Features and Types of the Economic Evaluation

There are basically two features characterizing the economic evaluation: 1) both the costs and consequences of alternative treatments will be estimated and considered in an economic evaluation; 2) comparison of the alternative treatments and economic evaluation will be conducted with the specific set of criteria established for making decision among them. And with these two characteristics, the economic evaluations can be categorized in the following Table (Table 1) [6]. As shown in Table 1, the research without comparing alternatives can only be called "descriptions of the outcome/cost/cost-outcome". The research which has compared different alternatives but addresses only either costs or consequences is defined as "cost analysis" or "evaluation on efficacy/effectiveness". Only the research which makes comparison among different alternatives and also consider both costs and consequences simultaneously can be called “full economic evaluation”. There are three types of full economic evaluation: cost-effectiveness analysis (CEA), cost-utility analysis (CUA), and cost-benefit analysis (CBA). The main similarities and differences between these three types of economic evaluations have been summarized from references and textbooks in this area and are shown in the following table (Table 2) [6,8]. As shown in the above table, all of these three types of evaluations use monetary units to measure the costs of alternatives treatments. However, CUA and CBA use the measurement of quality-adjusted life years (QALYs) and monetary units which can summarize the multiple effects into one single unit, so even alternatives with different effects can be compared. While CEA only use the natural units such as life lost or disability-days saved to measure the effects, therefore, it cannot compare alternatives with different effects.

**Table 1. Distinguishing characteristics of health care evaluation**

<table>
<tr><td colspan="2" rowspan="2"></td><td colspan="3">Are both costs and consequences of the alternative examined?</td></tr>
<tr><td colspan="2">No</td><td>Yes</td></tr>
<tr><td rowspan="5">Is there comparison of the two or more alternatives?</td><td rowspan="3">No</td><td>only consequences</td><td>only costs</td><td rowspan="3">Partial evaluation<br>Cost-outcome description</td></tr>
<tr><td colspan="2">Partial evaluation</td></tr>
<tr><td>Outcome description</td><td>Cost description</td></tr>
<tr><td rowspan="2">Yes</td><td colspan="2">Partial evaluation</td><td rowspan="2">Full economic evaluation<br>Cost-effectiveness analysis (CEA)<br>Cost-utility analysis (CUA)<br>Cost-benefit analysis (CBA)</td></tr>
<tr><td>Efficacy or effectiveness evaluation</td><td>Cost analysis</td></tr>
</table>

Additionally, there is a variant of CEA called cost-consequence analysis (CCA) which only presents all the relevant consequences and costs of the various alternative treatments without the aggregation of them, such as calculating the incremental cost effectiveness ratio (ICER). The trade-off of costs and consequences needs to be made by the readers themselves [9].

**Table 2. The main similarities and differences between CEA, CUA and CBA**

| **Type of study** | **Measurement of costs in both alternatives** | **Identification of consequences** | **Measurement of consequences** | **Comparison between alternatives with different health outcomes** |
|---|---|---|---|---|
| CEA | Monetary units | Single effect of interest, common to both alternatives | Nature units (e.g. life-years gained, disability-days saved, points of blood pressure reduction, etc.) | Impossible |
| CUA | Monetary units | Single or multiple effects, not necessarily common to both alternatives | Healthy years (typically measured as quality-adjusted life-years) | Possible |
| CBA | Monetary units | Single or multiple effects, not necessarily common to both alternatives | Monetary units | Possible |

# 4. Pharmacoeconomic Evaluation on Kampo Medicine

Kampo medicine (Japanese traditional herbal medicine) is used by over 80% of doctors and recognized as an important medical approach in modern medicine in Japan [10]. Some characteristics of Kampo medicine are its unique therapeutic approach, certain effectiveness in specific therapeutic areas, and comparatively low cost. These characteristics may make Kampo medicine be more cost-effective than other alternative treatments in some situations of health practices and may make it a promising means of inhibiting the fast increase in health expenditures while maintaining the quality of health practices in Japan. There is already published research which has reported the comparative cost-effectiveness of Kampo medicine in the prevention of MRSA infection and the treatment of common cold syndrome [11,12].

However, the effectiveness and cost-effectiveness of Kampo medicine are still always doubted and in recent years there was a hot argument on whether or not Kampo medicine should be excluded from National Health Insurance. According to the survey of actual condition of Kampo medicine prescription conducted by Japan Kampo Medicines Manufacturers Association (JKMA) in 2011, the second biggest reason why Kampo medicine is not used among doctors is "lack of evidence" [10]. What's more, 66.3% of the doctors in the survey thought that the establishment of scientific evidence for Kampo medicine is necessary for its future development. Given these facts, the scientific evaluation including the pharmacoeconomic evaluation on Kampo medicine and establishing more evidence to prove Kampo medicine's effectiveness and cost-effectiveness in health practices are considered to be critical tasks at present.

The Special Committee for Evidence-based Medicine of Japan Society for Oriental Medicine (JSOM) made a systematic review on the randomized controlled trials (RCTs) of Kampo formulations in Japan, and compiles structured abstracts (SAs) and publishes them as "Kampo Chiryo Ebidensu Repoto" (Evidence Reports of Kampo Treatment: EKAT). As the results of this review, the "Kampo Chiryo Ebidensu Repoto 2010 - 345 no RCT" (Evidence Reports of Kampo Treatment: 345 Randomized Controlled Trials (EKAT 2010) and "Evidence Reports of Kampo Treatment Appendix 2011" which includes 14 newly reported RCTs, thus totally 359 RCTs have already been published in both Japanese and English. These reports can be accessed from: http://www.jsom.or.jp/medical/ebm/index.html, as well as the Cochrane CENTRAL. On the other hand, to our knowledge, there is no review on the published pharmacoeconomic evaluations on Kampo medicine in Japan and this unclear situation demands to be analyzed.

# 5. Review of Pharmacoeconomic Evaluations on Kampo medicine and Development of Structured Abstracts (SA)

Here we introduce the research being conducted on the review of pharmaconomic evaluations on Kampo medicine in Japan which started since 2010. The purpose of this research is 1) to collect published pharmacoeconomic evaluations on Kampo medicine in

Japan; 2) to develop structured abstracts (SA) for full economic evaluations (FEE) of them; 3) to assess the number and quality of published pharmacoeconomic evaluations; 4) to identify topics for future research.

Generally, there are two types of abstracts: the indicative abstract and the informative abstract. The structured abstract (SA) is one kind of informative abstract with distinct, labeled sections (e.g., Introduction, Methods, Results and Discussion: IMRAD) for rapid comprehension and scrutiny. Also, the abstractor can review the research and add comments to SA. SA was developed in the late 1980s. *ACP Journal Club,* which is a journal consisting of SAs exclusively, has adopted the 8-item SA proposed by Altman DG for clinical trial since the first issue in 1991. The term of "Evidence-based Medicine" was coined by Guyatt GH. on the second issue of it. There are several merits in using SA: SA can help health professionals in selecting clinically relevant and methodologically valid journal articles. They also guide authors in summarizing the content of their manuscripts precisely and facilitate the peer-review process for manuscripts submitted for publication. Also the creation of SA can enhance computerized literature searching [13]. By now, many journals in the area of EBM have adopted the use of SA, and make SA accessible on internet.

The National Health Service Economic Evaluation Database (NHS-EED, http://www.crd.york.ac.uk/CRDWeb/AboutNHSEED.asp), which is a world famous database of clinical economic evaluations, began to create SA of clinical economic evaluations with comments and publish them online in 1994. At first there were too many (43) items in SA which made them hard to be understood. Since 2008, the SA has been simplified to contain only 18 items. And in the review of pharmacoeconomic evaluations on Japan, with reference to the format of SA used by NHS-EED, a new format of SA was developed and used.

In the following text, we report the methods and results of the research reviewing pharmacoeconomic evaluations on Kampo medicine. Two examples of SA created in the review are showed to be reference for readers who are interested in them.

## 1) Methods

### *Search Strategy*

We searched the database Ichushi Web Ver.5(http://www.jamas.or.jp/), using search terms of "漢方" (Kampo medicine) and "経済" (keizai, economics). Searching date: 8 Feb 2012. Ichushi (医中誌, *Japana Centra Revuo Medicina,* since 1903) is the largest database of medical literature in Japan, and Ichushi Web covers the period of data since 1983 and indexes currently c.a. 3,000 journals.

### *Screening*

A double-stage screening on the search results was conducted. In the primary screening the case reports in 'publication type' field were excluded. And by the title and abstract, the articles which are not studies on Kampo medicine were excluded from the search results. The excluded articles in the secondary screening by full text include: 1) no detailed report on cost information; 2) duplicate or secondary publication; 3) case reports which are not tagged as "case reports" in original database; 4) inadequate information about the studies; 5) the object of study was not Kampo medicine. 6) studies with little value for decision-making; 7) other narrative reviews or explanations. By this two-stage screening, those pharmacoeconomic evaluations on Kampo medicine which are proper for analysis and the creation of SA were identified.

### *Development of the Format of SA*

With the reference to the format of SA used by NHS-EED since 2008, a new format of SA for the pharmacoeconomic evaluation on Kampo medicine was developed, with 8 items including research question, interventions, location/setting, methods, results, author's conclusions and abstractor's comments, abstractor and date.

## 2) Results

The results of searching and screening are displayed in **Figure 1**.

117 articles were identified with the search strategy mentioned before. Then the two-stage screening was performed. Finally, 10 articles of economic evaluations were identified while others were excluded. Among those 10 articles, 5 are considered as cost-effectiveness analyses (CEA), while 5 cost-consequence analyses (CCA) were also identified. No cost-utility analysis (CUA) or cost-benefit analysis (CBA) was identified.

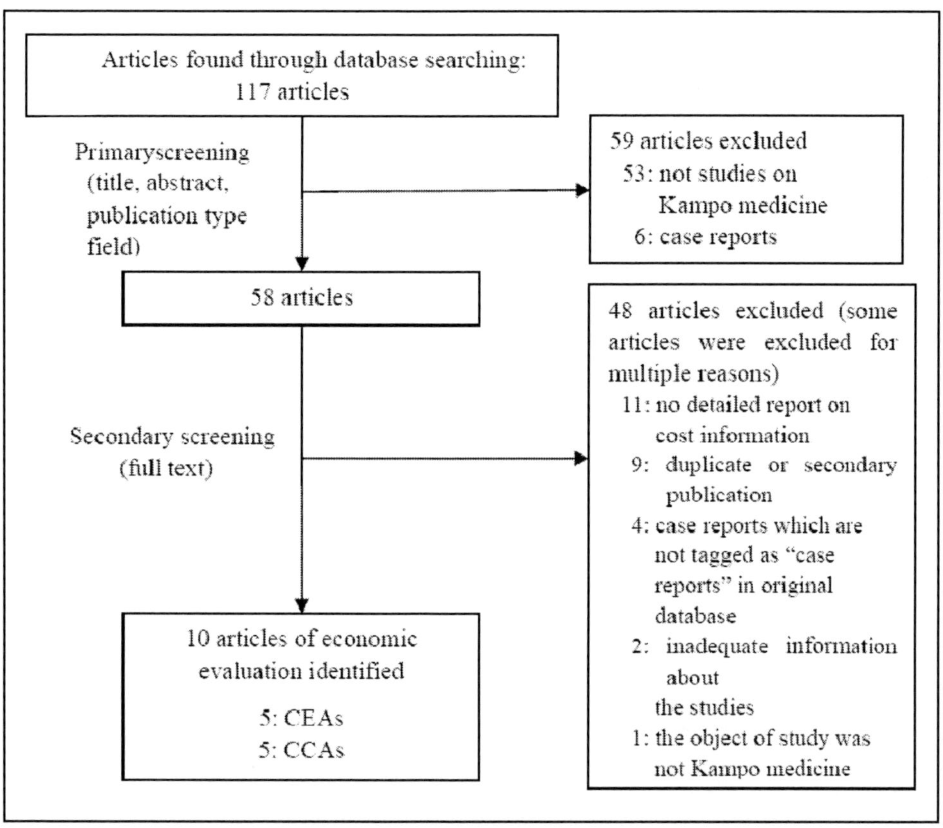


Figure 1. Screening of pharmacoeconomic evaluations on Kampo medicine.

# 6. Two Exemplary Structured Abstracts (SA) of Pharmacoeconomic Evaluations on Kampo Medicine

Two examples of SAs of pharmacoeconomic evaluations on Kampo medicine were created in this review. One of them is a cost-effectiveness analysis (CEA) and the other one conducted a cost-consequence analysis (CCA). Details of each Kampo formula can be found in KCONSORT (http:// kconsort.umin.jp).

**Example 1. Cost-effectiveness analysis (CEA) of boiogito in the treatment of knee osteoarthritis**

*Reference*

Koinuma M. et al. Henkeisei Shitsukansetsu Syo no Hozon teki Yakubutsu Ryoho ni taisuru boiogito no Yakuzaikeizai Bunseki (Pharmacoeconomic analysis on boiogito in conservative drug therapy for knee osteoarthritis). *Iryoyakugaku* (*Japanese Journal of Pharmaceutical Health Care and Sciences*) 2006: 32(8): 729-39 (in Japanese).

**1. Research Question**

Evaluate the cost-effectiveness of boiogito (防巳黄耆湯) in the treatment of patients with knee osteoarthritis (K-OA), compared with internal use of NSAIDS by cost-effectiveness analysis.

Perspective of analysis: payer

**2. Interventions**

Study population : 84 Patients diagnosed as primary K-OA and meeting all of the 4 criteria such as the observed edema in the patella ballottement test.

Intervention : 1) Kampo medicine (boiogito) 31 patients 2) Integration of Kampo medicine and western medicine (boiogito+NSAIDS) 33patients

Control : NSAIDS 20patients

**3. Location/setting**

Japan, outpatient departments of 12 hospitals

**4. Methods**

Cost : Direct cost of medical expenses calculated according to the Shinryo Hosyu Tensuhyo (List of Remuneration Points for Medical Services) and National Health Insurance Drug Price Standard.

Period of data collection: 8 weeks

Outcome : The number and rate of patients reaching the presumed endpoint which was defined as "Improvement of subjective symptoms of K-OA" Period of data collection: Feb 2002 - Jan 2003

Discount rate : not reported

**5. Results**

| | Cost per person (JPY) | | | Outcome | |
|---|---|---|---|---|---|
| | Cost for medical practice and dispensation | Cost of drugs | Total costs | Rate of reaching endpoint (%) | ICER (JPY/person) |
| Kampo medicine | 6,860 | 5,197 | 12,057 | 54.8 | 5,250 |
| Kampo medicine+NSAIDS | 8,460 | 10,142 | 18,602 | 63.6 | 49,978 |
| NSAIDS | 6,860 | 4,945 | 11,805 | 50.0 | - |

- Compared with the treatment using only NSAIDS, the incremental cost effectiveness ratios (ICER) of the other two treatments were calculated as: 1) the treatment using Kampo medicine: 5250 yen; 2) the intergration treatment of Kampo medicine plus NSAIDS: 49,978 yen to get one more patient reach the endpoint.
- In whether the baseline analysis or the sensitive analysis, the same trend of the necessary medical expense for getting one patient to reach the endpoint was observed and showed in the following order: Integration treatment of Kampo medicine plus NSAIDS>NSAIDS treatment>Kampo medicine treatment

**6. Authors' Conclusions**

In order to carry out cost-effective treatment to the K-OA patient accompanied with edema, the Kampo medicine of boiogito should be used alone in principle, and the medication of NSAIDS when necessary to relieve the pain could be recommended for producing better effectiveness.

**7. Abstractor's Comments**

- Based on the data from the clinical trial studying on the effectiveness of boiogito in the treatment of K-OA which was published in 2004, this research conducted a second analysis focusing on the cost-effectiveness of boiogito in the treatment of K-OA.
- The results of the statistical test on the endpoint-reaching rates of various groups in this research were not reported. Therefore, still some doubts remain regarding the results of the incremental analysis and calculated ICER.
- The object of sensitivity analysis was limited to cost-effectiveness ratio (CER), without considering ICER. Considering that the uncertainty of ICER has a more important influence on the conclusion of economic evaluation and decision-making. The sensitivity analysis of ICER is expected to be performed in future.

8. Abstractor and date:

**Tang / Igarashi 5 Mar 2012**

**Example 2. Cost-consequence analysis (CCA) of tokishakuyakusan in the treatment of iron-deficiency anemia**

*Reference*

Akase T. et al. Ekiga kuteki Syuho wo mochiita Kampo-Yaku no Yakko oyobi Keizaisei no Hyoka: Tetsu Ketsubosei Hinketsu ni taisuru tokishakuyakusan no Koka (The effectiveness and economic evaluation of Kampo medicine using the epidemiological technique: The effectiveness of tokishakuyakusan in the treatment of iron-deficiency anemia). *Sanfujinka Kampo Kenkyu no Ayumi* (*Recent Progress of Kampo Medicine in Obstetrics and Gynecology*) 1996: 13: 62-5 (in Japanese).

## 1. Research Question

Evaluate the cost-effectiveness of tokishakuyakusan (当帰芍薬散) in the treatment of female patients diagnosed as iron-deficiency anemia, compared with sodium ferrous citrate (Ferromia) by cost-consequence analysis.
Perspective of analysis: not reported (payer of medical expenses?)

## 2. Interventions

Study population: 364 Patients diagnosed as iron-deficiency anemiain the two years from Jan 1993 to Dec 1994 and with the saved records of laboratory examination available (Patients with other complications were excluded)
Intervention : tokishakuyakusan 147 patients (Averageage: 41.4 ± 3.8 years)
Control : Ferromia 217 patients (Average age: 39.3 ± 4.6 years)

## 3. Location/setting

Japan, no more detail

## 4. Methods

Cost : Direct cost (Cost of drugs for treating anemia and digestive drugs alleviating the side effects caused in digestive organs. Calculated with drug price at Dec 1994) Period of data collection: Jan 1993-Dec 1994
Outcome : Indicators of laboratory examination (RBC, Hb, Hct) Period of data collection: Jan 1993-Dec 1994.
Discount rate : not reported

## 5. Results

| | Cost per person | | | | | Outcome |
|---|---|---|---|---|---|---|
| | Average treatment period (day) | Cost of drugs for anemia (JPY) | Rate of combined use of digestive drugs (%) | Cost of digestive drugs (JPY) | Total drug costs (JPY) | Indicators of laboratory examination |
| Intervention | 43 | 4,655 | 16.3 | 818 | 4,788 | Restored to normal level |
| Control | 66 | 2,309 | 68.2 | 4,588 | 6,896 | Restored to normal level |
| Difference | -23 | 2,346 | -51.9 | - | -2,108 | - |

- As a result of calculating the total costs of the intervention group (tokishakuyakusan) and control group (Ferromia), the cost per person in the intervention group is about 30% lower than that in the control group, which means that the therapy of the intervention group can be conducted more economically.

**6. Authors' Conclusions**

According to the comparative research on the effectiveness of tokishakuyakusan and the iron preparation in the treatment of iron-deficiency anemia, the high usefulness of tokishakuyakusan from any point of view of effectiveness, safety or economics was indicated.

**7. Abstractor's Comments**

- The authors conducted a retrospective investigation through the medical records and the conclusion of the economical evaluation obtained by them is considered to be appropriate.
- However, the subjects for this research were restricted to the patients whose records of laboratory examination were saved and available. Prospective research with wider studying population is desired in future.

8. Abstractor and date: **Tang / Igarashi 5 Mar 2012**

# Conclusion

In this chapter, we analyzed the current state of increasing demand for health services and scarce health resources in Japan and the importance of conducting economic evaluations on health services. Considering the certain role of Kampo medicine in the health system in Japan and its potential for being more cost-effective than other interventions, the pharmacoeconomic evaluations on Kampo medicine and the establishment of scientific evidence for it are critical tasks at present. Research reviewing the pharmacoeconomic evaluations on Kampo medicine in Japan is being conducted and the new format of structured abstract (SA) is being used to summarize those evaluations. The results of this review and developed SAs will be summarized as Evidence Reports of Economic Evaluation of Kampo Treatment (EREK) and published soon. They are also available from: http://jhes.umin.ac.jp/team.html. This review and the use of SA are believed to contribute to the future establishment of the evidence from pharmacoeconomic evaluations on Kampo medicine, and a database assisting in the management and utilization of the evidence.

# References

[1] Motoo Y, et al. Traditional Japanese medicine, Kampo: its history and current status. *Chin J Integr Med.* 2011;17(2): 85-7.

[2] Koseirodosyo (Ministry of Health, Labour and Welfare), Heisei 21 Nendo Kokumin Iryohi no Gaikyo (in Japanese, the situation of National Medical Expenditures in 2009. [http://www.mhlw.go.jp/ toukei/saikin/hw/k-iryohi/09/ kekka1.html, accessed 6 Jan 2012]

[3] Sackett DL, Straus SE, Richardson WS, et al. *Evidence-based medicine: how to practice and teach EBM.* 2nd Edition. Edinburgh: Churchill Livingstone; 2000.

[4] Tsutani, K. Toyo Igaku to Ishiketteini Hitsuyona Mono: clinical evidence to economic evidence (What is needed for decision making in oriental medicine: clinical evidence and economic evidence). *Nihon Toyo Igaku Zasshi* (*Kampo Medicine*) 2002; 53(3): 189-98 (in Japanese).

[5] Tsutani K. Yakubutsu Chiryo no Keizai Hyoka Syuho wo Gaisetsu dekiru (The methods of economic evaluation on pharmacetutical treatment). Nihon Yakugakkai (The Pharmaceutical Society of Japan) ed. *Yakugaku to Syakai, dai 2 han (Pharmaceutics and Society, 2nd edition).* Tokyo: Tokyo Kagaku Dojin; 2008 (in Japanese).

[6] Drummond MF, Sculpher MJ, et al. *Methods for the economic evaluation of health care programmes.* 3rd Edition. Oxford: Oxford University Press; 2005.

[7] Thorpe KE, et al. A pragmatic-explanatory continuum indicator summary (PRECIS): a tool to help trial designers. *Can Med Assoc J.* 2009; 180(10): E47-57.

[8] Herman PM, Craig BM, Caspi O. Is complementary and alternative medicine (CAM) cost-effective? A systematic review. *BMC Complement Altern Med.* 2005; 5: 11.

[9] Berger ML, et al. (2003) Health care cost, quality and outcomes: ISPOR book of terms. (Herusu Kea Saiensu no tame no Iryo Keizaigaku no Yogosyu, Japanese translation supervised by Kamae I. Tokyo: Iyaku Syuppan Senta; 2011).

[10] Japan Kampo Medicines Manufacturers Association. Kampo-Yaku Shoho Jittai Cyosa (Survey of actual condition of Kampo medicine prescription) 2011. Available from: http://medicalkaihatu.nikkeibp.co.jp/medical-kaihatu/kampo/index.html (in Japanese, accessed 10 Jan 2012).

[11] Sakamaki, H. Rojin Byoin nado ni okeru Iryoukeizaigaku to Kampo-Yaku (Health economics and Kampo medicine in geriatric hospital). *Kampo to Saishin Chiryo* (*Kampo & the Newest Therapy*) 2001: 10(4): 338-42 (in Japanese).

[12] Akase, T. et al. Kaze Syokogun ni okeru Yakuzaihi no Yakuzai Ekigaku oyobi Keizaigaku teki Kento: Kampo-Yaku to Seiyo-Yaku no Keizaisei ni okeru Hikaku Kenkyu (A pharmacoepidemiological and economic study on the medicinal expenses for the treatment of colds: comparison between modern drugs and Kampo medicine). *Nihon Toyo Igaku Zasshi* (*Kampo Medicine*) 2000: 50(4): 655-63 (in Japanese).

[13] U.S. National Library of Medicine. Structured Abstracts. Available from: http://www.nlm.nih.gov/bsd/policy/structured_abstracts.html (accessed 8 Jan 2012).

In: Traditional Medicine: New Research
Editor: Yoshiharu Motoo

ISBN: 978-1-62257-448-3


*Chapter 14*

# Primo Vascular System

***Kwang-Sup Soh[1*], Sharon Jiyoon Jung[1], Yong Joo Kwon[1], Min-Ho Nam[2] and Seung-Hoon Choi[2]***

[1] Nano Primo Research Center, Advanced Institute of Convergence Technology, Seoul National University, Suwon, Korea

[2] Department of Pathology, College of Oriental Medicine, Kyung Hee University, Seoul, Korea

## Abstract

Bong-Han Kim discovered anatomical structures regarded as acupuncture meridians and acupoints in the early 1960's. However, there was no description of the method he used to observe and identify the structures in his series of reports. Also, there was no reproduction of his findings except by one Japanese anatomist, Satoru Fujiwara. The findings of both Kim and Fujiwara have been ignored for more than forty years.

Only very lately in 2002 was Kim's work re-illuminated by the Biomedical Physics Laboratory of Seoul National University, which started intensive investigation of his discoveries. The Bong-Han system was renamed the Primo Vascular System (PVS) at the First International Symposium on the Primo Vascular System (ISPVS), which was held at JeCheon, Korea, on September 17-18, 2010.

In this paper we reviewed the current state of research on the PVS: identification in the nervous system, cardiovascular system, lymphatic system, fascia in the abdominal cavity, adipose tissue, reproductive system (testis), skin and abdominal wall, primo fluid, microcells, and egg vitelline membrane. We also considered the role of the PVS on pathological conditions, particularly cancer metastasis. We also discussed the primo microcell, which is a kind of embryonic-like stem cell which is associated with the PVS.

**Keywords:** Acupuncture, primo vascular system, cancer, sanal, stem cell

* Correspondence: Kwang-Sup Soh, Email: kssoh1@gmail.com.

# 1. Introduction

## 1.1. A Brief History

Traditional Chinese Medicine (TCM) practice is based upon acupuncture points (AP;經穴) and acupuncture meridians (AM;經絡) which are distributed in the skin of humans and some domestic animals. AP and AM are displayed in figures, and directions for disease treatments have been taught for thousands of years in Far East Asia. Yet, no one has yet shown what these points and lines are anatomically, which impedes the scientific investigation into the processes of acupuncture.

There have been many efforts to find or identify the APs with anatomically characteristic features. The work of Heine [1] and Langevin [2] is especially notable in that they find some special features of the APs, but they conclude that there are no exclusive structures corresponding to APs or AMs.

Bong-Han Kim's claim to finding the anatomical structures corresponding to APs and AMs is therefore unique. He further maintains that the novel structure is a third circulatory system in addition to the well-known blood and lymph vessel systems [3, 4]. He identifies a network of what he calls Bonghan ducts, and what we term primo vessels, that correspond to AMs. These primo vessels run not only through the skin but also throughout the body, including inside blood vessels and lymph vessels. Fluid inside flows very slowly and contains important biochemicals such as hormones [5]. He also identifies structures that he calls Bonghan corpuscles, and that we call primo nodes, which correspond to APs.

Medically, Kim's most striking claim is about what he calls Sanal, which literally means living eggs. He describes their behavior as acting identical to the modern concept of embryonic-like stem cells in modern terms. He displays data showing the hematopoietic function of Sanal [6].

He mentions that the essential technique to reveal the primo vessels and primo nodes is to use a certain blue dye which specifically flows into and traces the primo vessels [3]. However, he kept the details of the dye secret, and this is the reason why other people could not reproduce his well-documented results. Only one group in Japan under the direction of Dr. Fujiwara, an anatomist in Osaka City University, was able to confirm some parts of Kim's claims in 1967 [7, 8]. His results did not garner much attention and the Bong-Han Theory has been neglected for some time.

It was in the year 2002 that a systematic reinvestigation of the Bong-Han Theory began at the Biomedical Physics Laboratory of Seoul National University. Primo vessels and primo nodes were indeed observed inside the blood vessels of rabbits and rats in 2002, confirming Kim's claims [9-12]. However, no further progress was made in the effort to detect primo vessels and nodes in other organs for about a year. Then Dr. KS Soh contacted and met Dr. Satoru Fujiwara in Osaka to get help. The advice and information Dr. Soh received from Dr. Fujiwara was critical to reproduce Fujiwara's earlier experiments to observe the primo vessels and nodes on the surface of the stomach, liver, and small intestine of rabbits and rats [13-15]. Observation of primo vessels inside lymph vessels was subsequently performed [16, 17, 18, 19].

An important technical breakthrough was made in the year 2008 when the Trypan blue staining technique was developed to specifically reveal the primo vascular system (PVS) among blood or lymph vessels, nerves, and connective tissue [20]. It led most importantly to the discovery of the PVS around tumor tissue and also in adipose tissue [21, 22].

With the finding of the PVS around tumor tissue, many researchers in the US and China showed interest in this subject, and an international symposium on PVS with special topics on cancer and stem cells was held in 2010 [23], where the International Society for Primo Vascular System was organized. In March 2011, the Nano Primo Research Center was established in the Advanced Institute of Convergence Technology of Seoul National University.

### 1.2. Organs where the Primo Vascular System Was Observed

The PVS was first observed in the blood vessels of rabbits and rats without any staining dyes, but the question was raised of how to distinguish the primo vessels from similar-looking coagulated fibrin strings. The question was answered by applying the fluorescent dye Acridine orange, which stained the nuclei of cells. String of coagulated fibrin did not have nuclei, while the primo vessel had endothelial cell nuclei that were stained by Acridine orange [10]. The primo vessels inside mouse blood vessels were detected using another kind of dye, Alcian blue [12]. The network of the PVS inside the heart of a cow was observed using the Trypan blue technique [24].

The presence of the PVS inside lymph vessels was first confirmed in rabbits using Alcian blue [16] and in rats with fluorescent magnetic nanoparticles [17]. With the enhanced optical coherence method, the moving the PVS inside lymph vessels was demonstrated in vivo and in situ in the abdominal cavity of a rabbit [19].

Professor YK Hong's group at the University of Southern California studied the lymphatic vascular biology and was interested in the primo vessels present within the thoracic lymph duct, the largest caliber lymphatic vessel. They reported an endeavor to study the primo vessels present in the thoracic ducts of rodents. Prox1-GFP BAC transgenic mice were used to visualize the thoracic ducts. Consistent with previous studies on rabbits [16, 19], they were able to detect primo vessels within the thoracic ducts of mice and rats. Based on H&E staining, in both species the primo vessels appeared to be highly elastic and to contain extracellular matrix materials with residing cells. Because both thoracic ducts and primo vessels were significantly shrunken upon dissection, only a few frozen sections of the thoracic ducts contained the primo vessel and most of the sections were found to not have the primo vessel. Techniques for optimal tissue preparation should be developed for further studies [25].

Many people raised doubts about whether or not Dr. Kim and others had mistaken lymph vessels for primo vessels. The above work showing the presence of the PVS inside lymph vessels is a strong answer to such skepticism, because there have been no reports about any lymph vessels floating in the lymphatic fluid of another lymph vessel.

The PVS on the surface of internal organs such as the liver, stomach, bladder, small intestine, and large intestine of various animals like rabbits [13], rats [26], mice [27], pigs [27], and dogs [28] was extensively investigated. They were recognizable even without any staining dye, but were difficult to distinguish from similar-looking torn membranes or blood-coagulated fibrin that formed due to bleeding during surgery. Detection became somewhat easier using the Trypan blue technique [20].

The PVS in the brain ventricles and in the central canal of the spinal cord of rabbits was observed using chrome-hematoxylin after surgery [29]. An improvement of technique was followed by injection of Trypan blue into the lateral ventricle of a rat so that the PVS was stained before surgery [30]. Further progress was achieved by replacing Trypan blue with fluorescent nanoparticles [31]. Detection or imaging of the PVS in the brain is envisioned with a combination of MRI and the nanoparticles as contrast agents.

A fine network of the PVS in the peritonea and in adipose tissues among the abdominal organs was also detectable with the Trypan blue staining method [20, 22]. A putative primo vessel in the mesentery between the colon and the root of the mesentery of a mouse was identified using 4',6-diamidino-2-phenylindole (DAPI) staining of nuclei and phalloidin staining of f-actin in cells [32]. A thread-like structure in the vital line membrane of a chicken egg was observed with the Trypan blue technique, which seemed to be a primo vessel precursor [33].

### 1.3. Morphological and Immunohistochemical Characteristics of the PVS

Primo vessels are extremely difficult to identify in ordinary hematoxylin and eosin (H&E) staining of thin cross-sections. It is, however, straightforward to distinguish the PVS from blood or lymph vessels by observing the nuclei distributions in longitudinal sections. The nuclei of endothelial cells of the primo vessels are arranged in the fashion of parallel broken lines. They are rod-shaped and about 10-20 micrometers in length. These hallmarks of the primo vessels are easily checked with DAPI, Acridine Orange, or Feulgen reaction staining of nuclei [10, 13, 16]. Another characteristic of the primo vessel is the bundle structure which is composed of several sub-ducts. This bundle structure is a hallmark of the primo vessel, which uniquely distinguishes it from blood or lymph vessels [13, 34]. Still one more distinguishing feature is the f-actin distribution pattern of the primo vessel, which is quite different from that of blood or lymph vessels. This feature can be shown using phalloidin staining [32]. The ultra-fine structure of primo vessels was studied to show the multi-bundle structure using scanning electron microscopy (SEM), transmission electron microscopy (TEM) and focused ion beam scanning electron microscopy (FIB-SEM). Even though the electron microscopic images of cross sections were consistent with a multi-bundle structure, they were not distinctive enough compared to the longitudinal views [34, 35, 36]. Immunohistochemical studies using antibodies were partially successful in identifying the primo vessels. Primo vessels showed positive expression to VWF, but negative to CD31 and LYVE-1 [26, 37]. Thus primo vessels are quite different from blood vessels (positive to both VWF and CD31) and lymph vessels (positive to LYVE-1). Primo vessels also showed positive expression to fibronectin [26], but more extensive research in this direction is necessary.

### 1.4. Physiological Characteristics

Only limited studies on the physiological characteristics of the PVS have been performed. The flow speed of the fluid in the PVS on the surface of internal organs of rabbits was measured as slower compared to blood or lymph flow speed at $0.3 \pm 0.1$ mm/sec [36].

The flow of Alcian blue injected into the acupuncture point BL23 on the dorsal skin of a rat was traced to the PVS on the stomach and other internal organs. But its path was not fully revealed, and the paths did not repeat. It may because the paths from BL23 were multiply divergent and required more precise control beyond the current technical level [38].

The flow of fluorescent nanoparticles and chrome-hematoxylin injected into the testis of a rat also demonstrated primo vascular paths from the testis toward the abdominal wall, but no unique route was established. There were many paths but repeated flow to the same path was not obtainable due to technical immaturity [39].

The presence of catecholamine-producing cells in the primo node on the surface of rabbit internal organs was shown by immunohistochemistry with an anti-adrenaline polyclonal antibody and anti-noradrenaline polyclonal antibody [40]. Cells of a mixed type with a relatively high concentration of adrenaline in relation to noradrenalin were present in the primo node. Cells containing only adrenaline or noradrenaline were not found. For the quantitative analysis of the catecholamine content in the primo node, ELISA was employed. The adrenaline content was significantly greater ($20.6 \pm 8.8$ ng/g) than the noradrenaline content ($5.8 \pm 2.6$ ng/g). In other control tissues and fluids (adrenal gland, heart, and urine) the adrenal concentrations were significantly lower than those of noradrenaline. The meaning of this rather surprising result is not understood yet. The presence of catecholamine in the PVS was previously studied [41]. Catecholamine-storing cells were again observed in putative primo nodes in the skin of rabbits [42]. Yet a more definite conclusion requires further extensive experiments.

Proteomic analysis of the primo vessels on the surface of rabbit intestines and the primo fluid was performed using nano LC-ESI MS/MS. In the primo vessel, 207 different proteins were identified, and 70 in the primo vessel and fluid. The result showed a high concentration of proteins involved in metabolism that are not usually found in blood, lymph, or blood vessels. They are associated with stem cells, especially mesenchymal stem cells, cancer cells, and myeloid cells [43]. This result is consistent with our previous immunohistochemical study that suggested the presence of mesenchymal stem cells in primo nodes [37]. Primo nodes on the organ surface may have a role as a temporary depot and point of differentiation of stem cells for tissue regeneration.

# Cancer and Primo Vascular System

## 2.1. PVS Developed around a Tumor Tissue

Proteomic analysis suggested an intimate relationship between cancer and the PVS, and encouraged a search for the PVS around cancer tissues. However, it was only possible to find the PVS around tumor tissue after the development of the Trypan blue technique of PVS detection [44].

The tumor tissues were grown on the skin after subcutaneous inoculation of human lung cancer cells (NCI-H460) into nude mice. The lateral sides of the tumor skin were incised, and the skin on the tumor was carefully removed to expose the tumor with an intact membrane. A 0.1% Trypan blue solution filtered through 0.22-μm pore-sized filter paper was poured on the membrane of the exposed tumor, drop by drop. After Trypan blue had been washed off with warm saline, identification of the PVS was assessed using direct visualization with a surgical microscope (SZX12, Olympus). A histological analysis of the PVS with H&E showed sinuses and rod-shaped nuclei, which are characteristic hallmarks of a primo vessel.

In a subsequent study [26], primo vessels were again found inside the abdominal cavity of NCI-H460 lung cancer murine xenograft models. These vascular threads were largely distributed on the surfaces of various organs and were often connected to peritoneal tumor nodules. Histological and immunofluorescent investigations showed the characteristic features of the primo vessels, that is, the rod-shaped nuclei aligned longitudinally along the channels. These endothelial cells of the primo vessels, did not express the LYVE-1, a specific marker of lymphatics, which indicated a clear difference from lymphatic endothelial cells.

Simple criteria to distinguish primo vessels from blood vessels, lymph vessels, or nerves in the subcutaneous layer of skin around a tumor xenografted on the dorsal side of a mouse were developed. It used phalloidin to reveal f-actin and DAPI to show the pattern of nuclei distributions of these vessels and nerves. This simple technique demonstrated the characteristic differences in distribution of f-actins and nuclei in the relevant tissues [45]. This practical criterion can be useful in a clinical situation to search for and identify the PVS in patients.

The PVS was also found in melanoma models of female nude mice (BALB-c-nu/nu) with B16F10 melanoma cells. The compositional differences were investigated between the PVS and lymph vessels in murine melanoma models by immunofluorescence staining and ultra performance liquid chromatography-quadrupole time-of-flight mass spectrometry (UPLC-Q-TOF MS). Primo vessels and primo nodes were identified on the surface of cutaneous melanoma using Trypan blue staining. Immufluorescent study revealed that the PVS did not express against LYVE-1, a specific endothelial antigen of lymphatics. UPLC-Q-TOF MS chromatograms showed different levels of ion mass peak between two vascular systems [46].

PVS study with other melanoma models with C57BL6 mice and B16BL6 murine melanoma cells were done by Hong et al., an independent group led by Professor M. Suh of Sungkyunkwan University. They showed higher concentrations of tissue oxygen in the PVS compared with neighbor tissues [47]. In another study, this group used GFP transgenic mice to demonstrate that the PVS on the surface and within melanoma xenografts are derived from the parent mouse. They provided convincing data that the PVS in this system originated from the host mouse, not the tumor. The significance of their work is that this system is a good model system in which to address questions about the role of the PVS in cancer development and metastasis [48].

Still another group led by Professor S. Achilefu at the Washington University in the US found primo vessels extended to and from abdominal viscera, often disappearing into layers of adipose tissue before resurfacing in a more distal region. Female Swiss Webster mice, 6-8 weeks old, were used for identification of primo vessels in mice. They injected 4T1 mouse mammary carcinoma cells suspended in PBS subcutaneously in the right flanks. Flank tumors grown from mouse mammary carcinoma cells implanted subcutaneously are a rudimentary but useful model of cancer growth and development. Based on Trypan blue staining, several primo structures on the tumor surface were observed. Blue-stained primo vessels and nodes on the tumor surface were distinct in color, location, and structure from neighboring blood vessels. Unlike the primo vessels associated with the surface of abdominal organs, these primo vessels were more within the clear serosal tissues. They appeared to be attached to the tumors, invading into them [49].

## 2.2. PVS and Cancer Metastasis

Since the PVS is known to make up a circulatory system corresponding to acupuncture meridians or collaterals, we propose a hypothesis that besides the currently known blood or lymph vessels the PVS on the fascia of tumor tissue may be a novel path of metastasis.

Metastasis is the process whereby cancer cells spread from a primary site to form new tumors in distant organs [50, 51]. Inhibition and control of metastases are critical approaches for complete cancer therapy, and the study of cancer metastasis has grown exponentially [52]. Tumor metastases are usually thought to occur via blood vessels and lymphatic vessels, referred to as the hematogenous and lymphatic routes, respectively. However, suppressing angiogenesis and lymphangiogenesis has not always proven to be effective in clinical trials and the understanding of the processes and the mechanisms of metastasis remains far from complete.

A notable research on metastatic events, i.e., the formation of matrix-rich vasculogenic-like networks by highly aggressive tumor cells in a number of different tumor types including melanomas and breast, prostate, ovarian, and lung carcinomas has gotten much attention. Vasculogenic mimicry (VM) is found in aggressive tumor tissues [53–55]. This indicates a reversion of tumor cells to an undifferentiated, embryonic-like phenotype. In addition, VM in melanomas was involved in several signaling molecules that are also involved in embryonic vasculogenesis, including vascular endothelial cadherin, erythropoietin-producing hepatocellular carcinoma-A2, and laminin 5 $\gamma$2-chain. This primitive micro-circulation may act as an additional route for metastasis.

The PVS is a new kind of conduit, and, like VM, they are distinctively different from blood or lymph vessels. It is remarkable that these newly-discovered conduits are present both outside and inside the tumor tissue. Whether VM and the PVS are correlated is an open question at the present time.

To witness metastasis through the PVS, a set of new technologies amenable to *in vivo* imaging of cancer cells were developed: near-infrared quantum dot (NIR QD) electroporation and multispectral fluorescence imaging. NIR QD electroporation has been shown to be capable of high-throughput cancer cell tagging for long-term imaging with rapid clearance of released QDs. Multispectral fluorescence imaging can account for tissue auto-fluorescence and variation in the tissue's optical properties to resolve fluorescence reliably in living animals. By performing *in vivo* imaging of QD labeled lung cancer cells inside the PVS around a superficially grown tumor and abdominal organs, evidence for the functional relevance of the primo vessels as an additional independent metastasis route was obtained. All *in vivo* observations were further confirmed by post-inspection of histological analyses [56].

Migration of cancer cells along primo vessels on the surface of internal organs was observed, and the function and mechanism of the primo vessel as a guide path of cancer cells are important subjects to be studied in the future. These studies were done with GFP labeled cancer cells for tracking their migration [57].

Besides being a metastasis path, the PVS may play other roles in connection with tumor tissues. The fluid flowing in the PVS may play important roles in tumor growth as it contains hyaluronic acid, adrenalin and noradrenalin hormone, albumin, and microcells. In addition, a proteomic analysis of the tissues and liquids from primo vessels on rabbit intestinal surfaces revealed a chemical composition similar to that usually associated with stem cells [58, 59], cancer cells [60], and differentiated myeloid cells [61]. These vigorously-proliferating cells show a similar abundance of carbohydrate or energy-related processes [58-61]. The tumor tissues likely take advantage of the chemicals supplied through the PVS.

Another hypothetical significance of the PVS connected to tumor tissues is its possible use as a drug delivery path for anti-cancer medicine or even as a route for acupuncture stimulation, because the PVS is an anatomical structure of acupuncture collaterals. A host of items such as migration, invasion, relation to angiogenesis, proliferation, and growth of cancer tissue have immediate importance in connection with the PVS.

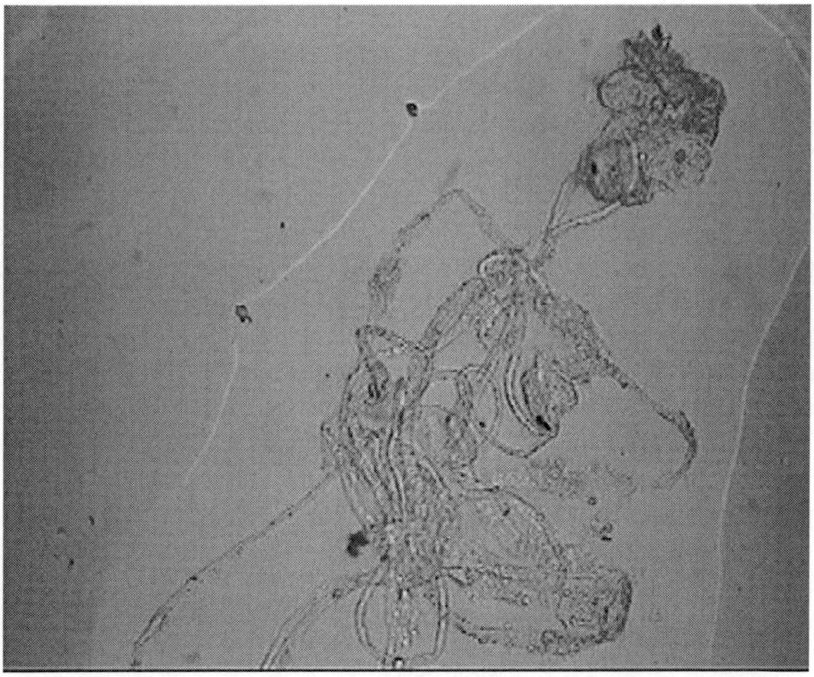

Figure 1. Phase-contrast microscope image of the Primo Vessel from an artery of a rat. The total length is about 4 cm [Baik KY et al., *The Newest Medical J* 2004;47:18-22].

# Primo Microcell and Stem Cell

## 3.1. Morphology of Primo Microcell

A primo microcell, or sanal, is of spherical or oval shape. Its diameter is about 1.5 um and ranges from 0.8 μm to 2.4 μm. It is wrapped with a thin membrane, has DNA in it, and cytoplasm as well, according to BH Kim [5].

Sanals were obtained from primo nodes by homogenization and differential centrifugation [62, 63, 64]. Their DNA content was confirmed with Acridine orange staining and confocal microscopy. In order to study surface structures SEM was used, and surface structures with round bumps were shown (Figure 3B). With TEM the nuclei with DNA was observed (Figure 3B)

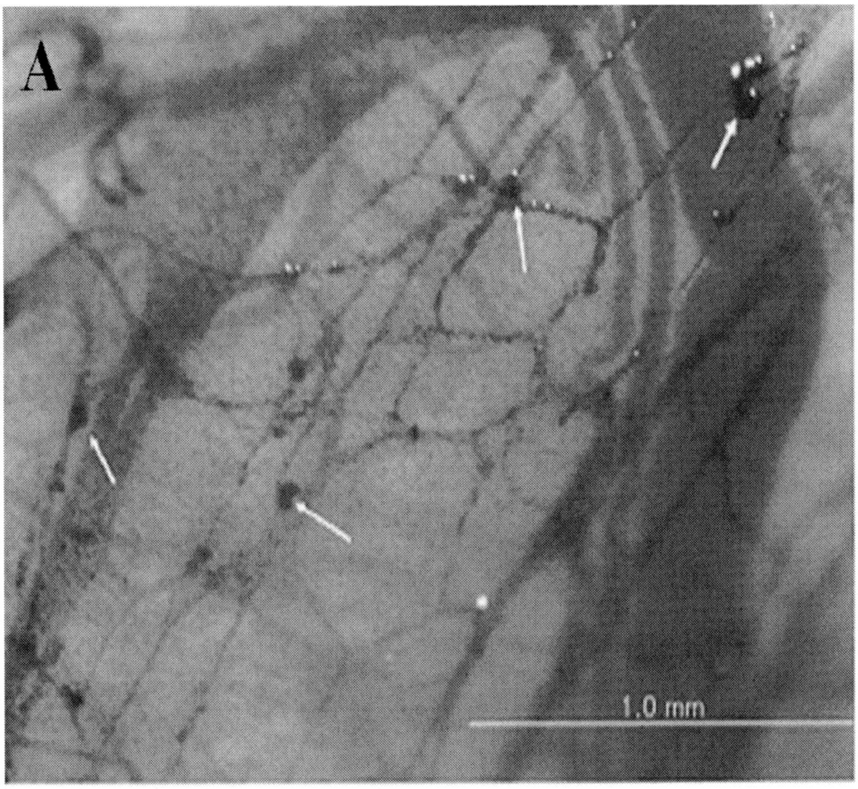


Figure 2. Weblike network of PVS revealed by using Trypan blue. A web of PVS on the visceral peritoneum around the stomach near the spleen of a rat. There were several small primo nodes at crossing points, as indicated by the arrows. The blood capillaries were not stained. [Lee BC et al., *J Acup Mer Stud* 2009;2: ].

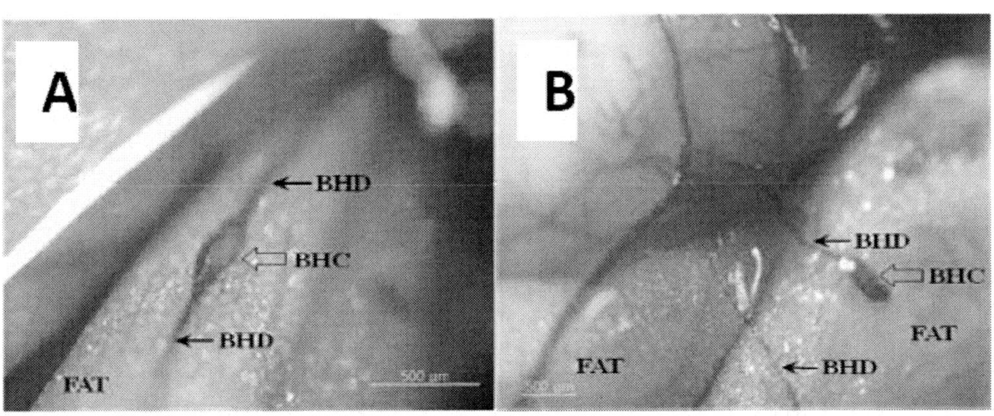


Figure 3. Trypan blue staining of a primo vessel and a primo node inside adipose tissues. A: A primo node and connected primo vessel inside adipose tissue around the small intestine of a rat. B: A primo node and two primo vessels near a small intestine of the same rat. Notice that the blood vessels and the adipose tissues were not stained [Lee BC et al., *J Acup Mer Stud* 2009;2: ].

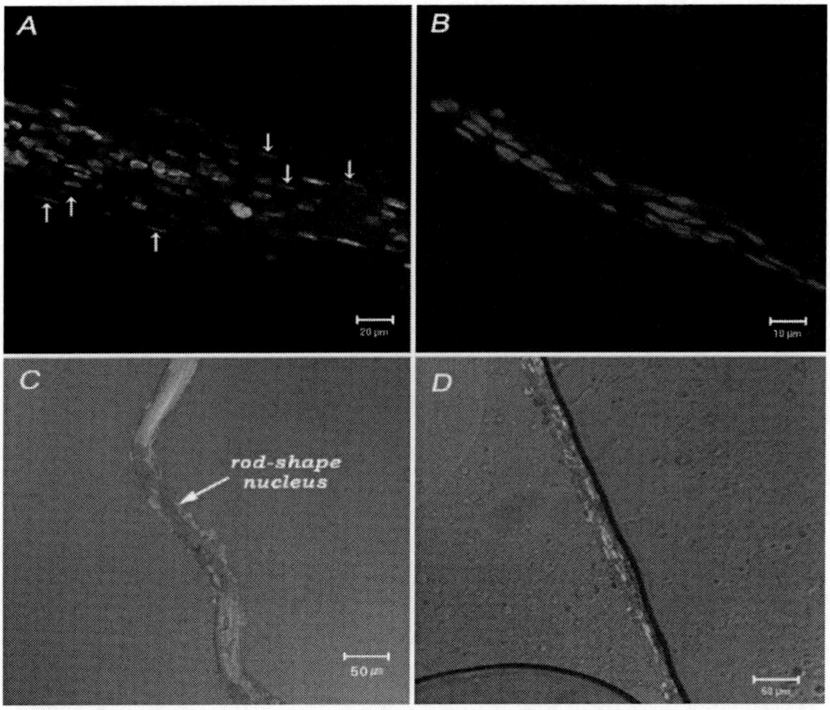


Figure 4. Confocal laser scanning microscopic images of primo vessels showing rod-shaped nuclei (arrows) distributed in a broken-lined striped fashion. **A:** The primo vessel was stained by YoYo-1, DNA-specific dye, after having been taken from an Alcian-blue-injected lymphatic vessel of a rabbit [Lee C et al., *Lymph Res Biol* 2006;4:181-190]. **B:** The BHD was stained by using Acridine orange, another DNA staining dye, after having been taken from a Janus-Green-B-injected lymphatic vessel of a rabbit [Lee BC et al., *Anat Rec* 2005;286B;1-7]. **C:** The primo vessel was stained by using a Feulgen reaction, a DNA-specific dye, after taken from the organ surfaces of rabbits [Shin HS et al., *Anat Rec* 2005;284B;35-40]. **D:** The primo vessel was stained by using Acridine orange after having been taken from the caudal vena cava of a rabbit [Lee BC et al., *Anat Rec* 2004;278B;27-30]. The shapes, lengths, and distributions of the rod-shaped nuclei are similar to each other for the four cases. This suggests that the primo vessel in lymph vessels, in blood vessels, and on organ surfaces belong to the same system.

### 3.2. Motion

Sanals extracted with a centrifuge from the primo nodes on the surface of rabbit internal organs exhibited a jittering motion as observed with an inverted microscope or phase contrast microscope [65]. The jittering motion was apparently Brownian random motion, not thermal motion as BH Kim said. Kim claimed it was most active at 37-38 C [5], but this has not yet been confirmed. The effects of UV-A and visible light on the motion of sanals were studied. The average velocity and acceleration increased significantly after irradiation with UV-A light (355-375 nm), but there was no noticeable change with visible light [66]. The DNA molecules, which are known to be reactivated by the light of 365 nm [67], may absorb the irradiated photons on sanals. The viscosity of μL volumes of primo fluid obtained from the PVS on the surfaces of rabbit internal organs was measured. The fluid was mechanically micro-extracted *in situ* from the primo nodes with a glass capillary connected to an extractor. From the Brownian motion of the sanals in the extracted fluid, the fluid viscosity was determined to be 1.4±0.1 mPa·s at room temperature. This viscosity is comparable to the viscosity of rabbit blood plasma [68].

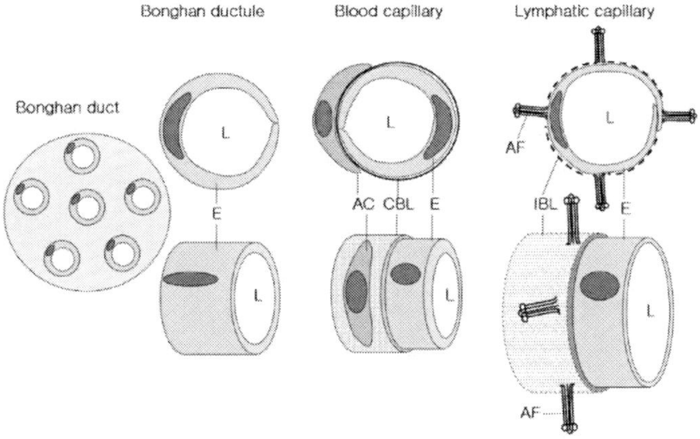


Figure 5. Structural properties of the primo vessel (Bonghan duct and ductile), blood and lymphatic capillary. E means endothelium; L, lumen; AC, accessory cell; CBL, complete basal lamina; IBL, incomplete basal lamina; and AF, anchoring filaments.

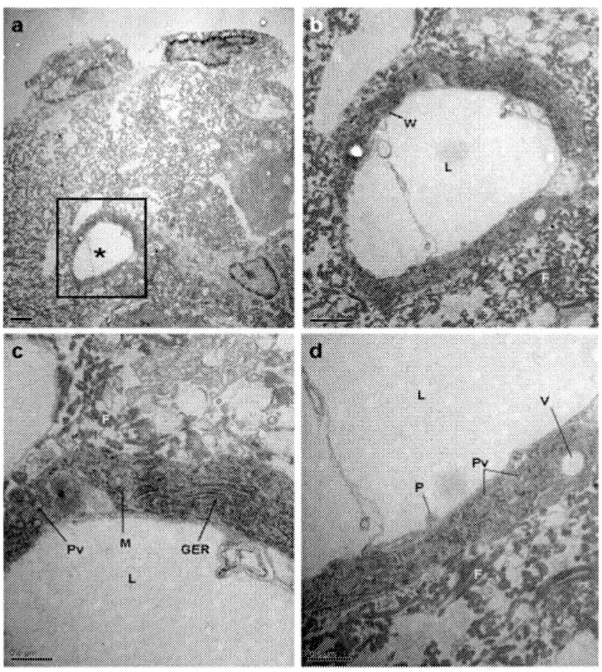


Figure 6. Ultrastructural organization of the ductule of primo vessel. **a:** Electron micrograph clearly showing the presence of the ductule (asterisk) in a cross section through the primo vessel. Scale bar, 2 μm. **b:** Magnified image of the rectangular area in Figure 4a shows that the wall (W) of the ductule consists of a single layer of endothelial cells surrounded by fibrin-like fibers. Scale bar, 1μm. **c** and **d:** Highly-magnified electron micrographs showing the ultrastructural characteristics of the endothelial cells of the ductule. L means lumen; M, mitochondria; RER, rough endoplasmic reticulum; P, cytoplasmic protrusion; ICP, interdigitated cytoplasmic processes; Pv, pinocytotic vesicles; V, vacuole; and F, fibrin-like fibers. Scale bar, 0,5 μm.

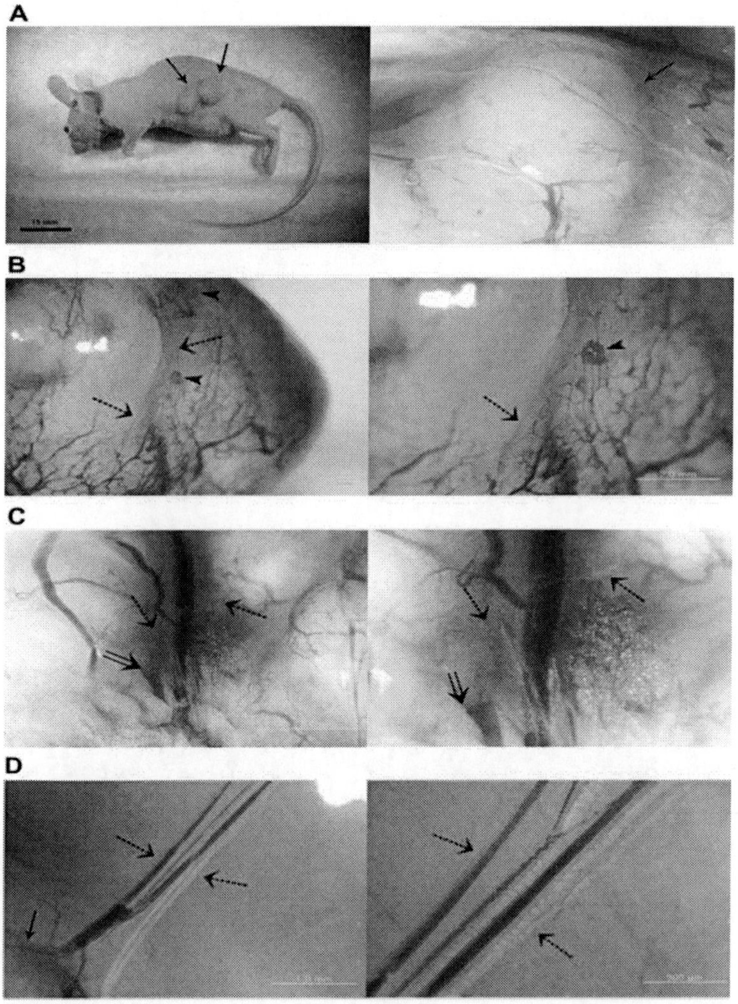


Figure 7. Visualization of a PVS on the fascia surrounding a tumor tissue in the skin of a mouse. A: Images of the tumor tissue indicated by arrows. Left, a camera image of the mouse with two tumor tissues grown for two weeks after subcutaneous inoculation of human lung cancer cells. Right, part of the surface of the tumor tissue after skin resection. the presence of the PVS is hardly noticeable. B: *In-situ* Trypan blue staining revealed primo vessel (dotted arrows) and corpuscles (arrow heads) on the fascia surrounding a tumor tissue. The right panel is a magnified view of the left panel. Trypan blue did not stain the blood vessels. C: Another sample showing multiple a primo vessel (dotted arrows) on the fascia surface of a tumor tissue. The right panel is a magnified view of the left panel. There is a branching of the primo vessel. It is also significant that the primo vessel enters the nearby fat layer (double arrow). D: The Trypan blue technique revealed primo vessel (dotted arrows) along a bundle of blood vessels and nerves. The magnified view in the right panel clearly shows the duct along the blood vessel. The bundle of blood vessels and nerves connect the tumor tissue (arrow) at the lower left corner to the outside skin. Samples A, B, C, and D were from different mice [Yoo JS et al., *J Acup Mer Stud* 2009;2: ].

The viscosity of the primo fluid was significantly lower than that of whole blood and was similar to that of blood plasma. Since it is known that the PVS can transport liquid, the comparable viscosities of primo fluid and plasma is an important piece of evidence implicating the PVS in micro-circulation. It is conceivable that the PVS viscosity might be germane in certain circulatory diseases.

### 3.3. Proliferation and Cultivation

The cultivation of sanals was described by BH Kim, which is controversial because it is completely different from ordinary cell division processes. It resembles a budding of yeast that a protrusion of a bud grows to form a daughter sanal [5]. A cell is formed by repetition of this budding process which is not known in standard animal biology. Whether or not his claim is accurate needs to be checked in the future.

Nevertheless, preliminary observation of sanals extracted from primo nodes showed consistent results with his claim. In particular, SEM and atomic force microscopic (AFM) images clearly showed the budding and the mother-daughter pair of sanals formed by budding as shown in Figure III.2 [64].

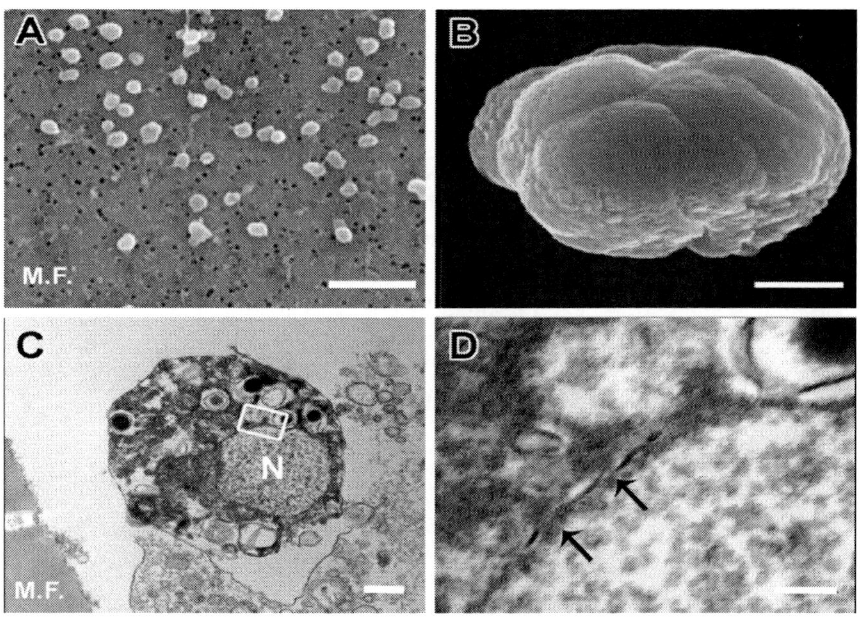


Figure 8. SEM and TEM images of BH-MCs (primo microcells) adhering to a 0.2-μm-pore-sized polycarbonate membrane filter (M.F.). (A) The SEM image shows that most of the primo micro-cells are round and about 1 μm in diameter. The scale bar is 5 um. (B) Higher magnification shows a bumpy surface structure. The scale bar is 200 nm. (C) The DNA-containing primo micro-cell was selected by staining and was observed by using TEM after ultrathin sectioning. Its largest part was assumed to be the micronucleus "N" based on the fact that it was stained with acridine orange. Several 250-nm-sized granules and many smaller-sized granules are inside the membrane. All the granules are surrounded by a lipid membrane and contain electron dense contents. The scale bar is 500 nm. (D) In square part of (C), the border of the micronucleus "N" is magnified. The membrane has discontinuous parts (arrows) whose size is about 20 nm, the same as nuclear pores, but the membrane is not a double structure as is a nuclear membrane. The scale bar is 100 nm.

A similar process of microcell proliferation was reported by Bukiki et al. Some microcells in cancer tissues were metabolically active and intensely accumulated nucleoproteins into their nuclei and cytoplasm. The microcells grew rapidly and transformed into young undifferentiated cells. This implied that stem cells could arise from microcells. They called this cytological mechanism for the immortality of tumor cell populations sporosis [68]. Sanals may proliferate through sporosis, which will bring a revolutionary outcome in regenerative medicine and cancer biology.

### 3.4. Sanal and Stem Cell

Small cells with pluripotent characteristics in different adult tissues and organs of humans and animals have recently been gaining much attention [69]. Small stem cells have been found in the bone marrow, brain, umbilical cord blood, cartilage, ovarian surface epithelium, kidney, and liver [70-74]. However, most detailed studies were performed for a rare population of very small embryonic-like (VSEL) stem cells that were found by Ratajczak et al. in bone morrow, spinal cord blood, and other adult tissues [75, 76]. The size of VSEL stem cells is about 3.6 μm, and they express several markers for pluripotent stem cells (PSCs) that are characteristic of epiblast/germ line-derived stem cells. These cells may participate in cellular turnover and the rebuilding pool of tissue-specific stem cells, especially under urgent circumstances such as tissue injury [77].

A rare population of small stem-like cells in the primo nodes of adult rats was obtained, and these small cells express stem cell marker CD133 and pluripotent transcription factors such as Oct4 and Nanog. It was suggested that a rare population of small cells found in the PVS have broad tissue differentiation potential and that these cells are capable of differentiation into all specialized cells in the adult body [78]. These are consistent with the results of proteomic analysis [43] and immunohistochemical study [37].

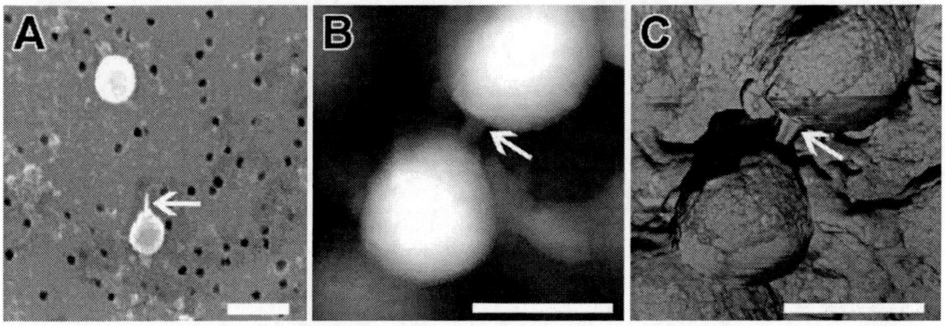


Figure 9. The unique threadlike structure of primo micro-cells dried at the critical points was observed in (A) a SEM image, (B) an AFM height image, and (C) an AFM phase image. The first step of budding, protrusion of a threadlike structure from a primo micro-cell, is shown by the arrows. The bi-thread shape can be seen in detail in the AFM phase image. The scale bars are 2 μm, 1 μm, and 1 μm, respectively.

Important questions about whether or not sanals are the same as, or related in some other ways to, VSEL stem cells remain to be resolved. BH Kim claimed that sanals had a sort of hematopoietic function and also regenerated damaged liver tissues [5, 6]. In other words, a sanal is a kind of embryonic-like stem cell.

# 4. Discussion

TCM has been used for thousands of years without anatomical knowledge. It remains a technical art without accumulating knowledge to understand its mechanism and to develop more systematic strategies for acupuncture treatment beyond old prescriptions. The language and concepts in TCM are not communicable with modern science or medicine at all.

With the discovery of the PVS, acupuncture will become a scientific subject and can take advantage of many modern scientific concepts, methods, and technology as Western medicine does. Imaging techniques can especially provide a means to visualize the primo vessels (acupuncture meridians) and primo nodes (acupuncture points) in the skin, and monitor their change in activities when stimulated in various ways with acupuncture needles, moxibustion, laser light, electricity, magnets, or others.

With monitoring techniques of the PVS in the skin, one can evaluate the personal fit of specific foods, drugs, cosmetics, clothes, and other accessories. Medicine and industrial goods for each individual can be evaluated and thus the era of personalized industry will come.

Visualization of the PVS in the skin would bring a revolution in diagnosis, as the PVS will reflect the health states of connected internal organs. It can replace traditional pulse diagnoses and can provide new techniques to see the state of internal organs from the skin. The primo path can also be used for drug delivery so that diagnosis and therapy can become closely related.

Primo microcells flowing in the PVS may revolutionize regenerative medicine because it is a kind of embryonic-like stem cell according to BH Kim. It is natural in the sense that it flows in the PVS normally. It can be used in fighting disease by taking samples of sanals and cultivating and re-injecting them into the patient. There will be no adverse immune problems. It is similar to using one's own umbilical cord blood.

Many incurable diseases like cancer and Alzheimer's diseases will get new light from the study of PVS, so that completely different diagnoses and therapy can be developed based upon the new knowledge. Other diseases like obesity, diabetes, and anemia will also be viewed with from a PVS perspective. In addition, many practices for health management like exercise, breathing, Qigong, and meditation will be affected by the advent of the PVS monitoring technique.

# Conclusion

In this review we presented the current state of the PVS research in connection with cancer and stem cell after a brief history and summary of Bong-Han theory. Bong-Han Kim's claims on the network of the third circulatory system corresponding to acupunctures meridians were confirmed in various pasts of animal body like blood or lymph vessels, on the surfaces of internal organs in the adipose tissues, heart, brain and spine.

New developments in the PVS-research occurred with the discovery of a Trypan blue technique that stained the PVS but not other tissues like blood vessel, nerve, or membranes. With this technique the PVS around tumor tissue were found which opened a host of topics about the role of PVS in the cancer biology. One role is already being investigated. The primo vessel is an additional metastatic path of cancer besides the blood or lymph path. A possible use of the primo vessel is a drug delivery path for the anti-cancer drug that can be administered through the skin at the acupuncture points.

Primo microcells or sanals flowing in the PVS are hypothesized to be fundamental embryonic-like stem cells. This was originally claimed by Bong-Han Kim and looked unbelievable at that time. However, recent discovery of very small embryonic-like(VSEL) stem cells by Ratjczak naised a high probability on the realizability of Kim's claim. It is worthy of serious in vestigation to compare sanals with VSEL stem cells.

## Acknowledgments

This research was supported in part by the grant from the Traditional Korean Medicine R&D Project, Ministry of Health and Welfare, Korea (B110076)

## References

[1] Heine H. Anatomical structure of acupoints. *J Tradit Chin Med* 1988;8(3):207-12.

[2] Langevin HM, Yandow JA. Relationship of acupuncture points and meridians to connective tissue planes. *Anat Rec Part B, New Anatomist* 2002;269:257-65.

[3] Kim BH. On the Kyungrak system. *J Acad Med Sci DPR Korea* 1963;90:1-41.

[4] Kim BH. The Kyungrak system. *J Jo Sun Med* 1965;108(6):1-38 [Korean].

[5] Kim BH. Sanal theory. *J Jo Sun Med* 1965;108(6):39-62 [Korean].

[6] Kim BH. Sanal and hematopoiesis. *J Jo Sun Med* 1965;108(12):1-6 [Korean].

[7] Fujiwara S, Yu SB. 'Bonghan theory' morphological studies. *Igaku no Ayumi* 1967;60:567-77.

[8] Fujiwara S, Yu SB: *A Follow-up Study on the Morphological Characteristics in Bong-Han Theory: An Interim Report, in The Primo Vascular System: Its Role in Cancer and Regeneration.* Eds. Soh KS, Kang K, and Harrison D. Springer, New York, pp. 19-22, 2010

[9] Jiang X, Kim HK, Shin HS, Lee BC, Choi C, Soh KS, Cheun BS, Baik KY, Soh KS. *Method for observing* intravascular Bonghan duct. *Korean J Orient Prevent Med Soc* 2002;6:162–6.

[10] Shin HS, Soh KS. Electrical method to detect a Bonghan duct inside blood vessels. *New Phys* 2002; 45:376-8.

[11] Lee BC, Baik KY, Cho S, Min C, Johng HM, Hahm J, Choi C, Yi SH, Soh KS, Park DH, Ahn SY, Cheun BS, Soh KS. Comparison of Intravascular Bonghan Ducts from Rats and Mice. *J Kor Orien Preven Med Soc* 2003;7:47-53.

[12] Lee BC, Baik KY, Johng HM, Nam TJ, Lee J, Sung B, Choi C, Park WH, Park ES, Park DH, Yoon YS, Soh KS. Acridine orange staining method to reveal the characteristic features of an intravascular threadlike structure. *Anat Rec B (New Anat)* 2004;278:27-30.

[13] Shin HS, Johng H, Lee BC, Cho S, Baik KY, Yoo JS, Soh KS. Feulgen reaction study of novel threadlike structures on the surface of rabbit livers. *Anat Rec B (New Anat)* 2005;284:35-40.

[14] Johng HM, Shin HS, Yoo JS, et al. Bonghan Ducts on the Surface of Rat Liver, *J. Int. Soc. Life Information Science,* 2004; 22(2): 469-72.

[15] Lee KJ, Kim S, Jung TE, et al. Unique Duct System and the Corpuscle-Like Structures Found on the Surface of the Liver, J. Int. Soc. Life Information Science, 2004; 22(2): 460-2.

[16] Lee BC, Yoo JS, Baik KY, Kim KW, Soh, KS. Novel Threadlike structures (Bonghan ducts) inside lymphatic vessels of rabbits visualized with a Janus Green B staining method. *Anat Rec B (New Anat)* 2005;286:1-7.

[17] Lee C, Seol SK, Lee BC, Hong YK, Je JH, Soh KS. Alcian blue staining method to visualize Bonghan threads inside large caliber lymphatic vessels and X-ray microtomography to reveal their microchannels. *Lymphat Res Biol* 2006;4:181-90.

[18] Johng HM, Yoo JS, Yoon TJ, Shin HS, Lee BC, Lee C, Lee JK, Soh KS. Use of magnetic nanoparticles to visualize threadlike structures inside lymphatic vessels of rats. *Evid Based Complement Alternat Med* 2007;4:77-82.

[19] Lee BC, Soh KS. Contrast-enhancing optical method to observe a Bonghan duct floating inside a lymph vessel of a rabbit. *Lympholgy* 2008;41:178-85.

[20] Lee BC, Kim KW, Soh KS. Visualizing the network of Bonghan ducts in the omentum and peritoneum by using Trypan blue. *J Acupunct Meridian Stud* 2009; 2:66-70.

[21] Yoo JS, Kim HB, Ogay V et al. Bonghan ducts as possible metastasis-paths of cancer. *J Acupunct Meridian Stud* 2009;2:118-23.

[22] Lee BC, Bae KH, Jhon GJ et al. Bonghan system as mesenchymal stem cell niches and pathways of macrophages in adipose tissues. *J Acupunct Meridian Stud* 2009;2:79-82.

[23] The Primo Vascular System*: Its Role in Cancer and Regeneration.* Eds. Soh KS, Kang K, and Harrison D. Springer, New York, 2010

[24] Lee BC, Kim HB, Sung B, Kim KW, Sohn J, Son B, Chang BJ, Soh KS Network of endocardial vessels, *Cardiology.* 2011;118(1):1-7.

[25] Choi IH, Chung HK, Hong YK, Detection of the Primo-Vessels in the Rodent ThoracicLymphatic Ducts, in *The Primo Vascular System: Its Role in Cancer and Regeneration.* Eds. Soh KS, Kang K, and Harrison D. Springer, New York, pp. 121-126, 2010.

[26] Yoo JS, Hossein Ayati M, Kim HB et al. Characterization of the Primo-Vascular System in the Abdominal Cavity of Lung Cancer Mouse Model and Its Differences from the Lymphatic System. *PLos One* 2010;5:e9940.

[27] Hossein Ayati MH, Yu-ying T, Tao H et al. Finding a Novel Threadlike Structure on the Intra-abdominal Organ Surface of Small Pigs by Using In-vivo Trypan Blue Staining, in *The Primo Vascular System: Its Role in Cancer and Regeneration.* Eds. Soh KS, Kang K, and Harrison D. Springer, New York, pp. 63-70, 2010.

[28] Jia Z, Soh KS, Zhou Q et al. Observation of the Primo Vascular System on the Fascia of Dogs, in *The Primo Vascular System: Its Role in Cancer and Regeneration.* Eds. Soh KS, Kang K, and Harrison D. Springer, New York, pp. 71-76, 2010.

[29] Lee BC, Kim SK, Soh KS. Novel anatomic structures in the brain and spinal cord of rabbit that may belong to the Bonghan system of potential acupuncture meridians. *J Acupunct Meridian Stud* 2008;1:29-35.

[30] Dai JX, Lee BC, Soh KS et al, In *vivo in situ staining of the primo vascular system in ventricles and subarachnoid space of brain by injecting Trypan blue into the lateral ventricle,* Neural Regeneration Research, 2011 (accepted).

[31] Jaekwan Lim, Jong Hyun Jung, Sungwoo Lee, Zhendong Su, Zhou Qiang. Estimating the density of fluorescent nanoparticles in the primo vessels in the fourth ventricle and the spinal cord of a rat. *J Biol Opti*, 2011 (in press).

[32] An P, Dai J, Su Z, Yoo JS, Qu R, Lee SW, Eom KH, Bae KH, Luo H, Soh KS. Putative primo-vascular system in mesentery of rats. *J Acupunct Meridian Stud.* 2010; 3(4):232-40.

[33] Lee SY, Lee BC, Soh KS et al. Development of the Putative Primo Vascular System before the Formation of Vitelline Vessels in Chick Embryos, in *The Primo Vascular System: Its Role in Cancer and Regeneration.* Eds. Soh KS, Kang K, and Harrison D. Springer, New York, pp. 77-82, 2010.

[34] Lee BC, Yoo JS, Ogay V, Kim KW, Dobberstein H, Soh KS, Chang BS. Electron microscopic study of novel threadlike structures on the surfaces of mammalian organs *Microsc Res Tech* 2007;70:34-43.

[35] Sung B, Kim MS, Lee BC, Yoo JS, Lee SH, Kim YJ, Kim KW, Soh KS. Measurement of flow speed in the channels of novel threadlike structures on the surfaces of mammalian organs. *Naturwissenschaften* 2008;95:117-24.

[36] Yoo JS, Kim MS, Sung B, Lee BC, Soh KS, Lee SH, Kim YJ, Dobberstein H. Cribriform Structure with Channels in the Acupuncture Meridian-like System on the Organ Surfaces of Rabbits. *Acup Electrother Res* 2007;32(1/2):130-2.

[37] Kim MS, Hong JY, Hong S, Lee BC, Nam CH, Woo HJ, Kang DI, Soh KS. Bong-Han corpuscles as possible stem cell niches on the organ-surfaces. *J Kor Pharmacopunct Inst* 2008;11(1):5-12.

[38] Han HJ, Sung B, Ogay V et al. The Flow Path of Alcian Blue From the Acupoint BL23 to the Surface of Abdominal Organs. *J Acupunct Meridian Stud* 2009;2:182-9.

[39] Han HJ, Ogay V, Park SJ et al. Primo vessels as new flow paths for intratesticular injected dye in rats. *J Acupunct Meridian Stud* 2010;3:81-8.

[40] Kim JD, Ogay V, Lee BC, Kim MS, Lim I, Woo HJ, Park HJ, Kehr J, Soh KS. Catecholamine producing novel endocrine organ: Bonghan system. *Med Acupunct* 2008;20:97-102.

[41] Yoo JS, Choi K, Baik KY et al. Liquid-phase microextraction method in capillary electrophoresis to detect adrenaline in Bonghan lipid *J Int Soc life inf Sci* 2005;23:292-5.

[42] Ogay V, Kim MS, Seok HJ, Choi CJ, Soh KS. Catecholamine-storing cells at acupuncture points of rabbits. *J Acup Mer Stud* 2008;1:83-90.

[43] Lee SJ, Lee BC, Nam CH, Lee WC, Jhang SU, Park HS, Soh KS. Proteomic analysis for tissues and liquid from Bonghan ducts on rabbit intestinal surfaces. *J Acup Mer Stud* 2008;1:97-109.

[44] Lee SW, Lim JK, Soh KS et al, *Primo Vascular System Accompanying a Blood Vessel from Tumor Tissue and a Method to Distinguish It from the Blood or the Lymph System*, 2011 (in preparation).

[45] Lee SW, Lim JK, Jung JH, Soh KS et al, *Flow characteristics of nanoparticles through blood, lymph, and primo vessels from tumor,* 2011 (in preparation).

[46] Yoo JS, Oyungerel B, Han TY et al, Molecular Compositional Differences of the Primo and the Lymphatic Vascular Systems in Murine Melanoma Models, in *The Primo Vascular System: Its Role in Cancer and Regeneration.* Eds. Soh KS, Kang K, and Harrison D. Springer, New York, pp. 185-92, 2010.

[47] Hong MY, Suh MA et al, The primo vascular system (PVS) of murine melanoma and the heterogeneity of tissue oxygenation of the melanoma *J Acup Mer Stud* 2011;4:in press.

[48] Hong MY, Suh MA et al, The study of primo-vascular system (PVS) by utilizing melanoma tumor model with green fluorescence protein (GFP) expressing mouse.J *J Acup Mer Stud* 2011;4: in press.

[49] Akers W, Liu Y, Achilefu S et al, Identification of Primo-Vascular System in Murine Tumors and Viscera, in *The Primo Vascular System: Its Role in Cancer and Regeneration.* Eds. Soh KS, Kang K, and Harrison D. Springer, New York, pp. 179-184, 2010.

[50] Bacac M, Stamenkovic I. Metastatic cancer cell. *Annu Rev Pathol* 2008;3:221–47.

[51] Chambers AF, Groom AC, MacDonald IC. Dissemination and growth of cancer cells in metastatic sites. *Nat Rev Cancer* 2002;2(8):563–72.

[52] Fidler IJ. Timeline—the pathogenesis of cancer metastasis: the 'seed and soil' hypothesis revisited. *Nat Rev Cancer* 2003;3(6):453–8.

[53] Hess AR, Margaryan NV, Seftor EA, Hendrix MJC. Deciphering the signaling events that promote melanoma tumor cell vasculogenic mimicry and their link to embryonic vasculogenesis: role of the Eph receptors. *Dev Dyn* 2007;236(12):3283–96.

[54] Maniotis AJ, Folberg R, Hess A et al. Vascular channel formation by human melanoma cells *in vivo* and *in vitro*: vasculogenic mimicry. *Am J Pathol* 1999;155(3):739–52.

[55] Hendrix MJC, Seftor EA, Hess AR, Seftor REB. Vasculogenic mimicry and tumour-cell plasticity: lessons from melanoma. *Nat Rev Cancer* 2003;3(6):411–21.

[56] Yoo JS, Kim HB, Won N et al. Evidence for an Additional Metastatic Route: In vivo Imaging of Cancer Cells in the Primo-vascular System around Tumors and Organs. *Mol Imag Biol* 2010; DOI: 10.1007/s11307-010-0366-1

[57] Han HJ, Soh KS et al, *Cancer migration through primo vessels,* 2011 (in preparation)

[58] Chen EI, Hewel J, Krueger JS, Tiraby C, Weber MR, Kralli A, et al. Adaptation of energy metabolism in breast cancer brain metastases. *Cancer Res* 2007;67:1472−86.

[59] Lian Z, Kluger Y, Greenbaum DS, Tuck D, Gerstein M, Berliner N, et al. Genomic and proteomic analysis of the myeloid differentiation program: global analysis of gene expression during induced differentiation in the MPRO cell line. *Blood* 2002;100:3209−20.

[60] Forte G, Minieri M, Cossa P, Antenucci D, Sala M, Gnocchi V, et al. Hepatocyte growth factor effects on mesenchymal stem cells: proliferation, migration, and differentiation. *Stem Cells* 2006;24:23−33.

[61] Wuchter P, Boda-Heggemann J, Straub BK, Grund C, Kuhn C, Krause U, et al. Processus and recessus adhaerentes: giant adherens cell junction systems connect and attract human mesenchymal stem cells. *Cell Tissue Res* 2007;328:499−514.

[62] Ogay V, Baik KY, Lee BC, Soh KS. Characterization of DNA-containing granules flowing through the meridian-like system on the internal organs of rabbits. *Acup Electrother Res* 2006;31(1-2):13-31.

[63] Kwon JH, Baik KY, Lee BC, Soh KS, Lee NJ, Kang CJ. Scanning probe microscopy study of microcells from the organ surface Bonghan corpuscle. *App Phys Lett* 2007;90:173903,1-3.

[64] Baik KY, Ogay V, Jeoung SC, Soh KS. Hypothesis on the origin of adult stem cells and Bonghan microcells observed with an electron microscope and an atomic force microscope. *J Acup Mer Stud* 2009;2: in press.
[65] Sung B, Kim MS, Corrigan A, Donald A, Soh KS. In situ microextraction method to determine the viscosity of biofluid in threadlike structures on the surfaces of mammalian organs. *Phys Rev E* 2009;79:022901,1-3.
[66] Sung B, Ogay V, Yoo JS, Yu HR, Lee BC, Chung C, Jung G, Soh KS, UV-A-induced activation of Bonghan granules in motion. *J Int Soc Life Inf Sci* 2005;23(2):297-301.
[67] J. Jagger, *Bacteriol. Rev.* 1958;22: 99-142.
[68] Buikis I, Harju L, Freivalds T. Origin of microcells in the human sarcoma cell line HT-1080. *Anal Cell Pathol* 1999;18(2):73-85.
[69] Zuba-Surma EK, Kucia M, Ratajczak J et al. "Small stem cells" in adult tissues: very small embryonic stem cells stand up!, *Cytometry Part A* 2009;75A:4-13.
[70] Vacanti MP, Roy A, Cortiea J et al. Identification and initial characterization of spore-like cells in adult mammals. *J Cell Biochem* 2001;80(3):455-60.
[71] Chen MH, Lin S, Hsieh CH et al. Identification and initial characterization of small cells in adult cartilage and bone marrow. *J Formos Med Assoc* 2004;103(4):264-73.
[72] McGuckin C, Jurga M, Ali H et al. Culture of embryonic-like stem cells from human umbilical cord blood and onward differentiation to neural cells in vitro. *Nat Protoc* 2008;3(6):1046-55.
[73] Virant-Klun I, Zech N, Rozman P et al. Putative stem cells with embryonic character isolated from ovarian surface epithelium of women with no naturally present follicules and oocytes. *Differentiation* 2008;76:843-56.
[74] Kucia M, Reca R, Campbell FR et al. A population of very small embryonic-like (VSEL) CXCR4(+)SSEA-1(+)Oct-4+stem cells identified in adult bone marrow. *Leukemia* 2006;20(5):857–69.
[75] Ratajczak MZ, Kucia M, Ratajczak J et al. A multi-instrumental approach to identify and purify very small embryonic like stem cells (VSELs) from adult tissues. *Micron* 2009;40:386-93.
[76] Ratajczak MZ, Zuba-Surma EK, Machalinski B et al. Very small embryonic-like (VSEL) stem cells: purification from adult organs, characterization, and biological significance. *Stem Cell Rev* 2008;4:89-99.
[77] Ratajczak MZ, Machalinski B, Wojakovski W et al. A hypothesis for an embryonic origin of pluripotent Oct4+ stem cells in adult bone marrow and other tissues. *Leukemia* 2007;21:860-7.
[78] Vyacheslav Ogay, Kwang-Sup Soh. Identification and characterization of small stem-like cells in the primo vascular system of adult animals, in *The Primo Vascular System: Its Role in Cancer and Regeneration.* Eds. Soh KS, Kang K, and Harrison D. Springer, New York, pp. 149-156, 2010.

In: Traditional Medicine: New Research
Editor: Yoshiharu Motoo

ISBN: 978-1-62257-448-3


*Chapter 15*

# A Sustainable Approach to Traditional Medicine for a Future beyond the Conflict with Nature Conservation

***Ryunosuke Kikuchi****

Faculty of Science and Technology, Ryukoku University,
Yokotani, Oe-cho, Seta, Otsu, Japan
Centro de Estudos de Recursos Naturais, Ambiente e Sociedade (CERNAS) – Instituto Politécnico de Coimbra, Bencanta, Coimbra, Portugal

## Abstract

About 80% of the developing world's rural population depends on traditional medicines for its primary healthcare needs; moreover, since application of medicines has been scaled up from a regional to a global level, concerns over the quality and standardization of traditional medicines have also been on the rise; however, international standardization of production methods and applications of such medicines has yet to catch up. Case studies show the severe conflict between traditional medicine and nature conservation: (i) in a survey area of South Africa, the forest biome is the vegetation type found to be most threatened by over-harvesting and 97% of the species are harvested unsustainably; (ii) the tiger is currently classified as endangered in the Red List, but many different parts of the tiger have been used to produce remedies for a wide range of complaints in traditional medicine – its population has decreased by about 95 percent since 1900; and (iii) among several threats facing Asiatic black bears, the major threat is the commercial trade in bear parts such as bile and gall bladders. Up to 13,000 adult bears are kept in cages little bigger than their own bodies and captive bears are suffering extreme pain due to daily bile extractions in such confinement.

Therefore, the current mode of traditional medicine is not ecologically sustainable. As traditional medicine relies on the benefits of nature, it is fundamental to preserve the health of Earth's ecosystem and harmonize with nature. It is considered that current traditional medicine may need to be fused with the concept of ecological medicine. This is a new field of inquiry and action to reconcile the care and health of ecosystems, populations, communities, and individuals.

# 1. Introduction

About 80% of the developing world's rural population depends on traditional medicines for its primary healthcare needs [1]. Traditional medicine encompasses a large number of practices, approaches, knowledge and beliefs that include remedies drawn from raw materials, in addition to spiritual, manual or psychological techniques such as massage, meditation and acupuncture. Traditional medical knowledge and practice are intrinsically linked in most societies to other domains and traditions, and such knowledge is transmitted through the oral network in many communities in the world [2].

In the past few decades, there has been a new interest in the use of traditional treatments for a wide range of diseases that affect urban populations (review in ref. [3]): according to a review by Rath [4], (a) China is the world's top exporter of medicinal herbs, with the amount reaching about US$200 million per year; (b) the global market for herbal medicines/products is estimated at US$62 billion annually, and (c) this market will hit US$5 trillion by 2050. Since application of traditional medicines has been scaled up from a regional to a global level, concerns over the quality and standardization of traditional medicines have also been on the rise; however, international standardization of how such medicines are produced and used has yet to catch up (review in ref. [3]).

The contradiction between nature conservation and people's enjoyment of the benefits of the very same nature sometimes leads to conflicts (i.e. ref. [5]). If a specific nature area is vulnerable, having people entering that area will lead to (partial) destruction of that area. This is something both nature conservators and nature enthusiasts do not want. Sometimes this conflict is resolved and leads to something where both nature and people enjoying the same nature benefit. Man himself is a sort of ecosystem: each human being is physiologically and physically (as a habit) connected with an immense number of species of living nature [5]. Traditional medicine is an approach to healthcare where patients are treated using natural plant, mineral and animal-based ingredients (figure 1). Most traditional medicines are herbal and are derived from sustainable sources, but some are made from endangered animals and plants [6].

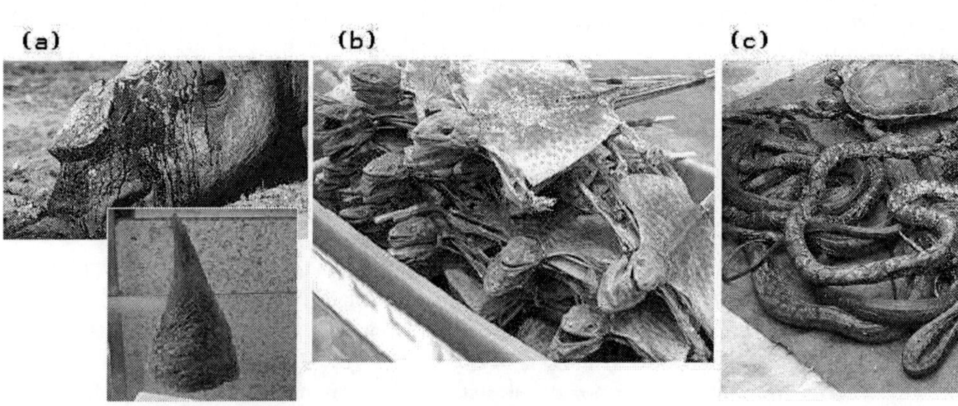


Figure 1. Animals used for traditional Asian medicine (courtesy Facts & Details Project): (a) a rhino is killed to take away its horn. In certain Asian countries, ground rhino horn is used to cure almost every disease (cf. ref. [6]); (b) Lizards are taken for high blood pressure and the skulls of gazelles are ground into powder to make people strong; and (c) turtle heads are consumed for labor pains, and snake oil is a traditional Chinese medicine used to treat joint pain [7].

The trade in these medicines not only threatens the survival of endangered species all over the world but is illegal under the Convention on International Trade in Endangered Species (CITES) [8]. Products that include ingredients from these species can be found in markets across the world. Among the animals used in traditional medicine are tigers, leopards, sharks, elephants, rhinoceros, pangolins, tortoises, seahorses, musk deer, as well as 7 of the 8 species of bear [7 & 8].

The Asiatic Black Bear (more commonly known as the Moon Bear) are kept in captivity on bear bile farms to enable the regular extraction of their bile acid [9-11]. Tiger bones, skin, fat, whiskers, tail, penises and gall bladders among other parts are believed to cure ailments, keep black magic at bay and possess aphrodisiac properties [7]. It is estimated that there are approximately 5,000 wild tigers. About 75 percent are in India while less than 50 are believed to be found in China's forests. The United States is home to some 10,000 captive tigers, owned by zoos, sanctuaries and private individuals (review in ref. [8]).

The purpose of this chapter is not to criticize traditional medicine but to describe essential information and discuss the harmonization of traditional medicine with nature in order to make present traditional medicine ecologically sustainable.

## 2. Necessity of Ecological Sustainability

As mentioned in section 1, application of traditional medicines has been scaled up from a regional to a global level, and concerns over the quality and standardization of traditional medicines have also been on the rise. Since already endangered species are being sacrificed for this incremental demand [6], it can be concluded that the current mode of traditional medicine is unsustainable.

The concept of sustainability has been recognized since the 1992 Earth Summit attended by 152 world leaders and ~1,400 non-governmental organizations in Rio de Janeiro (review in ref. [12]), and it has been strengthened worldwide by the 2002 World Summit in Johannesburg. As the concept of sustainability warns that human health care continues to consume more of Earth's natural resources [13], sustainable medicine is today the emerging concern in both modern pharmacy and traditional pharmacy. An approach to sustainable medicine advises us to take all participants in the product lifecycle into consideration – manufacturers, retailers, consumers and disposers – and share the responsibility for reducing negative impacts of pharmaceuticals [13].

The above-mentioned standardization is closely related to the concept of sustainable medicine. Constructive approaches to improving traditional therapies are to be welcomed. However, various country-based factors may inevitably be a great obstacle in bridging the gap between the Eastern and Western concepts of medicine. The criteria of ecosystem health (e.g. life quality of wild animals and plants) vary among countries because there are different cultures, histories, religions, policies, etc. in different countries.

To overcome this problem, it is essential to conceive international standards that will establish minimum agreed practices for traditional medicine, and urgent attempts should be made to define what is considered an acceptable mode of traditional medicine from the product lifecycle and ecological viewpoints.

# 3. Case Studies

Two reports from TRAFFIC, the world's largest wildlife trade monitoring network, on traditional medicine systems in Asia suggest that illegal wildlife trade, including entire tiger skeletons, and unsustainable harvesting is depleting the region's rich and varied biodiversity and putting the primary healthcare resource of millions at risk [14 & 15].

Relaxation of international trade barriers, the impact of free market economies and complex national government policies have led to an increase in the demand and supply for flora and fauna used in traditional medicine [14 & 15]. The growing illegal wildlife trade in the region is fuelled by the difficulty of sourcing prescribed ingredients, including parts, from globally threatened species. The supply of many wild animals and plants for medicine in these regions is becoming scarce due to overexploitation.

Case studies are given to help the reader to follow the unsustainable mode of traditional medicine and its global trends.

## Medicinal Plants in South Africa

The trade in traditional medicines forms part of a multi-million rand 'hidden economy' in southern Africa [16 & 17] stimulated by high population growth, rapid urbanization, unemployment, and the high cultural value of traditional medicines.

Demand generates a species-specific trade network that can extend across national boundaries [16 & 17]. Consequently, the trade in traditional medicines is now greater than at any time in the past and is certainly the most complex resource management issue facing conservation agencies, healthcare professionals and resource users in South Africa today [16 & 17].

It is estimated that there are 27 million indigenous medicine consumers in South Africa with a large supporting industry [16]. The use and trade of plants for medicine is therefore no longer confined to traditional healers but has entered both the informal and formal entrepreneurial sectors of the South African economy, resulting in an increase in the number of herbal gatherers and traders [16].

Demand for plant-derived medicines has created a trade in indigenous plants in South Africa currently estimated to be worth approximately R270 million (equivalent to ≈ US$ 37 million) a year [18]. More than 700 plant species are known to be actively traded for medicinal purposes throughout the country and intensive harvesting of wild material is acknowledged as a serious threat to biodiversity in the region. Increasing harvesting pressures on traditional supply areas are linked to a growing shortage in supply of popular medicinal plant species [16].

The Eastern Cape Province (see figure 2a), home to 15.5% (6.3 million) of South Africa's total population (40.6 million), incorporates two of the former 'homelands' of the apartheid period, where many aspects of traditional culture are still part of everyday life. Of the Eastern Cape population, 86% is African, 37% is urbanized, 49% is unemployed — with 31% of those employed earning less than R500 (≈ US$68) a month, and 41% of the households live in traditional dwellings [19].

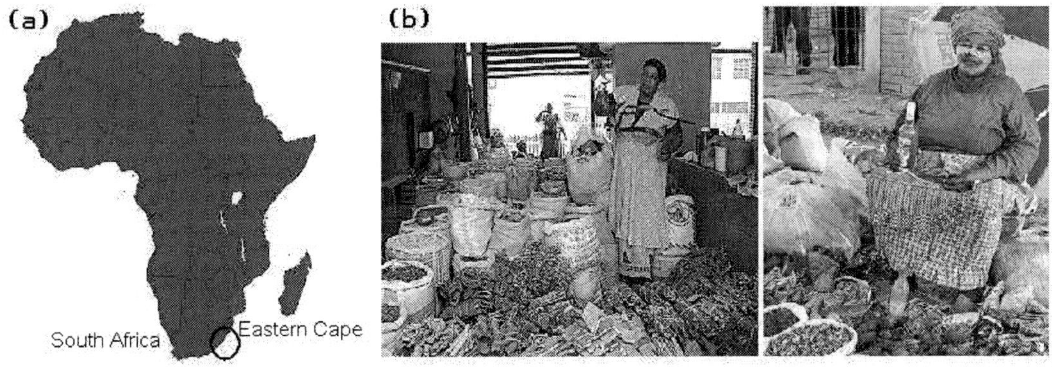


Figure 2. Medicinal plants in Africa (courtesy Africanalchemy): (a) localization of Eastern Cape; and (b) markets of traditional medicine in South Africa.

The people of the Eastern Cape tend to be more traditional and rural, but also significantly poorer and less developed, than those in other parts of South Africa [20]: a large proportion of the province's population is reliant to some extent on natural resources for direct subsistence use or, indirectly, for generating income [21]. A rapidly growing population coupled with increasing poverty and urbanization has a compound impact on the province's resource base.

Holdstock estimates that up to 80% of the African people in South Africa use traditional medicines [22], and Mander reports that there are more than 100 000 practicing traditional healers in the country, with a contingent industry worth about R500 million (≈ US$37 million) per annum [18]. The low socio-economic standing of the large, predominantly rural Eastern Cape population suggests that the great majority use traditional methods of health care. The shift to a cash economy and the emergence of commercial harvesters in what was largely a specialist activity restricted to traditional healers have resulted in medicinal plants becoming a common property resource with few incentives for resource management or traditional conservation practice.

Four key stakeholder groups are identified in the medicinal plant trade [23]: informal gatherer-hawkers (figure 2b), traditional healers, owners of *amayeza esiXhosa* stores (equivalent to the more widely known *muthi* stores found in KwaZulu-Natal), and consumers of traditional medicines.

Three species are treated in the current Red Data List of Southern African Plants [24]: *Bowiea volubilis* (insufficiently known), *Cassipourea flanaganii* (rare) and *Ocotea bullata* (vulnerable). The threat to *Cassipourea flanaganii* and *Ocotea bullata* due to medicinal plant harvesting has been documented in detail [25].

In addition to the above species, a further 31 species are highlighted for conservation and management attention based on the following criteria [25]: taxa that are harvested unsustainably and traded in large quantities of material are known to be rare or uncommon in the wild and/or are near-endemic, endemic or localized, and/or protected within the Eastern Cape Province. It can be concluded that the forest biome is the vegetation type found to be most threatened by over-harvesting; of the species documented, 93% are harvested unsustainably.

## Tiger Parts Used for Traditional Medicine in Asia

The tiger is the largest of the Asian big cats, and its population has decreased by about 95 percent since 1900. According to World Wildlife Fund [26], the greatest threats are loss of habitat due to human population expansion and activities such as logging; and trade in tiger bone for traditional medicines.

The International Union for Conservation of Nature (IUCN) is the world's main authority on the conservation status of species. The IUCN Red List of Threatened Species (also known as the IUCN Red List or Red Data List) is the world's most comprehensive inventory of the global conservation status of plant and animal species, and the tiger is currently classified as endangered in this list [27]. There are only around 4,000 tigers in the wild [26]. All commercial tiger trade has been banned since 1987 by an international treaty, but national trade is subject to each country's laws. China outlawed domestic tiger trade in 1993 (figure 3b), but entrepreneurs there have bred more than 5,000 tigers in captivity (figure 3a) – more than exist in the wild [26].

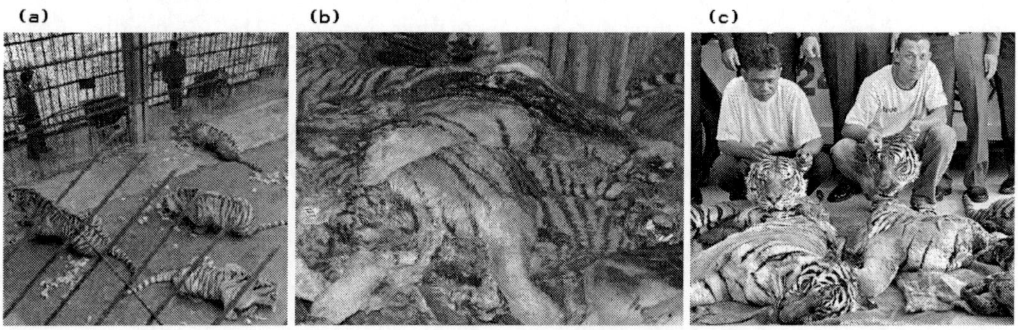


Figure 3. Illegal tiger trade in Asia (courtesy Gyandotcom and Tiger Voice): (a) tiger farming; (b) refrigerated tiger stockpile; and (c) confiscated bodies would have been used in traditional medicine.

The tiger, inspiration behind many folklore legends, has long been revered as "the king of the forest" (cf. ref. [15]). In traditional medicine, many different parts of the tiger have been used to produce remedies for a wide range of complaints (see ref. [15]). A number of tiger parts are used for their reported ability to treat arthritis. Tiger bones are boiled in water to produce a "bone gel" which is believed to enhance body strength and treat arthritis. Tiger paws are steeped in rice wine to produce a medicinal alcohol which will also treat arthritis and generally improve health (cf. ref .[15]). Tiger claws are worn as jewellery to help the wearer ward off the common cold, while it is said that the tiger's penis can improve a man's sexual prowess and treat impotence [28]. In addition to their medicinal qualities, tiger parts are also used for decoration: a tiger skin hung on a wall in a house can be used to express the power and prestige of the home owner (cf. ref. [15]). The believed "miracle" medicinal effects of tiger parts, and the prestige associated with purchasing tiger skins have meant that wealthy people are willing to buy tiger parts at very high prices. The trade in tiger parts generally occurs quite openly in Viet Nam (cf. ref. [15]). Purchasing genuine tiger parts is not difficult once a suitable price has been negotiated between trader and buyer (cf. ref. [15]). Based on published data [15], the prices of tiger parts are summarized in table 1; cf. 1 million Viet Nam Dong (VND) is equivalent to about US$63.

It is suggested that live tiger cubs, tiger skeletons, raw materials and processed medicinal products are mainly hunted in Cambodia, and then transported to Ho Chi Minh City to supply the southern medicinal trade market [15]. Some tigers may also enter the southern market from Malaysia. Lao People's Democratic Republic (PDR) is considered to be the main source of wild tiger products into northern Viet Nam [15]. It means that the tiger trade in the medicine market occurs on a large scale in South Asia.

**Table 1. Prices of tiger parts traded and used for traditional medicine in Viet Nam**

| Tiger parts | Price (VND) |
|---|---|
| Live cubs | 30-40 million |
| Skin (piece larger than 1.2m) | 20-30 million |
| Skin (piece smaller than 1.2m) | 15 million |
| Teeth | 1.6 million per tooth |
| Dried tendons | 700 thousand for one set of four leg tendons |
| Large claws | 1.5 million |
| Small claws | 700-800 thousand |
| Dried whole leg | 3 million |
| Complete skeleton | 200-300 million |
| Bone gel | 5-6 million per mg |

## Captive Bears Used in Bile Extraction

Consumption of animal bile to give strength to human beings is believed to have entered the Asian pharmacopeia 3000 years ago, and bear bile is still the most prized [29]: cf. the oversupply of bear bile is now used in products with no medical purpose such as shampoos, skin creams, and wine [30].

Japan is one of the biggest consumer countries of bear bile as well as gall: Japan has a long tradition of medicinal use of bear bile, and it is consumed both as a processed medicine and in unprocessed form [31] (see also figure 4). According to a questionnaire survey on the use of traditional medicine [32], more than 10% of Japanese people have purchased or acquired bear bile products. In 1994, 1997 and 1998, TRAFFIC East Asia-Japan studied the availability of bear bile and its derivatives in the Japanese market and found that about one-third of shops specializing in traditional medicine sold the products [33]; however, information on the origin of the material was very scarce.

Japan has virtually no regulation in the current Japanese legislation to restrict domestic trade in bear products [34]. As animal protection has historically not been a significant issue in Japan, legislation contains no definition of animal cruelty and has not often been invoked, so it is only natural that there is no government department that oversees animal issues in Japan (review in ref. [35]). Japan is a lucrative market for exotic pets, and it is possible to buy almost any animal such as ponies, pigs, civet cats, wallabies, eagles, owls, cockatoos, rare reptiles, monkeys and the like (review in ref. [35]). When these animals are no longer fun or become unmanageable, they are often dumped [36].

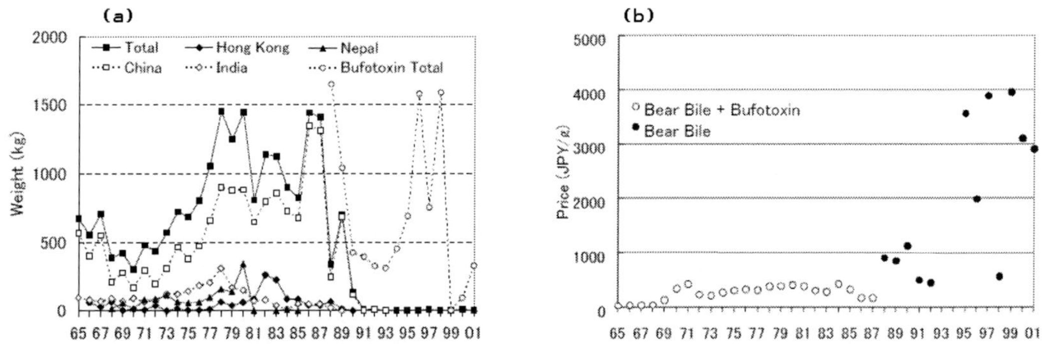


Figure 4. Bear bile imported by Japan (redrawn from ref. [37]): (a) amount trend, and (b) price trend.

### *The Number of Captive Bears*

The number of captive bears is roughly estimated at ~13,000 in Asia (review in ref. [38]): ~7,000 Asiatic black bears are legally kept on China's farms for bile extraction – cf. the number of illegal captive bears in China is unknown; ~2,000 Asiatic black bears are legally kept on Korea's farms for propagation; and ~4,000 bears (Asiatic black bears and Malayan sun bears) are illegally kept on Viet Nam's farms for bile extraction.

Thus, Asiatic black bear is the main species used in farming operations. According to a recent assessment [39], 75% of bear species are threatened with extinction. This assessment warns that Asia and South America are revealed as the areas most in need of urgent countermeasures. The world population of Asiatic black bears (*Ursus thibetanus*) has declined by 30-49% over the past 30 years, and this rate will continue over the next 30 years unless abated by the implementation of significant measures [38]. Sport hunting of Asiatic black bears is legal only in Japan (~500 bears per year) and Russia (~100 bears per year) [38]; however, among several threats facing Asiatic black bears (e.g., habitat loss, sport hunting, bear baiting, etc.), the major threat is the commercial trade in bear parts such as bile and gall bladders [39].

### *Bile Extraction from a Living Bear*

Once a bear reaches ~2.5 years old, it is used for bile extraction. Over a long period of captivity for bile extraction, the adult bears are kept in cages little bigger than their own bodies (see figure 5a), so they are often hurt from rubbing or hitting themselves against the iron bars of their tiny enclosures [40]. The bears are fed various mixtures such as rice, vegetables, cereals, and fishmeal twice a day. Instead of free access to water, most farms only hose the bears down once a day [40].

The bile extraction is generally carried out in a bear's permanent living cage that provides insufficient space for the bear's movements. The bears are fed twice a day to stimulate bile extraction. On most farms, the feeding tray is attached to the cage below the bear's chin because this forces bears to scrape the food into their cages while lying on their stomachs, which facilitates bile extraction (see figure 5b). Without anesthetics, bile extraction is surgically carried out by farm workers who have no veterinary experience in many cases [40]. The bears are kept in cages that are too small to allow their movements, and this immobility enables easy access to the bear's abdomen; thus, the painful extraction of bile is performed without difficulty. During the bile extraction, the bears twitch, gnash their teeth, bite the bars, and utter distress calls; they curl up after the extraction, shiver, and hold their paws to their stomachs. Bears can perceive terror and feel pain the same as we humankind do [39]. The above-mentioned behavioral signs therefore prove that bile extraction is an extremely painful procedure. As stated above, bears can perceive terror. This suggests that farm workers engaged in bile extraction need to approach the bears without fear of injury (i.e., the reduction of danger); hence, farm workers often subjugate and mutilate the bears by breaking their teeth (see figure 5c), pulling out claws, and sometimes removing whole digits.

When a bear can no longer produce sufficient bile, the bear is normally moved to another cage (i) to await death through major sickness such as cholecystitis, cholelithiasis, polyp formation, or liver cancer [41]; (ii) to be killed for its paws and gall bladder [40]: if customers of the bear farm so require, bear paws are cut off because the paws are eaten as a delicacy in Asia (China and South East Asia in particular) and the sale of bear parts provides an additional income for farms; or (iii) to be left to die of starvation.

Thus, it can be concluded that bile extraction from living bears is the worst scenario in terms of animal welfare.

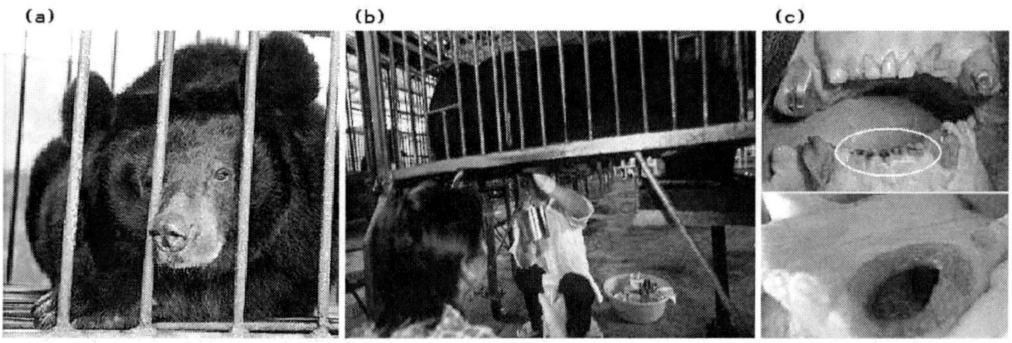


Figure 5. Asian bear farming for bile extraction (courtesy WSPA): (a) a captive bear for bile extraction spends most (~10 years) of its life in the cage; (b) farm workers extract bile from the gall bladder; and (c) broken teeth (upper picture) and open tooth roots (lower picture) can be constantly painful because the nerve inside the tooth may be damaged and exposed to the air, food and water.

# 4. Consideration

It is today important to maintain a proper balance between nature conservation and the security of Asian traditional medicine. However, there is doubt as to how to maintain this balance: changes in the production system of traditional medicine to improve ecosystem management often have an economic cost, which is ultimately met by consumers. An increase in medicine costs may be inconvenient because traditional remedies have been fostered by people who are unable to afford costly medicines or medical services [42].

## Medicinal Plants in Africa

The medicinal plant industry plays a critical role in empowering a large number of women, and lack of access to it would leave them and their families destitute. Present harvesting is indiscriminate, destructive, and unsustainable for many species, particularly those harvested from Afromontane Forest.

Of the traditional healers interviewed, 54% indicated an increase in the number of patients they had attended to over the last five years [43]; therefore, the current demand for medicinal plants is likely to increase and to have adverse consequences on the environment, particularly if wild plant material is not supplemented with cultivated material. To replace traditional medicines with modern Western medicines is neither practical nor appropriate [44]. It is significant for steps to be taken to accommodate the medicinal plant trade in South Africa. As formal and traditional conservation measures have been largely unsuccessful [43], cultivation initiatives and new management programs are essential regimes to conserve biodiversity and protect threatened species. The need for these regimes is acknowledged in developing countries throughout the world

## Careful Monitoring for Tiger Parts

Several Asian nations including China, Nepal, Japan, South Korea and Thailand have endorsed tough protections for tigers in the Convention on the International Trade in Endangered Species (CITES). Most traditional medicines are herbal and are derived from sustainable sources, but some are made from endangered animal and plant species. The trade in these medicines not only threatens the survival of endangered species all over the world, but is illegal under the CITES. The measures commit the countries to enact laws banning the trade of tiger derivatives, preserve tiger habitat, and form a regional network to halt tiger trade; however, lack of government resolve and corruption at the highest levels have thwarted enforcement of other wildlife agreements that the nations have signed [45] .

Most traditional medicine originally relied on herbs and other plants in Asia, but booming economies and growing wealth in the Asian region are increasing demand for the precious medicines made from animal parts [6]. Since already endangered species are being sacrificed for this incremental demand [6], it can be concluded that the current mode of traditional medicine is unsustainable. Trends in various traditional medicine systems should be monitored in an effort to understand the constantly changing use of wildlife species for medicinal purposes [46]. Such monitoring allows for more targeted and effective law enforcement and outreach efforts. These trends, as well as the conservation status of species used for medicinal purposes, will need to be carefully monitored in the future so that appropriate outreach efforts and legislative and enforcement actions can be undertaken.

## Alternatives to Bear Bile

The main effective component of bear bile consists of ursodeoxycholic acid (UDCA). Though other animals such as pigs and cows produce UDCA [47], bears are the only species to produce a significant amount of UDCA (review in ref. [48]); this is one reason that bears are used to extract bile. Nowadays, about 200 tons per year of UDCA is synthesized [47], and it has been widely used in the Western pharmacopeia (review in refs. [47 & 48]) . However, the synthesized product seems not to be in line with the philosophy of the traditional nature-based pharmacopeia that is an indispensable part of the cultural heritage in Asia.

Among the possible alternatives to bear bile, Coptis (*Huang lian* in Chinese) is a possible choice because both bear bile and Coptis can detoxify the body, purify the liver, and improve eyesight, as well as treat eclampsia, epilepsy, tics caused by heat, carbuncles, and pyocutaneous diseases: at present, prescriptions with Coptis (e.g., *Huang Lian Jie Du Tang, Qing Ying Tang, and An Gong Niu Huang Wan*) are widely used to treat symptoms such as coma, eclampsia, epilepsy, tics, and liver diseases [47]. Three types of Coptis are recognized for medical use: *Coptis chinensis Franch*, *Coptis deltoidea C.Y. Cheng et Hsiao*, and *Coptis teeta*; and all these types can be found in mainland China [49]. The cultivation of medicinal plant alternatives to bear bile makes it possible to (ii) phase out the practice of bear farming for the supply of bile and bear parts, and (ii) provide cruelty-free medicines to the market served by the traditional pharmacopeia.

## Conclusion

Case studies in section 3 show that the current mode of traditional medicine is not sustainable; and section 4 proposes some methodologies to ecologically reduce the conflict associated with nature conservation.

Traditional medicine relies on the benefits of nature, so it is fundamental to keep the health of Earth's ecosystem. It is considered that current traditional medicine may need to incorporate the concept of ecological medicine. This is a new field of inquiry and action to reconcile the care and health of ecosystems, populations, communities, and individuals [50]. Whether it is in the way we make and use medicines, conduct public health services, or choose the means of maintaining our own health, we must do so with a commitment to enhancing life on our planet. This ideal approach will make the current mode of traditional medicine more ecologically sustainable.

## Acknowledgments

Ryukoku University is founded on the spirit of caring for all living beings (i.e. equality of life). This university's "No Life No Animal" student group encouraged me to write the presented chapter. Parts of this work are supported by Centro de Estudos de Recursos Naturais, Ambiente e Sociedade (Coimbra). The author is grateful to Ms. C. Lentfer for English review.

## References

[1] Bannerman RH, Burton J, Chen WC. *Traditional medicine and health care coverage*. Geneva: World Health Organization; 1993.

[2] United Nations Educational, Scientific and Cultural Organization. *United Nations Year for Cultural Heritage, Traditional Medicine*. Paris: UNESCO Culture Sector; 2002.

[3] Shankar D, Venkatasubramanian P. *The evaluation of global standards for traditional medicine*. London: Science and Development Network; 2005.

[4] Rath B. *Globalisation, global trend in herbal market, and the impact thereof on medicinal plants in Orissa.* Orissa: VASUNDHARA; 2005.
[5] Yablokov AV, Ostroumov SA. *Conservation of living nature and resources – problems, trends and prospects.* Berlin: Springer-Verlag; 1991.
[6] Ellis R. *Tiger bone and rhino horn – the destruction of wildlife for traditional Chinese medicine.* Washington, DC: Island Press; 2005.
[7] Kunin RA. Snake oil. *Western Journal of Medicine.* 1989; 151(2): 208.
[8] International Animal Assistance Network. Animals Used in Traditional Medicine [online]. 2011. Available from: *www.internationalanimal net.org/?q=issues/medicine*
[9] Mills JA. Milking the bear trade. *International Wildlife.* 1992; 22: 38-45.
[10] Robinson J, Cocharane G, Loeffler K. Discussion regarding the impact of bear bile farming upon wild bears in China and Vietnam. In Williamson DF (ed.), *Proceedings of the 4th International Symposium on Trade in Bear Parts.* Tokyo: TRAFFIC East Asia-Japan; 2007; pp 67-73.
[11] Servheen C. 1993. The future of bears in the wild. pp. 212-221 In Stirling I (ed.), In Bears - Majestic Creatures of the Wild. Emmaus: Rodale press; 1993; pp 212-21.
[12] Nath B, Hens L, Devuyst D. *Textbook on Sustainable Development.* Brussels: VUB University Press; 1996.
[13] Teleosis Institute. *The green health care program – good for people and the environment.* Berkeley: Teleosis Institute; 2007.
[14] Ashwell D, Walston N. *An overview of the use and trade of plants and animals in traditional medicine systems in Cambodia.* Ha Noi: TRAFFIC Southeast Asia – Greater Mekong Program; 2008.
[15] Van NDN, Tap N. *An overview of the use of plants and animals in traditional medicine systems in Viet Nam.* Ha Noi: TRAFFIC Southeast Asia – Greater Mekong Program; 2008.
[16] Cocks ML, Dold AP. The role of African chemists in the health care system of the Eastern Cape Province of South Africa. *Social Science and Medicine.* 2000; 51: 1505-15.
[17] Cunningham AB. An Africa-wide overview of medicinal plant harvesting, conservation and health care. *Non-wood Forest Products.* 1997: 11: 116-29.
[18] Mander M. *Marketing of Indigenous Medicinal Plants in South Africa – a case study in KwaZulu-Natal. Rome*: Food and Agriculture Organization; 1998.
[19] South African Institute. *Fast Facts* 1. Johannesburg: South African Institute of Race Relations; 1999.
[20] Cocks, ML, Moller V. Use of indigenous and indigenized medicines to enhance personal well-being: a South African case study. *Social Science and Medicine. 2002:* 54; 387-97.
[21] Shackleton CM, Shackleton SE, Ntshudu M, Ntsebeza J. The role and value of savanna non-timber forest products to the rural households in the Kat River Valley, South Africa. *Tropical Animal Health and Production.* 2002: 8; 45-65.
[22] Holdstock, TL. *Economic aspects of indigenous healing.* Conference on the Economics of Health Care in Southern Africa. Cape Town: 1978.
[23] Cocks ML. *Towards an understanding of Amayeza esiXhosa (African chemists) stores – how they operate, and the services they offer in the Eastern Cape,* M.A. thesis, Grahamstown: Rhodes University; 1997.

[24] Hilton-Taylor C. *Red Data List of Southern African Plants.* Pretoria: National Botanical Institute; 1996.
[25] Cocks ML, Dold AP. The informal trade of *Cassipourea flanaganii* as a cosmetic in South Africa. In Stepp JR, Wyndham FS, Zarger RK (eds.), *Ethnobiology and Biocultural Diversity – proceedings of the 7th International Congress of Ethnobiology* Athens: International Society of Ethnobiology; 2002; pp 412-27.
[26] World Wildlife Fund. Tiger farms – a ticket to extinction [online]. 2001. Available from: *www.worldwildlife.org/what/globalmarkets/ wildlifetrade/tigerfarms.html*
[27] International Union for Conservation of Nature. IUCN Red List of Threatened Species [online]. 2006. Available from *www.iucnredlist.org*
[28] Loi, DT. *Vietnamese Medicinal Plants and Remedies/Substances* (12th edition), Ha Noi: Health Publishing House; 2004.
[29] Baron JH, Lim AG. Human bile for animals. *Lancet.* 1998: 531, 604.
[30] British Broadcasting Corporation. MEPs demand action on bear farms. London: *BBC News* (press release) on 10 January 2006.
[31] Ishihara A. *Bear gall trade in Japan.* Tokyo: TRAFFIC East Asia-Japan; 2005.
[32] Japan Wildlife Research Center. *FY1997 Survey report on the use of traditional medicine containing endangered species.* Tokyo: JWRC; 1998.
[33] Ishihara A. Bear gall bladder use and trade in Japan. In Japan Bear Network (ed.), *Understanding Asian bears to secure their future.* Tokyo: Japan Bear Network; 2006; pp 135-37.
[34] Togawa K, Sakamoto M. *Bear market in Japan.* Tokyo: Japan Wildlife Conservation Society; 2002.
[35] Mellor D, Yeow J, Hapidzal NFM, Yamamoto T, Yokoyama A, Nobuzane, Y. Childhood cruelty to animals – a tri-national study. *Child Psychiatry and Human Development.* 2009: 40; 527-41.
[36] Oliver E. Animal welfare in Japan. *Animal and People.* 2002: 11 (the November issue), 6.
[37] Ishii N. Management of bears and utilization of bear bile in Japan. In Williamson DF (ed.), *Proceedings of the 4th International Symposium on Trade in Bear Parts.* Tokyo: TRAFFIC East Asia-Japan; pp 27-36.
[38] Kikuchi R. Captive bears in human-animal welfare conflict – a case study of bile extraction on Asia's bear farms. *Journal of Agricultural and Environmental Ethics.* 2010: DOI 10.1007/s10806-010-9290-2.
[39] International Union for Conservation of Nature. *IUCN Red List of Threatened Species – Ursus thibetanus Asiatic Black Bear.* Gland: IUCN Bear Specialist Group; 2007.
[40] World Society for the Protection of Animals. *The bear bile business – supply and sources of bear products* (section #1). London: WSPA Office; 2005.
[41] Loeffler K, Robinson J, Cochrane G. *Compromised health and welfare of bears in China's bear bile farming industry, with special reference to the free-dripping bile extraction technique,* #Vet/Report/07. Hong Kong: Animals Asia Foundation; 2007.
[42] Griggs B. *Green pharmacy.* Rochester: Inner Traditions; 1999.
[43] Dold AP, Cocks MJ. The trade in medicinal plants in the Eastern Cape Province (South Africa). *South African Journal of Science.* 2002: 98; 589-97.
[44] Cunningham AB. Are we barking up the wrong tree? Medicinal plants and witch doctors. *African Wildlife.* 1984: 38; 247-249.

[45] Single Vision. *Trade in tiger parts*. Melrose: NPO Single Vision; 2010.

[46] Henry LA. *A Tale of Two Cities: A Comparative Study of Traditional Chinese Medicine Markets in San Francisco and New York City*. Washington DC: World Wildlife Fund; 2004.

[47] Nette T. Bear gallbladders to sell or not to sell. Nova Scotia Government [online]. 2009. Available from: *www.gov.ns.ca /natr/wildlife/large-mammals/beargalls.asp*

[48] Feng Y, Siul K, Wang N, Ng KM, Tsao SW, Nagamatsu T, Tong, Y. Bear bile Dilemma of traditional medicinal use and animal protection. J*ournal of Ethnobiology and Ethnomedicine*. 2009: DOI10.1186/1746-4269-5-2.

[49] State Pharmacopoeia Commission. *Pharmacopoeia of the People's Republic of China 2005* (English edition). Beijing: People's Medical Publishing; 2005.

[50] Raffensperger C. Editor's note – ecological medicine. *Networker.* 2002: 7; 4.

In: Traditional Medicine: New Research
Editor: Yoshiharu Motoo
ISBN: 978-1-62257-448-3


*Chapter 16*

# Have You Got Consent? An Overview of Human Research Ethics for East Asian Medicine

***Chris Zaslawski and Mary Garvey***
College of Traditional Chinese Medicine, University of Technology, Sydney, Australia

During the last four decades the requirement of a committee to oversee the ethical concerns of human research has become an integral part of the research process [1]. This review process is well established in many western countries such as the United States of America, United Kingdom, Europe and Australia and more recently in many Asian countries as well [2]. Indeed many countries have produced guidelines and developed national networks to deal with research governance and the oversight of human clinical research.

These committees are known as Institutional Review Boards (IRB) in the United States of America, or Research Ethics Committees (REC) as occurs in the United Kingdom. Their role is to ensure the protection of the welfare and rights of all participants in research [3], not only clinical research but also other types of research methodologies that involve humans such as surveys, interviews and focus groups. Generally there has been little interest in the ethical issues involved in conducting research into East Asian medicine (EAM) and in some respects this may have impeded the development of clinical evidence [4].

This chapter will discuss the principles of ethical research and how these can impact on the design and conduct of clinical EAM research. Arguments to address some common ethical concerns for EAM research will also be suggested and these will be helpful to those new to EAM research as well as those more experienced. Finally extracts from the latest version of the *Helsinki Declaration* (2008) [5] will be used to highlight some of the ethical requirements of human research and offer direction for some ethical challenges.

## History of Human Research Ethics

The beginnings of the consideration of ethics in human research can be traced back to the post World War II period, when claims of inhumane experimentation conducted on prisoners of war were contended. The Nuremberg military tribunal was charged with examining these claims and following their investigations ten principles for ethical medical research were established. The 'Nuremberg Code' was the first time that concepts such as individual autonomy and voluntary consent were articulated. This generated a great deal of discussion regarding ethical research issues, and led to the World Medical Assembly issuing the *Helsinki Declaration* in 1964. The *Helsinki Declaration* laid out the basic concepts and principles concerning ethical human medical research; it has undergone eight revisions since its first publication, the most recent in 2008 [5]. Of interest was the seventh revision (2000), which generated significant international discussion on whether the use of a placebo intervention was ethical when an established treatment was available as an active comparator.

Two other documents have also been important in establishing the principles of ethical human research: the *Belmont Report* issued in 1974 [6]; and the *Proposed International Guidelines for Biomedical Research Involving Human Subjects* in 1982 [7]. The latter was published by the World Health Organisation in collaboration with the Council for International Organisations of Medical Sciences. The *Proposed International Guidelines* outlined issues such as the assessment of risk, the requirements of scientific validity, and the justifiability of research design and informed consent. Several revisions were undertaken with the most current being published in 2002. While the United States of America had been pivotal in establishing the basic concepts of ethical human research, many nations undertaking EAM research currently have their own national guidelines for human research including Japan [8] South Korea [9] and China [10].

It is also interesting to note that while most of the ethical principles that have been developed were based on Western ethical values there has been acknowledgement of other culturally based ethics systems. Over the last decade several researchers and philosophers have been arguing for the need to incorporate Asian cultural and philosophical beliefs especially when using EAM in an Asian culture [11]. For example, in some cultures and communities, the intended research participants would regard the Western ethics-based notions as less important than their socio-cultural customs and obligations, while others would rather orally consent than sign their name on paper [12, 13]. Although a detailed examination of these issues is beyond the scope of this chapter, we will refer briefly to some of the concerns as they pertain to EAM and ethical research.

## Ethical Issues for Human Research

Today, any research that involves human beings, their tissue or personal details must consider the ethical implications of the project itself and the procedures and processes involved in conducting that research. Ethical issues arise in human research and clinical trials for many reasons: broadly speaking, all human research entails some level of risk of harm, either to the participants, the researchers, or both.

Research participants agree to enter into a research project for altruistic reasons, that is, for the common good. When they do they also enter into a relationship with the researchers who they may not know but need to trust. Government legislation and guidelines concerning ethical human research have been generated as an expression of this relationship and the responsibilities of researchers and institutions conducting human research. In this regard, legislation and guidelines are an expression of community standards as well as the ethos of ethical research.

Ethical human research guidelines address issues regarding the quality, safety and ethical acceptability of research involving humans. They specify researcher responsibilities concerning the design, implementation and reporting of their work, and institutional responsibilities concerning the review and monitoring of human research. The *Helsinki Declaration* (2008) for example sets out principles for the ethical design, review, conduct and publication of human research [5].

## Four Principles of Human Research Ethics

There are four principles that cover all forms of research involving humans, not only clinical trials. The four principles of ethical human research are research merit and integrity, justice, beneficence and respect [14]. Their purpose is to guide researchers to reflect on their research design and assist decision making. A mechanical application of the four principles is not required so much as is the researcher's deliberation of the values they encompass, the researcher's understanding of the research context, and their careful exercise of judgement. To the extent that researchers consider these principles they should be able to address most of the ethical issues associated with clinical research.

The principle of research 'merit and integrity' requires that the proposed research is a genuine search for knowledge, and that the researchers themselves have appropriate experience and expertise. Research 'integrity' furthermore touches on the problems concerning conflicts of interest. A researcher's judgements and interpretations may be affected by their collaborative associations, funding agreements or professional interests.

With regard to 'merit', the research issue, proposed design and possible outcomes must be justifiable by their potential benefits. Benefit may be, for example, a contribution to knowledge and understanding, or an improvement in patient care and well-being. One way to address the issue of research merit is to ensure that researchers have relevant qualifications and a record of peer reviewed publications in the field of inquiry relevant to their research.

The *Helsinki Declaration* (Clauses 12 and 16) is clear in enunciating these concerns.

> Medical research involving human subjects must conform to generally accepted scientific principles, be based on a thorough knowledge of the scientific literature, other relevant sources of information, and adequate laboratory and, as appropriate, animal experimentation. ...
>
> Medical research involving human subjects must be conducted only by individuals with the appropriate scientific training and qualifications. Research on patients or healthy volunteers requires the supervision of a competent and appropriately qualified physician or other health care professional [5].

The principle of 'justice' focuses on the welfare of research participants and on the public interest. In terms of human research, justice means that the researcher should not exploit vulnerable populations or perpetuate social inequality. This could include vulnerable populations such as people highly dependent on medical care who may be unable to give consent; people with cognitive impairment, intellectual disability or a mental illness; pregnant women as well as children and young people; and other persons in dependent or unequal relationships. Again the *Helsinki Declaration* is clear in enunciating this perspective.

> (Clauses 17 and 9) Medical research involving a disadvantaged or vulnerable population or community is only justified if the research is responsive to the health needs and priorities of this population or community and if there is a reasonable likelihood that this population or community stands to benefit from the results of the research. ...
>
> Some research populations are particularly vulnerable and need special protection. These include those who cannot give or refuse consent for themselves and those who may be vulnerable to coercion or undue influence [5].

Regarding the welfare of participants and the public interest, there are two aspects to research 'justice' — distributive and procedural justice. Distributive justice is the fair distribution of the benefits and burdens of the research. For example, some of the early HIV research studies that took place in Africa targeted local populations and then sold the pharmaceutical products that had been developed as an outcome of the research at a price that only developed nations could afford.

Procedural justice refers to the review of research in its development, implementation and concluding stages. Procedural justice also includes the fair treatment and recruitment of participants. For example, if English-speaking researchers exclude non-English speaking people from their study because of the cost or inconvenience of hiring a translator, the welfare of those populations and the public interest are not served, and the value of the research itself is compromised.

The principle of 'beneficence' asks that researchers assess the likely benefits of their study and to weigh them against any risks of harm or discomfort to their study participants. Benefits may be to the research participants themselves, and/or to the wider community. When considering risks and benefits, researchers must be sensitive to the welfare and interests of those involved, and they should reflect on the social and cultural implications of their research. In their account of the risks of harm and benefits researchers should place the welfare and interests of their participants and community before their research objectives. The need to evaluate the risks to the perceived benefits is reiterated in the *Helsinki Declaration*, Clauses 8 and 18.

> In medical practice and in medical research, most interventions involve risks and burdens. ...
>
> Every medical research study involving human subjects must be preceded by careful assessment of predictable risks and burdens to the individuals and communities involved in the research in comparison with foreseeable benefits to them and to other individuals or communities affected by the condition under investigation() [5].

The principle of beneficence requires as far as possible that human research minimises the risk of harm and maximises potential benefits. 'Risk' is the potential for harm, discomfort or inconvenience, and includes the possibility of damage or hurt to a person's well-being, interests or welfare. Hurt may be physical, psychological (feelings of embarrassment, stress or guilt for example), professional or social (the participant may experience anxiety over the possible or actual loss of career opportunity, or damage to professional or other relationships, or there may be legal risks). In some cases, research can involve power differences, as in for example the physician–patient relationship.

It is ethically acceptable for research to have risks for participants, with only benefit to wider community, so long as there is informed and truly voluntary consent. Processes to ensure that participants can voluntarily consent to their involvement and are fully informed about their role in the research are crucial for the principle of beneficence.

> *Helsinke Declaration*, Clause 24: In medical research involving competent human subjects, each potential subject must be adequately informed of the aims, methods, sources of funding, any possible conflicts of interest, institutional affiliations of the researcher, the anticipated benefits and potential risks of the study and the discomfort it may entail, and any other relevant aspects of the study [5].

Some research does deliberately withhold information from participants. Limited disclosure is an essential feature of the randomised controlled clinical trial for instance, which 'blinds' its participants and researchers to control for the placebo effect. The ethical use of limited disclosure simply requires that the researchers and participants are fully aware of the trial conditions and their role in the testing process. This is especially an issue for complex clinical interventions such as acupuncture and will be discussed later.

Finally, the principle of 'respect' acknowledges the autonomy and intrinsic value of human beings. In human research the recognition of their value is acknowledged by the researcher's consideration of the first three principles: research merit and integrity, justice and beneficence. Specifically, the principle of respect calls on researchers and research institutions to respect their participants' privacy and confidentiality. Clause 23 of the *Helsinki Declaration* highlights this issue.

> Every precaution must be taken to protect the privacy of research subjects and the confidentiality of their personal information and to minimize the impact of the study on their physical, mental and social integrity [5].

In addition, respect encourages researchers to empower people where possible, to protect those with diminished autonomy, and to respect cultural heritage and sensitivities, and the beliefs and customs of the persons involved and their communities. Informed consent is the chief mechanism by which individual autonomy is protected.

## Ethical Issues for EAM Research

The World Health Organization document, *Guidelines for Clinical Research on Acupuncture*, states that 'consideration should be given to the different value systems that are involved in human rights such as social, cultural and historical issues' [15]. Some of the issues for ethical EAM research arise because of differences in disciplinary methods, and cultural differences regarding contemporary notions of individual autonomy and informed consent [2]. From ancient times, Confucian and Daoist philosophies supported a conception of the individual as interdependent with others. Confucian values emphasised the active participation in the family and community and the quality of one's interactions with others. They were fundamentally concerned with the 'application of right action' by individuals who are 'mindful of their relational commitments' [16, 17]. To that extent, East Asian ethical values are not unlike the ethos behind contemporary guidelines promoting ethical human research. However, these same traditional values have meant that the private / public distinction that has historically been a feature of many Western cultures is largely absent in East Asian countries. For this reason, ethical review frameworks based on the Western principle of individual autonomy can be problematic for East Asian populations or contexts where the focus is likely to be more concerned with relationships and a person's responsibility to work for the good of others [18].

Today's international principles and guidelines on bioethics emphasise the scientific and bioethical value of the study. As well as abiding by scientific and bioethical standards, some observers argue that the ethics review of human clinical trial research should accord with EAM theories and philosophy. The principles of research integrity and merit and respect, for example, would support the argument that research design and methods should encompass EAM's theoretical and practice models. Moreover, researcher qualifications, experience and expertise would have to encompass an awareness of cultural values, as well as an appropriate level of clinical training and experience in EAM [18].

An important consideration for EAM clinical trial research is the skill and competence of the researchers administering the interventions. All clinical researchers should have experience in the field and in the treatment of the condition being studied. Unfortunately some acupuncture and herbal medicine studies, especially many early studies published in Western scientific journals, failed to use qualified, competent East Asian medical practitioners when designing their research and when administering treatment [19]. A research study using unqualified and inexperienced researchers contravenes the principle of research merit and integrity and compromises the research outcomes.

In EAM clinical trials, subjective assessments may be considered appropriate. As well as the measurement of objective medical variables (such as laboratory findings) indicators for efficacy could record pattern-based information and apply questionnaires to measure participants' subjective changes and experiences [18].

In countries such as Japan, China and Korea, acupuncture and herbal medicine are accepted as effective therapies. If the use of a placebo participant group is seen by potential participants as withholding a valuable treatment, they will be reluctant to enter a randomized trial for fear of not receiving their treatment choice. The large number of uncontrolled cohort studies and single case reports in the Chinese medical literature in translation is a reflection of this situation [19].

## Issues for Acupuncture Research

The issues for acupuncture clinical research design are well known. Acupuncture needling, as well as being difficult to mimic visually, also elicits distinct physical sensations.

The use of sham procedures such as the non-invasive retractable 'stage dagger' needle may make it increasing difficult to deceive experienced acupuncture participants over a period of time. Control interventions such as inactive transcutaneous electric nerve stimulator (TENS) or a placebo medication are likely to produce a different psychological response compared to acupuncture.

In addition, there are two major ethical issues for acupuncture clinical trials. The first concerns the need for limited disclosure when using a sham or placebo control. The second revolves around the use of a placebo control rather than an existing effective treatment as a comparator. Both are issues for informed consent, and raise the question of whether limited disclosure and partially informed consent can be ethical. However, if participants are alerted to the possibility of receiving a sham or a placebo treatment at the informed consent stage it becomes more difficult to reliably blind them to the control intervention.

General requirements for informed consent usually involve:

- voluntary participation that is based on sufficient information and understanding — this means that participants should be fully informed about all aspects of the research and be able to understand everything that the researcher imparts about the study;
- an outline of the purpose, methods, demands, risks, inconvenience, discomforts and possible outcomes of the research — participants need to be informed about the aims and goals of the research, what is required of them and how participation in the study may affect them, both physically and psychologically;
- voluntary participation that is not subject to coercion, or to inducement which can impair its voluntary character — no participant should be pressured or induced into being involved in the research;
- participation that is clearly established (this could be a signed form, the return of a survey or a recorded agreement) — there should be some form of evidence that the participant has been informed about the study and consents to their involvement;
- voluntary participation that allows for participants to revoke their consent and withdraw from the research at any time without having to provide an explanation and without attracting any negative consequences.

In many clinical trials informed consent is obtained by using a document that is signed by both the participant and the researcher. An interesting review by Linde and Dincer [20] assessed 47 sham controlled acupuncture trials. They reported that only ten studies included information on how participants were informed. They also found information strategies varied considerably and were often not fully explicit.

They cite several examples of information supplied in published trial reports where deception or limited disclosure occurred. For example, they identify a back pain study with eight sessions of acupuncture or mock TENS where the participants were informed that were "studying the long term effects of three different sensory stimulation methods that were thought would be equally effective..." [21]. Another study cited involving eight sessions of acupuncture that used a blunted cocktail stick in a guide tube for a tension headache trial. The researchers informed their participants that they would "have an equal chance of receiving either a standardised form of treatment which is known to work in a certain number of cases, or the test form of acupuncture which may or may not be more effective" [22].

More recently, Miller and Kaptchuk argued that "accurate disclosure, consistent with informed consent, should take precedent over deceptive disclosure for the sake of maximizing scientific validity, especially in the absence of rigorous data showing that accurate disclosure undermines satisfactory blinding of participants" [23]. If researchers want to use limited disclosure the argument for needs to be convincing and researchers need to consider the specific conditions of the trial to make a convincing ethical argument for limited disclosure when applying for ethical approval.

To address the first ethical concern, it is our contention that several arguments can be mounted to make a case for limited disclosure. These could include:

- informing participants explicitly (in the consent form) that they would not receive any information on the specific goals of the interventions;
- making sure the target illness does not demand urgent medical attention, thereby ensuring minimal risk to the participants;
- certifying the treatment is low risk again safeguarding risk to participants;
- confirming that all risks have been adequately assessed and can be satisfactorily managed;
- highlighting that the merit of the research does outweigh the risk to participants;
- determining that there is no known effective treatment available for the target illness; and,
- emphasizing that the internal validity of the study will be threatened because of failure to blind [24].

The second and associated ethical issue concerns the use of an inactive placebo as a control when an established treatment already exists. In other words is it ethical to use a placebo control and thereby withhold an existing proven treatment? Some opponents of the use of a placebo in a clinical trial argue that every participant in a clinical trial should be assured of the best possible proven treatment which would proscribe placebo use [25]. Others however would contend that the absence of a placebo control would compromise evidence, impede development and diminish therapeutic options [26]. In support of this perspective the authors of a systematic review of non-steroidal anti-inflammatory drug trials for arthritis treatment concluded, "if efficacy is the outcome of interest, placebo control trials may be the most appropriate study design because patients participating in placebo drug trials are more conservative in rating a drug as being effective" [27]. The *Helsinki Declaration* (Clause 32) clearly identifies the conditions where a placebo control can be ethically implemented. These are when no effective treatment exists, when there is minimal risk to the participants and for methodologically sound trial design reasons.

> The benefits, risks, burdens and effectiveness of a new intervention must be tested against those of the best current proven intervention, except in the following circumstances:
>
> - the use of placebo, or no treatment, is acceptable in studies where no current proven intervention exists; or
> - where for compelling and scientifically sound methodological reasons the use of placebo is necessary to determine the efficacy or safety of an intervention and the patients who

receive placebo or no treatment will not be subject to any risk of serious or irreversible harm. Extreme care must be taken to avoid abuse of this option [5].

## Issues for Herbal Medicine Research

One concern often voiced by ethics committees concerns the paucity of information presented on the pharmacological profile and toxicology, and reported adverse events concerning the herbal ingredients to be used in the trial [4, 28]. Unlike pharmaceutical substances that proceed through an in-vitro investigation, followed by animal studies, and then through staged phase one, two and three human studies, traditional herbal medicines rarely undergo any preclinical evaluation. While the argument can be made that many herbal substances have been used safely for centuries, evidence of their dose response relationship and safety data is often anecdotal. Research ethics committees require detailed and accurate evidence [29]. To assemble the information needed, the research team may have to consult a diverse range of sources. Fortunately there do exist online databases that have amassed technical and safety data on all aspects of EAM herbals including formulation, herbal composition, chemical composition, molecular structure and functional properties, therapeutic and toxicity effects, clinical indication and application, and related literatures. One such public database currently contains entries for 1197 formulae, 1098 medicinal herbs and 9852 herbal ingredients [30]. Assembling such data will assist the ethic committee in determining the risk/benefit comparison and demonstrate to the committee that the researchers have taken a responsible and scientifically rigorous approach to dealing with such risks. In addition maintaining good relations between the committee and the research team and providing additional information when requested is essential in fulfilling the ethical responsibilities from both the research team and the ethics committee's perspective [31]. Another related issue is the monitoring of adverse events during a trial. Even though this is mandatory for pharmaceutical trials, many herbal trials do not mention monitoring and commonly do not report any occurrence of an adverse event. This is despite the *Helsinki Declaration* (Clause 15) clearly identifying the need to do so.

> The researcher must provide monitoring information to the committee, especially information about any serious adverse events [5].

While traditional medicines are in widespread public use this does not mean they are completely safe to use and without side effects [32]. Side effects may be long or short term, they may involve hepatic and renal function as well as producing cardiovascular, digestive, dermatological and respiratory symptoms [28]. Care must be taken to ensure close monitoring of participants during a clinical trial and accurate and transparent reporting of events to the ethics committee when they do occur [33]. Another issue for EAM researchers to consider is the registration of clinical trials. Clinical trial registration ensures that all relevant information on the trial is publically available. The registration of pharmaceutical and medical research is routine, however this is not the case for many EAM trials.

The *Helsinki Declaration* (Clause 19) states that

> Every clinical trial must be registered in a publicly accessible database before recruitment of the first subject [5].

From an ethical perspective the registration of clinical trials ensures transparency and accountability. The registry often requires specific information on the trial objectives, design features, the sample size and recruitment status, what treatments are being investigated, what outcomes are being assessed as well identifying the principal investigator and contact details for further information on the trial. Several countries including China, Japan and South Korea have developed their own national registries which in turn conjoin the WHO International Clinical Trials Registry Platform [34]. EAM researchers should comply with this requirement as many medical journals now require clinical trial publications to report trial registration and if this has not done the editor can reject the manuscript based on this requirement alone.

The publication of results raises another related ethical concern that affects pharmaceutical, medical and EAM research. Researchers should publish not only positive clinical trials but also trials that have a negative or mixed outcome. Again the *Helsinki Declaration* (Clause 30) is clear in directing researchers:

> Authors, editors and publishers all have ethical obligations with regard to the publication of the results of research. Authors have a duty to make publicly available the results of their research on human subjects and are accountable for the completeness and accuracy of their reports. They should adhere to accepted guidelines for ethical reporting. Negative and inconclusive as well as positive results should be published or otherwise made publicly available. Sources of funding, institutional affiliations and conflicts of interest should be declared in the publication. Reports of research not in accordance with the principles of this Declaration should not be accepted for publication [5].

Only by reporting comprehensive and detailed clinical trials can the validity and merit of the research be assessed and EAM researchers should endeavour to use the accepted reporting guidelines at all times. In addition to the CONSORT statement used for randomised clinical trials there are several specific guidelines for reporting EAM, acupuncture and herbal medicine research. The revised STRICTA guidelines were recently published for acupuncture research [35] while several groups have published guidelines for herbal medicine [36, 37, 38].

Finally, EAM's unique diagnostic characteristics entail certain procedural issues, and these can impact upon the ethics review of the research design and methods, and the relevance and validity of the research outcomes. Procedural issues arise for example, because of EAM's widely adopted methods of 'treatment according to pattern differentiation' and 'multi-component mixtures', and also because modern extraction technologies are different from the traditional decoction methods [11]. Considerable effort needs to be made by the research team in developing rational EAM protocols and standard operating procedures, and in developing effective communication between EAM researchers and their research ethics committees. Effective communication may involve, for example, providing background information to assist understanding of EAM research [31], and answering questions and reservations from the ethics committee in a responsive and open manner.

# The Way Forward

This chapter has considered some of the ethical issues associated with EAM research and the potential impacts on research design and conduct. It has discussed reasons why it is important for researchers to reflect on the principles of ethical research. Human research ethics committees are composed of a range of individuals who evaluate research from a very individual and personal perspective. Researchers must be able to communicate and respond to their research ethics committees in a reasoned and objective manner by referring to ethical principles. By working with the principles outlined above, researchers can pre-empt ethical issues and address any potential risks of harm in the design of their research.

Only by understanding the principles of ethical human research can researchers engage in meaningful dialogue with their study populations, participants and research partners, incorporate the management and resolution of potential risks, and develop ethically responsible research with clear benefits to patients and healthcare. Many Asian countries are now undertaking EAM research and it is hoped that the ethical concerns of human research will be an important consideration when designing and conducting research [39, 40].

# References


[1] Zaslawski C. The impact of ethics on the design and conduct of acupuncture clinical trials. *Clin Acu Orient Med.* 2003;4:121-126.

[2] Tsai DF-C. The bioethical principles and Confucian moral philosophy. *J Med Ethics.* 2005;31:159-163.

[3] Califf RM, Morse MA, Wittes J, Goodman SN, Nelson DK, DeMets DL, et al. Toward protecting the safety. *Control Clin Trials.* 2003;24:256-271.

[4] Tilbert JC, Kaptchuk TJ. Herbal medicine research and global health: an ethical analysis. *B World Health Organ.* 2008;86:594-599.

[5] World Medical Association *Declaration of Helsinki (2008)* Available from: http://www.wma.net/en/30publications/10policies/b3/

[6] National Institutes of Health. *The Belmont Report: Ethical Principles and Guidelines for the protection of human subjects of research.* Available from *http://ohsr.od.nih.gov/guidelines*

[7] Council for International Organizations of Medical Sciences(CIOMS) *International Ethical Guidelines for Biomedical Research Involving Human Subjects* Available from *http://www.cioms.ch/publications/guidelines/guidelines_nov_2002_blubhtm*

[8] Slingsby BT, Nagao N, Akabayashi A. Administrative legislation in Japan: guidelines on scientific and ethical standards. *Camb Q Healthc* Ethics. 2004;13:245-53.

[9] International Compilation of Human Research Protections Available from: *http://www.brynmawr.edu/grants.*

[10] Li EC, Du P, Ji KZ, Wang ZG. Chinese Ethics Review System and Chinese Medicine Ethical Review: Past, Present, and Future, *Chin J Int Med.* 2011;17:867-872.

[11] Tai MC-T, Lin CS. Developing a culturally relevant bioethics for Asian people. *J Med Ethics.* 27;51-54.

[12] Li B-F. Informed Consent in Research Involving Human Subjects. *J Clin Ethics.* 2004;15:35-37.

[13] Yuan L. Clinical Trials in China: Protection of Subjects' Rights and Interests. *J Clin Ethics.* 2004;15:30-34.

[14] Macklin R. Applying the four principles. *J Med Ethics*. 2003;29:275-280.

[15] World Health Organization. *Guidelines for Clinical Research on Acupuncture.* WHO Regional Publications: Western Pacific Series, 1995.

[16] Hall DL, Ames RT. *Thinking From The Han: Self, Truth, and Transcendence in Chinese and Western Culture*. Albany: State University of New York Press, 1998.

[17] Lai K. *Learning from Chinese Philosophies: Ethics of Interdependent and Contextualised Self.* Hampshire UK: Ashgate Publishing Limited, 2006.

[18] Wang RT, Henderson GE. Medical Research Ethics in China. *The Lancet*. 2008;372:1867-8.

[19] Zaslawski C. Ethical Considerations for Acupuncture and Chinese Herbal Medicine Clinical Trials. *Evid Based Complement Alternat Med.* 2010;7:295-301.

[20] Linde K, Dincer F. How Informed Is Consent in Sham-Controlled Trials of Acupuncture? *J Altern Complement Med.* 2004;102: 379-385.

[21] Carlsson CPO and Sjolund BH. Acupuncture for Chronic Low Back Pain: A Randomised Placebo-Controlled Study with Long-Term Follow-Up. *Clin J Pain* 2001; 17: 296-305.

[22] White AR, Eddleston C, Hardie R, Resch KL, Ernst E. A Pilot Study of Acupuncture for Tension Headache, Using a Novel Placebo. *Acupunct Med.* 1996; 4: 11-15.

[23] Miller FG, Kaptchuk TJ. Acupuncture trials and informed consent. *J Med Ethics.* 2007;33:43-44.

[24] Spigt MG, Knipschild PG, van Schayck CP, Knottnerus JA. The validity and ethics of giving placebo in a randomised nopharamacological trial was evaluated. *J Clin Epidemiol.* 2005;58:350-356.

[25] Rothman KJ, Michels KB. The continuing unethical use of placebo controls. *New Engl J Med.* 1994;331:394-398.

[26] Kleijnen J. The Use and Abuse of Placebo in Clinical Trials. *Forsch Komplementmed.* 1998;5:125-127.

[27] Rochon PA, Binns MA, Litner JA, et al. Are Randomised Control Trial Outcomes Influenced by the Inclusion of a Placebo Group? A Systematic Review of Nonsteroidal Antiinflammatory Drug Trials for Arthritis Treatment. *J Clin Epidemiol.* 1999;52:113-122.

[28] Wang XY, Liang ZH, Huang HL, Liang WX. Principles of Ethics Review on Traditional Medicine and the Practice of Institute Review Board in China. *Chin J Int Med.* 2011;17:631-634.

[29] Smith CA, Priest R, Carmady B, Bourchier S and Bensoussan A. The Ethics of Traditional Chinese medicine and Western herbal medicine Research: Views of Researchers and Human Ethics Committees in Australia. *Evid Based Complement Alternat Med.* 2011;2011:256915. Epub 2010 Dec 13

[30] Wang JF, Zhou H, Han LY, Cao ZW, Chen X, Chen YZ. TCM-ID: Traditional Chinese Medicine information database. *Clin. Pharmacol. Ther.2005;*78:92-93.

[31] Zaslawski C, Davis S. The ethics *Monash Bioeth Rev*. 2005;24:52-60.

[32] Pittler MH, Ernst E. Systematic review: hepatotoxic events associated with herbal medicinal products. *Aliment Pharmacol Ther.* 2003;18:451-71.

[33] Wu T, Shang H, Bian Z, Zhang J, Li T, Li Y, et al. Recommendations for reporting adverse drug reactions *J Evid Based Med.* 2010;3:11-7.

[34] *World Health Organisation-International Clinical Trials Registry Platform (ICTRP)* Available from *www.who.int/ictrp/*

[35] MacPherson H, Altman DG, Hammerschlag R, Youping L, Taixiang W, White A, et al; STRICTA Revision Group. Revised STandards for Reporting Interventions in Clinical Trials of Acupuncture (STRICTA): Extending the CONSORT statement. *J Evid Based Med.* 2010;3:140-55.

[36] Bian Z, Liu B, Moher D, Wu T, Li Y, Shang H, et al. Consolidated standards of reporting trials (CONSORT) for traditional Chinese medicine *Front Med.* 2011;5:171-7.

[37] Gagnier JJ, Boon H, Rochon P, Moher D, Barnes J, Bombardier C; CONSORT Group. Recommendations for reporting randomized controlled trials *J Clin Epidemiol.* 2006;59:1134-49.

[38] Bian ZX, Moher D, Li YP, Wu TX, Dagenais S, Cheng CW et al. Precise reporting of traditional Chinese medicine *Zhong Xi Yi Jie He Xue Bao.* 2008;6:661-7.

[39] Motoo Y, Seki T, Tsutani K. Traditional Japanese medicine, Kampo: its history and current status. *Chin J Integr Med.* 2011;17:85-7.

[40] Hu J, Zhang J, Zhao W, Zhang Y, Zhang L, Shang H. Cochrane systematic reviews of Chinese herbal medicines: an overview. *PLoS One.* 2011;6: e28696.

In: Traditional Medicine: New Research
Editor: Yoshiharu Motoo
ISBN: 978-1-62257-448-3


# Appendix: Standard Kampo Formula Nomenclature

***Kiichiro Tsutani,[1,2] Hiroaki Hikiami,[3] Motokichi Satake,[4] Kazuo Toriizuka[5] and Kazuo Yamada[6]***
[1] Graduate School of Pharmaceutical Sciences,
The University of Tokyo, Japan
[2] Uppsala Monitoring Centre (UMC) Signal Reviewer,
[3] The Committee on the Terminology, Medical and
Pharmaceutical Society for WAKAN-YAKU
[4] Committee on the International Affairs, The Japanese Society of Pharmacognosy
[5] the Committee on the Terminology, The Japan Society for Oriental Medicine
[6] the Committee on the Terminology, The Japan Society for Oriental Medicine
(all affiliation are as of 5 March 2005)

10 October 2010

## Introduction

The project on Standard Kampo Formula Nomenclature (SKFN) was launched against the following background.

In 2002, the Uppsala Monitoring Centre (UMC, WHO International Drug Monitoring Centre) started a project on Herbal Anatomical, Therapeutic and Chemical (HATC) classification. As part of the project, HATC classification of Kampo formulae and other herbal medicines in Japan was requested to develop. Thereafter, HATC codes together with SKFN were intended to use in the Vigibase when listing Adverse Drug Reactions (ADRs) of Japanese Kampo products.

In addition, Kampo products on the basis of classical Kampo formulae cover 85% of all herbal medicines used in Japan. Therefore, SKFN is also needed when Kampo formulae are listed on the Japanese Pharmacopoeia 15th edition scheduled for publication in 2006.

From 2003 to 2005, this project on SKFN was implemented as one of the subtopics of "the HATC classification of Kampo formulae" in one of the Ministry of Health, Labor and Welfare (MHLW) funded project, "The research on the usefulness evaluation (aiming to EBM) technique and the safety protection of general Kampo formulae" (principal investigator: Yukihiro GODA, the head of Division of Pharmacognosy, Photochemistry and Narcotics, National Institute of Health Sciences). As the HATC classification noted above, the purpose of the nomenclature were to standardize the name of 210 formulae listed on "The Guidance on general Kampo formulae" (1975) and the other 18 formulae marketed for ethical use as of 1 April 2004 in Japan. The total number of the formulae included in SKFN was 228. The development of this nomenclature was started by five expert members from April 2003. The final version of SKFN was released on 5 March 2005. Since then, SKFN was introduced and required in the Instructions for Authors of major scientific journals for traditional medicine in Japan such as *Nihon Toyo Igaku Zasshi* (*Kampo Medicine*), *Shoyakugaku Zasshi* (*The Japanese Journal of Pharmacognosy*), *Journal of Natural Medicines* and *Journal of Traditional Medicines*. SKFN was used in Japanese Pharmacopoeia 15th edition (2006), and also used in the data sent to the UMC from the Ministry of Health, Labour and Welfare (MHLW) and Pharmaceuticals and Medical Devices Agency (PMDA). The Japanese version of SKFN contains details of the methodology of this nomenclature and the final decision of the SKFN project (http://www.jsom.or.jp/pdf/standard_kampo.pdf).

**Table. Standard Kampo Formula Nomenclature (210 + 18 formulae, 2005); ver. 1.0 5 March 2005**

| No. | 漢字（Han character） | カタカナ（katakana） | ローマ字（Roman alphabet） |
|---|---|---|---|
| 1 | 安中散 | アンチュウサン | anchusan |
| 2 | 胃風湯 | イフウトウ | ifuto |
| 3 | 胃苓湯 | イレイトウ | ireito |
| 4 | 茵蔯蒿湯 | インチンコウトウ | inchinkoto |
| 5 | 茵蔯五苓散 | インチンゴレイサン | inchingoreisan |
| 6 | 温経湯 | ウンケイトウ | unkeito |
| 7 | 温清飲 | ウンセイイン | unseiin |
| 8 | 温胆湯 | ウンタントウ | untanto |
| 9 | 延年半夏湯 | エンネンハンゲトウ | en'nenhangeto |
| 10 | 黄耆建中湯 | オウギケンチュウトウ | ogikenchuto |
| 11 | 黄芩湯 | オウゴントウ | ogonto |
| 12 | 応鐘散 | オウショウサン | oshosan |
| 13 | 黄連阿膠湯 | オウレンアキョウトウ | oren'a k yoto |
| 14 | 黄連解毒湯 | オウレンゲドクトウ | orengedokuto |
| 15 | 黄連湯 | オウレントウ | orento |
| 16 | 乙字湯 | オツジトウ | otsujito |
| 17 | 化食養脾湯 | カショクヨウヒトウ | kashokuyohito |
| 18 | 藿香正気散 | カッコウショウキサン | kakkoshokisan |
| 19 | 葛根黄連黄芩湯 | カッコンオウレンオウゴントウ | kakkon'oren'ogonto |
| 20 | 葛根紅花湯 | カッコンコウカトウ | kakkonkokato |
| 21 | 葛根湯 | カッコントウ | kakkonto |
| 22 | 葛根湯加川芎辛夷 | カッコントウカセンキュウシンイ | kakkontokasenkyushin'i |

| No. | 漢字 (Han character) | カタカナ (katakana) | ローマ字 (Roman alphabet) |
|---|---|---|---|
| 23 | 加味温胆湯 | カミウンタントウ | kamiuntanto |
| 24 | 加味帰脾湯 | カミキヒトウ | kamikihito |
| 25 | 加味解毒湯 | カミゲドクトウ | kamigedokuto |
| 26 | 加味逍遙散 | カミショウヨウサン | kamishoyosan |
| 27 | 加味逍遙散合四物湯 | カミショウヨウサンゴウシモツトウ | kamishoyosangoshimotsuto |
| 28 | 加味平胃散 | カミヘイイサン | kamiheiisan |
| 29 | 乾姜人参半夏丸 | カンキョウニンジンハンゲガン | kankyoninjinhangegan |
| 30 | 甘草瀉心湯 | カンゾウシャシントウ | kanzoshashinto |
| 31 | 甘草湯 | カンゾウトウ | kanzoto |
| 32 | 甘麦大棗湯 | カンバクタイソウトウ | kambakutaisoto |
| 33 | 帰耆建中湯 | キギケンチュウトウ | kigikenchuto |
| 34 | 桔梗湯 | キキョウトウ | kikyoto |
| 35 | 帰脾湯 | キヒトウ | kihito |
| 36 | 芎帰膠艾湯 | キュウキキョウガイトウ | kyukikyogaito |
| 37 | 芎帰調血飲 | キュウキチョウケツイン | kyukichoketsuin |
| 38 | 芎帰調血飲第一加減 | キュウキチョウケツインダイイチカゲン | kyukichoketsuindaiichikagen |
| 39 | 響声破笛丸 | キョウセイハテキガン | kyoseihatekigan |
| 40 | 杏蘇散 | キョウソサン | kyososan |
| 41 | 苦参湯 | クジントウ | kujinto |
| 42 | 駆風解毒散 | クフウゲドクサン | kufugedokusan |
| 43 | 荊芥連翹湯 | ケイガイレンギョウトウ | keigairengyoto |
| 44 | 鶏肝丸 | ケイカンガン | keikangan |
| 45 | 桂枝加黄耆湯 | ケイシカオウギトウ | keishikaogito |
| 46 | 桂枝加葛根湯 | ケイシカカッコントウ | keishikakakkonto |
| 47 | 桂枝加厚朴杏仁湯 | ケイシカコウボクキョウニントウ | keishikakobokukyoninto |
| 48 | 桂枝加芍薬生姜人参湯 | ケイシカシャクヤクショウキョウニンジントウ | keishikashakuyakushokyoninj into |
| 49 | 桂枝加芍薬大黄湯 | ケイシカシャクヤクダイオウトウ | keishikashakuyakudaioto |
| 50 | 桂枝加芍薬湯 | ケイシカシャクヤクトウ | keishikashakuyakuto |
| 51 | 桂枝加朮附湯 | ケイシカジュツブトウ | keishikajutsubuto |
| 52 | 桂枝加竜骨牡蛎湯 | ケイシカリュウコツボレイトウ | keishikaryukotsuboreito |
| 53 | 桂枝加苓朮附湯 | ケイシカリョウジュツブトウ | keishikaryojutsubuto |
| 54 | 桂枝湯 | ケイシトウ | keishito |
| 55 | 桂枝人参湯 | ケイシニンジントウ | keishininjinto |
| 56 | 桂枝茯苓丸 | ケイシブクリョウガン | keishibukuryogan |
| 57 | 桂枝茯苓丸料加薏苡仁 | ケイシブクリョウガンリョウカヨクイニン | keishibukuryoganryokayokuin in |
| 58 | 啓脾湯 | ケイヒトウ | keihito |
| 59 | 荊防敗毒散 | ケイボウハイドクサン | keibohaidokusan |
| 60 | 桂麻各半湯 | ケイマカクハントウ | keimakakuhanto |
| 61 | 鶏鳴散加茯苓 | ケイメイサンカブクリョウ | keimeisankabukuryo |
| 62 | 堅中湯 | ケンチュウトウ | kenchuto |
| 63 | 甲字湯 | コウジトウ | kojito |
| 64 | 香砂平胃散 | コウシャヘイイサン | koshaheiisan |
| 65 | 香砂養胃湯 | コウシャヨウイトウ | koshayoito |
| 66 | 香砂六君子湯 | コウシャリックンシトウ | kosharikkunshito |

**Table. (Continued)**

| No. | 漢字（Han character） | カタカナ（katakana） | ローマ字（Roman alphabet） |
|---|---|---|---|
| 67 | 香蘇散 | コウソサン | kososan |
| 68 | 厚朴生姜半夏人参甘草湯 | コウボクショウキョウハンゲニンジンカンゾウトウ | kobokushokyohangeninjinkanzoto |
| 69 | 五虎湯 | ゴコトウ | gokoto |
| 70 | 牛膝散 | ゴシツサン | goshitsusan |
| 71 | 五積散 | ゴシャクサン | goshakusan |
| 72 | 牛車腎気丸 | ゴシャジンキガン | goshajinkigan |
| 73 | 呉茱萸湯 | ゴシュユトウ | goshuyuto |
| 74 | 五物解毒散 | ゴモツゲドクサン | gomotsugedokusan |
| 75 | 五淋散 | ゴリンサン | gorinsan |
| 76 | 五苓散 | ゴレイサン | goreisan |
| 77 | 柴陥湯 | サイカントウ | saikanto |
| 78 | 柴胡加竜骨牡蛎湯 | サイコカリュウコツボレイトウ | saikokaryukotsuboreito |
| 79 | 柴胡桂枝乾姜湯 | サイコケイシカンキョウトウ | saikokeishikankyoto |
| 80 | 柴胡桂枝湯 | サイコケイシトウ | saikokeishito |
| 81 | 柴胡清肝湯 | サイコセイカントウ | saikoseikanto |
| 82 | 柴芍六君子湯 | サイシャクリックンシトウ | saishakurikkunshito |
| 83 | 柴朴湯 | サイボクトウ | saibokuto |
| 84 | 柴苓湯 | サイレイトウ | saireito |
| 85 | 左突膏 | サトツコウ | satotsuko |
| 86 | 三黄瀉心湯 | サンオウシャシントウ | san'oshashinto |
| 87 | 酸棗仁湯 | サンソウニントウ | sansoninto |
| 88 | 三物黄芩湯 | サンモツオウゴントウ | sammotsuogonto |
| 89 | 滋陰降火湯 | ジインコウカトウ | jiinkokato |
| 90 | 滋陰至宝湯 | ジインシホウトウ | jiinshihoto |
| 91 | 紫雲膏 | シウンコウ | shiunko |
| 92 | 四逆散 | シギャクサン | shigyakusan |
| 93 | 四君子湯 | シクンシトウ | shikunshito |
| 94 | 滋血潤腸湯 | ジケツジュンチョウトウ | jiketsujunchoto |
| 95 | 七物降下湯 | シチモツコウカトウ | shichimotsukokato |
| 96 | 実脾飲 | ジッピイン | jippiin |
| 97 | 柿蒂湯 | シテイトウ | shiteito |
| 98 | 四物湯 | シモツトウ | shimotsuto |
| 99 | 四苓湯 | シレイトウ | shireito |
| 100 | 炙甘草湯 | シャカンゾウトウ | shakanzoto |
| 101 | 芍薬甘草湯 | シャクヤクカンゾウトウ | shakuyakukanzoto |
| 102 | 鷓鴣菜湯（三味鷓鴣菜湯） | シャコサイトウ（サンミシャコサイトウ） | shakosaito or sammishakosaito |
| 103 | 蛇床子湯 | ジャショウシトウ | jashoshito |
| 104 | 十全大補湯 | ジュウゼンタイホトウ | juzentaihoto |
| 105 | 十味敗毒湯 | ジュウミハイドクトウ | jumihaidokuto |
| 106 | 潤腸湯 | ジュンチョウトウ | junchoto |
| 107 | 蒸眼一方 | ジョウガンイッポウ | jogan'ippo |
| 108 | 生姜瀉心湯 | ショウキョウシャシントウ | shokyoshashinto |
| 109 | 小建中湯 | ショウケンチュウトウ | shokenchuto |
| 110 | 小柴胡湯 | ショウサイコトウ | shosaikoto |
| 111 | 小柴胡湯加桔梗石膏 | ショウサイコトウカキキョウセッコウ | shosaikotokakikyosekko |

| No. | 漢字 (Han character) | カタカナ (katakana) | ローマ字<br>( Roman alphabet) |
|---|---|---|---|
| 112 | 小承気湯 | ショウジョウキトウ | shojokito |
| 113 | 小青竜湯 | ショウセイリュウトウ | shoseiryuto |
| 114 | 小青竜湯加石膏 | ショウセイリュウトウカセッコウ | shoseiryutokasekko |
| 115 | 小青竜湯合麻杏甘石湯 | ショウセイリュウトウゴウマキョウ カンセキトウ | shoseiryutogomakyokansekit o |
| 116 | 椒梅湯 | ショウバイトウ | shobaito |
| 117 | 小半夏加茯苓湯 | ショウハンゲカブクリョウトウ | shohangekabukuryoto |
| 118 | 消風散 | ショウフウサン | shofusan |
| 119 | 升麻葛根湯 | ショウマカッコントウ | shomakakkonto |
| 120 | 逍遙散 | ショウヨウサン | shoyosan |
| 121 | 辛夷清肺湯 | シンイセイハイトウ | shin'iseihaito |
| 122 | 秦艽羗活湯 | ジンギョウキョウカツトウ | jingyokyokatsuto |
| 123 | 秦艽防風湯 | ジンギョウボウフウトウ | jingyobofuto |
| 124 | 参蘇飲 | ジンソイン | jinsoin |
| 125 | 神秘湯 | シンピトウ | shimpito |
| 126 | 参苓白朮散 | ジンリョウビャクジュツサン | jinryobyakujutsusan |
| 127 | 清肌安蛔湯 | セイキアンカイトウ | seikiankaito |
| 128 | 清湿化痰湯 | セイシツケタントウ | seishitsuketanto |
| 129 | 清上蠲痛湯 | セイジョウケンツウトウ | seijokentsuto |
| 130 | 清上防風湯 | セイジョウボウフウトウ | seijobofuto |
| 131 | 清暑益気湯 | セイショエッキトウ | seishoekkito |
| 132 | 清心蓮子飲 | セイシンレンシイン | seishinrenshiin |
| 133 | 清肺湯 | セイハイトウ | seihaito |
| 134 | 折衝飲 | セッショウイン | sesshoin |
| 135 | 川芎茶調散 | センキュウチャチョウサン | senkyuchachosan |
| 136 | 千金鶏鳴散 | センキンケイメイサン | senkinkeimeisan |
| 137 | 銭氏白朮散 | ゼンシビャクジュツサン | zenshibyakujutsusan |
| 138 | 疎経活血湯 | ソケイカッケツトウ | sokeikakketsuto |
| 139 | 蘇子降気湯 | ソシコウキトウ | soshikokito |
| 140 | 大黄甘草湯 | ダイオウカンゾウトウ | daiokanzoto |
| 141 | 大黄牡丹皮湯 | ダイオウボタンピトウ | daiobotampito |
| 142 | 大建中湯 | ダイケンチュウトウ | daikenchuto |
| 143 | 大柴胡湯 | ダイサイコトウ | daisaikoto |
| 144 | 大半夏湯 | ダイハンゲトウ | daihangeto |
| 145 | 竹筎温胆湯 | チクジョウンタントウ | chikujountanto |
| 146 | 治打撲一方 | ヂダボクイッポウ | jidabokuippo |
| 147 | 治頭瘡一方 | ヂヅソウイッポウ | jizusoippo |
| 148 | 中黄膏 | チュウオウコウ | chuoko |
| 149 | 調胃承気湯 | チョウイジョウキトウ | choijokito |
| 150 | 丁香柿蒂湯 | チョウコウシテイトウ | chokoshiteito |
| 151 | 釣藤散 | チョウトウサン | chotosan |
| 152 | 猪苓湯 | チョレイトウ | choreito |
| 153 | 猪苓湯合四物湯 | チョレイトウゴウシモツトウ | choreitogoshimotsuto |
| 154 | 通導散 | ツウドウサン | tsudosan |
| 155 | 桃核承気湯 | トウカクジョウキトウ | tokakujokito |
| 156 | 当帰飲子 | トウキインシ | tokiinshi |
| 157 | 当帰建中湯 | トウキケンチュウトウ | tokikenchuto |
| 158 | 当帰散 | トウキサン | tokisan |
| 159 | 当帰四逆加呉茱萸生姜湯 | トウキシギャクカゴシュユショウキョウトウ | tokishigyakukagoshuyushok yoto |

**Table. (Continued)**

| No. | 漢字（Han character） | カタカナ（katakana） | ローマ字（Roman alphabet） |
|---|---|---|---|
| 160 | 当帰四逆湯 | トウキシギャクトウ | tokishigyakuto |
| 161 | 当帰芍薬散 | トウキシャクヤクサン | tokishakuyakusan |
| 162 | 当帰湯 | トウキトウ | tokito |
| 163 | 当帰貝母苦参丸料 | トウキバイモクジンガンリョウ | tokibaimokujinganryo |
| 164 | 独活葛根湯 | ドッカツカッコントウ | dokkatsukakkonto |
| 165 | 独活湯 | ドッカツトウ | dokkatsuto |
| 166 | 二朮湯 | ニジュツトウ | nijutsuto |
| 167 | 二陳湯 | ニチントウ | nichinto |
| 168 | 女神散 | ニョシンサン | nyoshinsan |
| 169 | 人参湯 | ニンジントウ | ninjinto |
| 170 | 人参養栄湯 | ニンジンヨウエイトウ | ninjin'yoeito |
| 171 | 排膿散 | ハイノウサン | hainosan |
| 172 | 排膿湯 | ハイノウトウ | hainoto |
| 173 | 麦門冬湯 | バクモンドウトウ | bakumondoto |
| 174 | 八味地黄丸（八味丸） | ハチミジオウガン（ハチミガン） | hachimijiogan or hachimigan |
| 175 | 八味逍遙散 | ハチミショウヨウサン | hachimishoyosan |
| 176 | 半夏厚朴湯 | ハンゲコウボクトウ | hangekobokuto |
| 177 | 半夏瀉心湯 | ハンゲシャシントウ | hangeshashinto |
| 178 | 半夏白朮天麻湯 | ハンゲビャクジュツテンマトウ | hangebyakujutsutemmato |
| 179 | 白虎加桂枝湯 | ビャッコカケイシトウ | byakkokakeishito |
| 180 | 白虎加人参湯 | ビャッコカニンジントウ | byakkokaninjinto |
| 181 | 白虎湯 | ビャッコトウ | byakkoto |
| 182 | 不換金正気散 | フカンキンショウキサン | fukankinshokisan |
| 183 | 伏竜肝湯 | ブクリュウカントウ | bukuryukanto |
| 184 | 茯苓飲 | ブクリョウイン | bukuryoin |
| 185 | 茯苓飲加半夏 | ブクリョウインカハンゲ | bukuryoinkahange |
| 186 | 茯苓飲合半夏厚朴湯 | ブクリョウインゴウハンゲコウボクトウ | bukuryoingohangekobokuto |
| 187 | 茯苓沢瀉湯 | ブクリョウタクシャトウ | bukuryotakushato |
| 188 | 分消湯 | ブンショウトウ | bunshoto |
| 189 | 平胃散 | ヘイイサン | heiisan |
| 190 | 防已黄耆湯 | ボウイオウギトウ | boiogito |
| 191 | 防已茯苓湯 | ボウイブクリョウトウ | boibukuryoto |
| 192 | 防風通聖散 | ボウフウツウショウサン | bofutsushosan |
| 193 | 補気建中湯 | ホキケンチュウトウ | hokikenchuto |
| 194 | 補中益気湯 | ホチュウエッキトウ | hochuekkito |
| 195 | 補肺湯 | ホハイトウ | hohaito |
| No. | 漢字（Han character） | カタカナ（katakana） | ローマ字( Roman alphabet) |
| 196 | 麻黄湯 | マオウトウ | maoto |
| 197 | 麻杏甘石湯 | マキョウカンセキトウ | makyokansekito |
| 198 | 麻杏薏甘湯 | マキョウヨクカントウ | makyoyokukanto |
| 199 | 麻子仁丸 | マシニンガン | mashiningan |
| 200 | 楊柏散 | ヨウハクサン | yohakusan |
| 201 | 薏苡仁湯 | ヨクイニントウ | yokuininto |
| 202 | 抑肝散 | ヨクカンサン | yokukansan |
| 203 | 抑肝散加陳皮半夏 | ヨクカンサンカチンピハンゲ | yokukansankachimpihange |
| 204 | 立効散 | リッコウサン | rikkosan |

| No. | 漢字 (Han character) | カタカナ (katakana) | ローマ字 (Roman alphabet) |
|---|---|---|---|
| 205 | 六君子湯 | リックンシトウ | rikkunshito |
| 206 | 竜胆瀉肝湯 | リュウタンシャカントウ | ryutanshakanto |
| 207 | 苓姜朮甘湯 | リョウキョウジュツカントウ | ryokyojutsukanto |
| 208 | 苓桂甘棗湯 | リョウケイカンソウトウ | ryokeikansoto |
| 209 | 苓桂朮甘湯 | リョウケイジュツカントウ | ryokeijutsukanto |
| 210 | 六味丸 | ロクミガン | rokumigan |

## Annex. Appendix 18 Formulae Marketed in Japan (2005)

| No. | 漢字 (Han character) | カタカナ (katakana) | ローマ字 (Roman alphabet) |
|---|---|---|---|
| 211 | 越婢加朮湯 | エッピカジュツトウ | eppikajutsuto |
| 212 | 葛根加朮附湯 | カッコンカジュツブトウ | kakkonkajutsubuto |
| 213 | 桔梗石膏 | キキョウセッコウ | kikyosekko |
| 214 | 九味檳榔湯 | クミビンロウトウ | kumibinroto |
| 215 | 桂芍知母湯 (桂枝芍薬知母湯) | ケイシャクチモトウ (ケイシシャクヤクチモトウ) | keishakuchimoto or keishishakuyakuchimoto |
| 216 | 梔子柏皮湯 | シシハクヒトウ | shishihakuhito |
| 217 | 芍薬甘草附子湯 | シャクヤクカンゾウブシトウ | shakuyakukanzobushito |
| 218 | 真武湯 | シンブトウ | shimbuto |
| 219 | 大柴胡湯去大黄 | ダイサイコトウキョダイオウ | daisaikotokyodaio |
| 220 | 大承気湯 | ダイジョウキトウ | daijokito |
| 221 | 大防風湯 | ダイボウフウトウ | daibofuto |
| 222 | 腸癰湯 | チョウヨウトウ | choyoto |
| 223 | 当帰芍薬散加附子 | トウキシャクヤクサンカブシ | tokishakuyakusankabushi |
| 224 | 排膿散及湯 | ハイノウサンキュウトウ | hainosankyuto |
| 225 | 附子理中湯 (附子人参湯) | ブシリチュウトウ (ブシニンジントウ) | bushirichuto or bushininjinto |
| 226 | 麻黄附子細辛湯 | マオウブシサイシントウ | maobushisaishinto |
| 227 | 木防已湯 | モクボウイトウ | mokuboito |
| 228 | 苓甘姜味辛夏仁湯 | リョウカンキョウミシンゲニントウ | ryokankyomishingeninto |

# Index

## B

## C

## D



## E

## F

## G



## H

## I

## J



## K

## N

## O



## P

## T

## U



## V



## W

## X



## Y



## Z